UNEQUAL
TREATMENT

CONFRONTING RACIAL AND ETHNIC
DISPARITIES IN HEALTH CARE

Brian D. Smedley, Adrienne Y. Stith, and
Alan R. Nelson, Editors

Committee on Understanding and Eliminating
Racial and Ethnic Disparities in Health Care

Board on Health Sciences Policy

INSTITUTE OF MEDICINE
OF THE NATIONAL ACADEMIES

THE NATIONAL ACADEMIES PRESS
Washington, D.C.
www.nap.edu

THE NATIONAL ACADEMIES PRESS • 500 Fifth Street, N.W. • **Washington, D.C. 20001**

NOTICE: The project that is the subject of this report was approved by the Governing Board of the National Research Council, whose members are drawn from the councils of the National Academy of Sciences, the National Academy of Engineering, and the Institute of Medicine. The members of the committee responsible for the report were chosen for their special competences and with regard for appropriate balance.

Support for this project was provided by the Office of Minority Health, U.S. Department of Health and Human Services. Additional support for data collection activities was provided by The Commonwealth Fund and the Henry J. Kaiser Family Foundation. The views presented in this report are those of the Institute of Medicine Committee on Understanding and Eliminating Racial and Ethnic Disparities in Health Care and are not necessarily those of the funding agencies.

Library of Congress Cataloging-in-Publication Data

Unequal treatment : confronting racial and ethnic disparities in health care / Brian D. Smedley, Adrienne Y. Stith, and Alan R. Nelson, editors ; Committee on Understanding and Eliminating Racial and Ethnic Disparities in Health Care, Board on Health Sciences Policy, Institute of Medicine.
    p. ; cm.
Includes bibliographical references and index.
    ISBN 0-309-08265-X (hardcover with CD-ROM); ISBN 0-309-08532-2 (hardcover)
    1. Discrimination in medical care. 2. Health services accessibility. 3. Minorities—Medical care. 4. Race discrimination. 5. Racism—Cross-cultural stdies. 6. Social medicine.
    [DNLM: 1. Health Services Accessibility—United States. 2. Ethnic Groups—United States. 3. Minority Groups—United States. 4. Quality of Health Care—United States. WA 300 U515 2002] I. Smedley, Brian D. II. Stith, Adrienne Y. III. Nelson, Alan R. (Alan Ray) IV. Institute of Medicine (U.S.). Committee on Understanding and Eliminating Racial and Ethnic Disparities in Health Care.
    RA563.M56 U53 2002
    352.1'089—dc 21
                                                                    2002007492

Additional copies of this report are available for sale from the National Academies Press, 500 Fifth Street, N.W., Box 285, Washington, D.C. 20055. Call (800) 624-6242 or (202) 334-3313 (in the Washington metropolitan area); Internet, **http://www.nap.edu.**

For more information about the Institute of Medicine, visit the IOM home page at: **www.iom.edu.**

The serpent has been a symbol of long life, healing, and knowledge among almost all cultures and religions since the beginning of recorded history. The serpent adopted as a logotype by the Institute of Medicine is a relief carving from ancient Greece, now held by the Staatliche Museen in Berlin.

*"Knowing is not enough; we must apply.
Willing is not enough; we must do."*
—Goethe

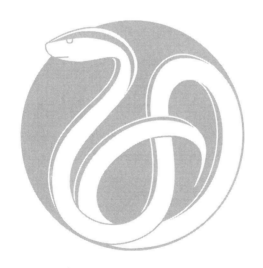

INSTITUTE OF MEDICINE
OF THE NATIONAL ACADEMIES

Shaping the Future for Health

THE NATIONAL ACADEMIES
Advisers to the Nation on Science, Engineering, and Medicine

The **National Academy of Sciences** is a private, nonprofit, self-perpetuating society of distinguished scholars engaged in scientific and engineering research, dedicated to the furtherance of science and technology and to their use for the general welfare. Upon the authority of the charter granted to it by the Congress in 1863, the Academy has a mandate that requires it to advise the federal government on scientific and technical matters. Dr. Bruce M. Alberts is president of the National Academy of Sciences.

The **National Academy of Engineering** was established in 1964, under the charter of the National Academy of Sciences, as a parallel organization of outstanding engineers. It is autonomous in its administration and in the selection of its members, sharing with the National Academy of Sciences the responsibility for advising the federal government. The National Academy of Engineering also sponsors engineering programs aimed at meeting national needs, encourages education and research, and recognizes the superior achievements of engineers. Dr. Wm. A. Wulf is president of the National Academy of Engineering.

The **Institute of Medicine** was established in 1970 by the National Academy of Sciences to secure the services of eminent members of appropriate professions in the examination of policy matters pertaining to the health of the public. The Institute acts under the responsibility given to the National Academy of Sciences by its congressional charter to be an adviser to the federal government and, upon its own initiative, to identify issues of medical care, research, and education. Dr. Harvey V. Fineberg is president of the Institute of Medicine.

The **National Research Council** was organized by the National Academy of Sciences in 1916 to associate the broad community of science and technology with the Academy's purposes of furthering knowledge and advising the federal government. Functioning in accordance with general policies determined by the Academy, the Council has become the principal operating agency of both the National Academy of Sciences and the National Academy of Engineering in providing services to the government, the public, and the scientific and engineering communities. The Council is administered jointly by both Academies and the Institute of Medicine. Dr. Bruce M. Alberts and Dr. Wm. A. Wulf are chair and vice chair, respectively, of the National Research Council.

www.national-academies.org

CAROLINA REYES, M.D., Vice President, Planning and Evaluation, The California Endowment, Woodland Hills, CA, and Associate Clinical Professor, UCLA School of Medicine, Los Angeles, CA

DONALD STEINWACHS, Ph.D., Chair and Professor of the Department of Health Policy and Management, Johns Hopkins School of Hygiene and Public Health, and Director, Johns Hopkins University Health Services Research and Development Center, Baltimore, MD

DAVID R. WILLIAMS, Ph.D., M.P.H., Professor of Sociology and Research Scientist, Institute for Social Research, University of Michigan, Ann Arbor, MI

HEALTH SCIENCES POLICY BOARD LIAISON

GLORIA E. SARTO, M.D., Ph.D., Professor, University of Wisconsin Health, Department of Obstetrics and Gynecology, Madison, WI

IOM PROJECT STAFF

BRIAN D. SMEDLEY, Study Director
ADRIENNE Y. STITH, Program Officer
DANIEL J. WOOTEN, Scholar-in-Residence
THELMA L. COX, Senior Project Assistant
SYLVIA I. SALAZAR, Edward Roybal Public Health Fellow, Congressional Hispanic Caucus Institute

IOM STAFF

ANDREW M. POPE, Director, Board on Health Sciences Policy
ALDEN CHANG, Administrative Assistant
CARLOS GABRIEL, Financial Associate
PAIGE BALDWIN, Managing Editor

COPY EDITOR

JILL SHUMAN

REVIEWERS

This report has been reviewed in draft form by individuals chosen for their diverse perspectives and technical expertise, in accordance with procedures approved by the NRC's Report Review Committee. The purpose of this independent review is to provide candid and critical comments that will assist the institution in making its published report as sound as possible and to ensure that the report meets institutional standards for objectivity, evidence, and responsiveness to the study charge. The review comments and draft manuscript remain confidential to protect the integrity of the deliberative process. We wish to thank the following individuals for their review of this report:

LU ANN ADAY, Professor of Behavioral Sciences, University of Texas-Houston Science Center, TX

JOHN F. ALDERETE, Professor of Microbiology, University of Texas Health Science Center at San Antonio, TX

NAIHUA DUAN, Professor-in-Residence, Center for Community Health, UCLA Wilshire Center, Los Angeles, CA

DEAN M. HASHIMOTO, Associate Professor, Boston College Law School, Newton, MA

SHERMAN A. JAMES, Director, Center for Research on Ethnicity Culture & Health, School of Public Health, University of Michigan, Ann Arbor, MI

JEROME P. KASSIRER, Yale University School of Medicine, New Haven, CT

WOODROW A. MYERS, Executive Vice President, Wellpoint Health Networks, Thousand Oaks, CA

FRANK A. SLOAN, Director, Center for Health Policy, Law & Management, Duke University, Durham, NC

KNOX H. TODD, Adjunct Associate Professor, The Rollins School of Public Health, Emory University School of Medicine, Atlanta, GA

WILLIAM A. VEGA, Director, Behavioral and Research Training Institute, Universit of Medicine and Dentistry of New Jersey, New Brunswick, NJ

EUGENE WASHINGTON, Professor and Chair, Department of Ob/Gyn & Reproductive Sciences, University of California, San Francisco, CA

Although the reviewers listed above have provided many constructive comments and suggestions, they were not asked to endorse the conclusions or recommendations nor did they see the final draft of the report before its release. The review of this report was overseen by HAROLD C. SOX, Editor, *Annals of Internal Medicine*, Philadelphia, PA, appointed by the Institute of Medicine, and ELAINE L. LARSON, Professor of Pharmaceutical & Therapeutic Research, Columbia University School of Nursing, New York, NY. Appointed by the NRC's Report Review Committee, these individuals were responsible for making certain that an independent examination of this report was carried out in accordance with institutional procedures and that all review comments were carefully considered. Responsibility for the final content of this report rests entirely with the authoring committee and the institution.

Acknowledgments

Many individuals and groups made important contributions to the study committee's process and to this report. The committee wishes to thank all of these individuals and organizations, but recognizes that attempts to identify all and acknowledge their contributions would require more space than is available in this brief section.

To begin, the committee would like to thank the sponsors of this report. Core funds for the committee's work were provided by the Office of Minority Health, U.S. Department of Health and Human Services, in response to a Congressional request. The committee thanks Joan Jacobs and Olivia Carter-Pokras of this office, who served as the Task Order Officers on this grant. Additional funding for data collection efforts was provided by the Henry J. Kaiser Family Foundation of Menlo Park, California, and The Commonwealth Fund, a New York City-based private, independent foundation. The committee thanks Marsha Lillie-Blanton of the Henry J. Kaiser Family Foundation, and Karen Scott Collins and Dora L. Hughes of The Commonwealth Fund for their support.

The committee found the perspectives of many individuals and organizations to be valuable in understanding the complex problem of racial and ethnic disparities in healthcare. Several individuals and organizations provided important information at open workshops of the committee. These include, in order of appearance, Nathan Stinson, Ph.D., M.D., M.P.H., Deputy Assistant Secretary for Minority Health, U.S. Department of Health and Human Services; Charles Dujon, Legislative Assistant, Office of the Honorable Jessie Jackson, Jr., U.S. House of Representatives; Rodney Hood, M.D., National Medical Association; Adolph Falcon, M.P.P., National Alliance for Hispanic Health; Jeanette Noltenius, Ph.D., Latino Council on Alcohol and Tobacco, representing the Multicultural Action Agenda for Eliminating Health Disparities; Yvonne Bushyhead, J.D., and Beverly Little Thunder, R.N., National Indian Health Board; H. Jack Geiger, M.D., City University of New York; Deborah Danoff, M.D., Assistant Vice President, Division of Medical Education, American Association of Medical Colleges; Paul M. Schyve, M.D., Senior Vice President, Joint Commission on Accreditation of Healthcare Organizations; Sindhu Srinivas, M.D., President, American Medical Student Association; Mary E. Foley, R.N., MS, President, American Nurses Association; Randolph D. Smoak, Jr., M.D., President, American Medical Association; Terri Dickerson, Assistant Staff Director, U.S. Commission on Civil Rights; Carolyn Clancy, M.D., Agency for Health Care Research and Quality; James Youker, M.D., President, American Board of Medical Specialties; Ray Werntz, Consumer Health Education Council; Vickie Mays, Ph.D., Chair, National Committee on Vital and Health Statistics Subcommittee on Populations; Robyn Nishimi, Ph.D., Chief Operating Officer, National Quality Forum; Lovell Jones, Ph.D., Intercultural Cancer Council; David Satcher, M.D., Ph.D., U.S. Surgeon General; Richard Epstein, J.D., James Parker Hall Distinguished Service Professor of Law, University of Chicago Law School; Clark C. Havighurst, J.D., Wm. Neal Reynolds Professor of Law, Duke University School of Law; Marsha Lillie-Blanton, Dr. P.H., Vice President in Health Policy, The Henry J. Kaiser Family Foundation; June O'Neill, Ph.D., Director, Center for the Study of Business and Government, Baruch College of Public Affairs; Thomas Perez, J.D., M.P.P., Assistant Professor and Director of Clinical Law Programs, University of Maryland Law School; and Thomas Rice, Ph.D., Professor and Vice-Chair, Department of Health Services, UCLA School of Public Health.

The committee also gratefully acknowledges the contributions of the many individuals who participated as members of one of four liaison panels, which were assembled to serve as a resource to the committee, to provide advice and guidance in identifying key information sources, to provide recommendations to the study committee regarding intervention strategies, and to ensure that relevant consumer and professional perspectives were represented. These individuals are listed in Appendix A. Similarly, the committee thanks the many individuals who provided input to study staff during "roundtable discussions" held at the Asian and Pacific Islander American Health Forum (APIAHF) conference on April 27 and 28, 2001, and the Indian Health Service (IHS) Research Conference on April 22 and 23, 2001. The committee extends its gratitude to Gem Daus of APIAHF and Leo Nolan, William Freeman, and Cecelia Shorty of IHS for their assistance in arranging these roundtable discussions.

Data from focus group discussions involving racial and ethnic minority healthcare consumers and healthcare providers helped to put a "human face" on the problem of disparities in care. The committee extends its gratitude to the many individuals who participated in these focus group discussions and shared their experiences, which included both positive as well as negative experiences in healthcare systems. These focus groups were convened and conducted by Westat, Inc., and a summary of the major themes is presented in Appendix D. Tim Edgar and Meredith Grady of Westat deserve special thanks for their work to convene these groups and provide a synthesis of the data.

Joe R. Feagin of the University of Florida, Nicole Lurie of RAND, Vickie Mays of UCLA, and Richard Allen Williams of UCLA and the Minority Health Institute served as technical reviewers on aspects of the report. These individuals provided technical comments only, and are not responsible for the final content of the report. Ruth Zambrana of the University of Maryland also provided valuable assistance regarding health care needs of Hispanic populations, and Elizabeth Marchak of the *Cleveland Plain Dealer* provided the study committee with informative and well-researched news articles from her research on healthcare disparities. Michael Sapoznikow designed the graphic illustration that appears as Figure 3-1 in Chapter 3. The committee thanks each of these individuals.

Finally, the committee would also like to thank the authors whose paper contributions contributed to the evidence base that the committee examined. These include H. Jack Geiger of the City University of New York; W. Michael Byrd and Linda A. Clayton of the Harvard School of Public Health; Lisa A. Cooper and Debra L. Roter of Johns Hopkins University; Jennie R. Joe, with the assistance of Jacquetta Swift and Robert S. Young of the Native American Research and Training Center, University of Arizona; Mary-Jo DelVecchio Good, Cara James, Byron J. Good, and Anne E. Becker, Department of Social Medicine, Harvard Medical School; Sara Rosenbaum of the School of Public Health and Health Services, George Washington University; Thomas Perez of the University of Maryland Law School; Madison Powers and Ruth Faden of the Kennedy Institute of Ethics, Georgetown University; and Thomas Rice of the Department of Health Services, UCLA School of Public Health.

Contents

xiii

---

*Pages 417-738 are not printed in this book but are on the CD-ROM attached to the inside back cover.

Summary

ABSTRACT

Racial and ethnic minorities tend to receive a lower quality of healthcare than non-minorities, even when access-related factors, such as patients' insurance status and income, are controlled. The sources of these disparities are complex, are rooted in historic and contemporary inequities, and involve many participants at several levels, including health systems, their administrative and bureaucratic processes, utilization managers, healthcare professionals, and patients. Consistent with the charge, the study committee focused part of its analysis on the clinical encounter itself, and found evidence that stereotyping, biases, and uncertainty on the part of healthcare providers can all contribute to unequal treatment. The conditions in which many clinical encounters take place—characterized by high time pressure, cognitive complexity, and pressures for cost-containment—may enhance the likelihood that these processes will result in care poorly matched to minority patients' needs. Minorities may experience a range of other barriers to accessing care, even when insured at the same level as whites, including barriers of language, geography, and cultural familiarity. Further, financial and institutional arrangements of health systems, as well as the legal, regulatory, and policy environment in which they operate, may have disparate and negative effects on minorities' ability to attain quality care.

A comprehensive, multi-level strategy is needed to eliminate these disparities. Broad sectors—including healthcare providers, their patients, payors, health plan purchasers, and society at large—should be made aware of the healthcare gap between racial and ethnic groups in the United States. Health systems should

1

base decisions about resource allocation on published clinical guidelines, insure that physician financial incentives do not disproportionately burden or restrict minority patients' access to care, and take other steps to improve access—including the provision of interpretation services, where community need exists. Economic incentives should be considered for practices that improve provider-patient communication and trust, and reward appropriate screening, preventive, and evidence-based clinical care. In addition, payment systems should avoid fragmentation of health plans along socioeconomic lines.

The healthcare workforce and its ability to deliver quality care for racial and ethnic minorities can be improved substantially by increasing the proportion of underrepresented U.S. racial and ethnic minorities among health professionals. In addition, both patients and providers can benefit from education. Patients can benefit from culturally appropriate education programs to improve their knowledge of how to access care and their ability to participate in clinical-decision making. The greater burden of education, however, lies with providers. Cross-cultural curricula should be integrated early into the training of future healthcare providers, and practical, case-based, rigorously evaluated training should persist through practitioner continuing education programs. Finally, collection, reporting, and monitoring of patient care data by health plans and federal and state payors should be encouraged as a means to assess progress in eliminating disparities, to evaluate intervention efforts, and to assess potential civil rights violations.

Looking gaunt but determined, 59-year-old Robert Tools was introduced on August 21, 2001, as a medical miracle—the first surviving recipient of a fully implantable artificial heart. At a news conference, Tools spoke with emotion about his second chance at life and the quality of his care. His physicians looked on with obvious affection, grateful and honored to have extended Tools' life. Mr. Tools has since lost his battle for life, but will be remembered as a hero for undergoing an experimental technology and paving the way for other patients to undergo the procedure. Moreover, the fact that Tools was African American and his doctors were white seemed, for most Americans, to symbolize the irrelevance of race in 2001. According to two recent polls, a significant majority of Americans believe that blacks like Tools receive the same quality of healthcare as whites (Lillie-Blanton et al., 2000; Morin, 2001).

Behind these perceptions, however, lies a sharply contrasting reality. A large body of published research reveals that racial and ethnic minorities experience a lower quality of health services, and are less likely to receive even routine medical procedures than are white Americans. Relative to whites, African Americans—and in some cases, Hispanics—are less likely to receive appropriate cardiac medication (e.g., Herholz et al., 1996) or to undergo coronary artery bypass surgery (e.g., Ayanian et al., 1993; Hannan et al., 1999; Johnson et al., 1993; Petersen et al., 2002), are less likely to receive peritoneal dialysis and kidney transplantation (e.g., Epstein et al., 2000; Barker-Cummings et al., 1995; Gaylin et al., 1993), and are likely to receive a lower quality of basic clinical services (Ayanian et al., 1999) such as intensive care (Williams et al., 1995), even when variations in such factors as insurance status, income, age, co-morbid conditions, and symptom expression are taken into account. Significantly, these differences are associated with greater mortality among African-American patients (Peterson et al., 1997; Bach et al., 1999).

STUDY CHARGE AND COMMMITTEE ASSUMPTIONS

These disparities prompted Congress to request an Institute of Medicine (IOM) study to assess differences in the kinds and quality of healthcare received by U.S. racial and ethnic minorities and non-minorities. Specifically, Congress requested that the IOM:

• Assess the extent of racial and ethnic differences in healthcare that are not otherwise attributable to known factors such as access to care (e.g., ability to pay or insurance coverage);
• Evaluate potential sources of racial and ethnic disparities in healthcare, including the role of bias, discrimination, and stereotyping at the individual (provider and patient), institutional, and health system levels; and,
• Provide recommendations regarding interventions to eliminate healthcare disparities.

This Executive Summary presents only abbreviated versions of the study committee's findings and recommendations. For the full findings and recommendations, and a more extensive justification of each, the reader is referred to the committee report. Below, findings and recommendations are preceded by text summarizing the evidence base from which they are drawn. For purposes of clarity, some findings and recommendations are presented in a different sequence than they appear in the full report; however, their numeric designation remains the same.

Defining Racial and Ethnic Healthcare Disparities

The study committee defines *disparities* in healthcare as racial or ethnic differences in the quality of healthcare that are not due to access-

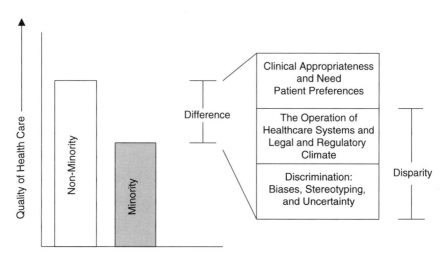

FIGURE S-1 Differences, disparities, and discrimination: Populations with equal access to healthcare. SOURCE: Gomes and McGuire, 2001.

related factors or clinical needs, preferences,[1] and appropriateness of intervention (Figure S-1). The committee's analysis is focused at two levels: 1) the operation of healthcare systems and the legal and regulatory climate in which health systems function; and 2) discrimination at the individual, patient-provider level. Discrimination, as the committee uses the term, refers to differences in care that result from biases, prejudices, stereotyping, and uncertainty in clinical communication and decision-making. It should be emphasized that these definitions are not legal definitions. Different sources of federal, state and international law define discrimination in varying ways, with some focusing on intent and others emphasizing disparate impact.

---

[1]The committee defines patient *preferences* as patients' choices regarding healthcare that are based on a full and accurate understanding of treatment options. As discussed in Chapter 3 of this report, patients' understanding of treatment options is often shaped by the quality and content of provider-patient communication, which in turn may be influenced by factors correlated with patients' and providers' race, ethnicity, and culture. Patient preferences that are not based on a full and accurate understanding of treatment options may therefore be a source of racial and ethnic disparities in care. The committee recognizes that patients' preferences and clinicians' presentation of clinical information and alternatives influence each other, but found separation of the two to be analytically useful.

EVIDENCE OF HEALTHCARE DISPARITIES

Evidence of racial and ethnic disparities in healthcare is, with few exceptions, remarkably consistent across a range of illnesses and healthcare services. These disparities are associated with socioeconomic differences and tend to diminish significantly, and in a few cases, disappear altogether when socioeconomic factors are controlled. The majority of studies, however, find that racial and ethnic disparities remain even after adjustment for socioeconomic differences and other healthcare access-related factors (for more extensive reviews of this literature, see Kressin and Petersen, 2001; Geiger, this volume; and Mayberry, Mili, and Ofili, 2000).

Studies of racial and ethnic differences in cardiovascular care provide some of the most convincing evidence of healthcare disparities. The most rigorous studies in this area assess both potential underuse and overuse of services and appropriateness of care by controlling for disease severity using well-established clinical and diagnostic criteria (e.g., Schneider et al., 2001; Ayanian et al., 1993; Allison et al., 1996; Weitzman et al., 1997) or matched patient controls (Giles et al., 1995). Several studies, for example, have assessed differences in treatment regimen following coronary angiography, a key diagnostic procedure. These studies have demonstrated that differences in treatment are not due to clinical factors such as racial differences in the severity of coronary disease or overuse of services by whites (e.g., Schneider et al., 2001; Laouri et al., 1997; Canto et al., 2000; Peterson et al., 1997). Further, racial disparities in receipt of coronary revascularization procedures are associated with higher mortality among African Americans (Peterson et al., 1997).

Healthcare disparities are also found in other disease areas. Several studies demonstrate significant racial differences in the receipt of appropriate cancer diagnostic tests (e.g., McMahon et al., 1999), treatments (e.g., Imperato et al., 1996), and analgesics (e.g., Bernabei et al., 1998), while controlling for stage of cancer at diagnosis and other clinical factors. As is the case in studies of cardiovascular disease, evidence suggests that disparities in cancer care are associated with higher death rates among minorities (Bach et al., 1999). Similarly, African Americans with HIV infection are less likely than non-minorities to receive antiretroviral therapy (Moore et al., 1994), prophylaxis for pneumocystic pneumonia, and protease inhibitors (Shapiro et al., 1999). These disparities remain even after adjusting for age, gender, education, CD4 cell count, and insurance coverage (e.g., Shapiro et al., 1999). In addition, differences in the quality of HIV care are associated with poorer survival rates among minorities, even at equivalent levels of access to care (Bennett et al., 1995; Cunningham et al., 2000).

Racial and ethnic disparities are found in a range of other disease and health service categories, including diabetes care (e.g., Chin, Zhang, and Merrell, 1998), end-stage renal disease and kidney transplantation (e.g., Epstein et al., 2000; Kasiske, London, and Ellison, 1998; Barker-Cummings et al., 1995; Ayanian et al., 1999), pediatric care and maternal and child health, mental health, rehabilitative and nursing home services, and many surgical procedures. In some instances, minorities are *more* likely to receive certain procedures. As in the case of bilateral orchiectomy and amputation, however (which African Americans undergo at rates 2.4 and 3.6 times greater, respectively, than their white Medicare peers; Gornick et al., 1996), these are generally less desirable procedures.

> **Finding 1-1: Racial and ethnic disparities in healthcare exist and, because they are associated with worse outcomes in many cases, are unacceptable.**

> **Recommendation 2-1: Increase awareness of racial and ethnic disparities in healthcare among the general public and key stakeholders.**

> **Recommendation 2-2: Increase healthcare providers' awareness of disparities.**

RACIAL ATTITUDES AND DISCRIMINATION
IN THE UNITED STATES

By way of context, it is important to note that racial and ethnic disparities are found in many sectors of American life. African Americans, Hispanics, American Indians, and Pacific Islanders, and some Asian-American subgroups are disproportionately represented in the lower socioeconomic ranks, in lower quality schools, and in poorer-paying jobs. These disparities can be traced to many factors, including historic patterns of legalized segregation and discrimination. Unfortunately, some discrimination remains. For example, audit studies of mortgage lending, housing, and employment practices using paired "testers" demonstrate persistent discrimination against African Americans and Hispanics. These studies illustrate that much of American social and economic life remains ordered by race and ethnicity, with minorities disadvantaged relative to whites. In addition, these findings suggest that minorities' experiences in the world outside of the healthcare practitioner's office are likely to affect their perceptions and responses in care settings.

> **Finding 2-1: Racial and ethnic disparities in healthcare occur in the context of broader historic and contemporary social and economic**

inequality, and evidence of persistent racial and ethnic discrimination in many sectors of American life.

ASSESSING POTENTIAL SOURCES OF DISPARITIES IN CARE

The studies cited above suggest that a range of patient-level, provider-level, and system-level factors may be involved in racial and ethnic healthcare disparities, beyond access-related factors.

Patient-Level Variables:
The Role of Preferences, Treatment Refusal, and the
Clinical Appropriateness of Care

Racial and ethnic disparities in care may emerge, at least in part, from a number of patient-level attributes. For example, minority patients are more likely to refuse recommended services (e.g., Sedlis et al., 1997), adhere poorly to treatment regimens, and delay seeking care (e.g., Mitchell and McCormack, 1997). These behaviors and attitudes can develop as a result of a poor cultural match between minority patients and their providers, mistrust, misunderstanding of provider instructions, poor prior interactions with healthcare systems, or simply from a lack of knowledge of how to best use healthcare services. However, racial and ethnic differences in patient preferences and care-seeking behaviors and attitudes are unlikely to be major sources of healthcare disparities. For example, while minority patients have been found to refuse recommended treatment more often than whites, differences in refusal rates are small and have not fully accounted for racial and ethnic disparities in receipt of treatments (Hannan et al., 1999; Ayanian et al., 1999). Overuse of some clinical services (i.e., use of services when not clinically indicated) may be more common among white than minority patients, and may contribute to racial and ethnic differences in discretionary procedures. Several recent studies, however, have assessed racial differences relative to established criteria (Hannan et al., 1999; Laouri et al., 1997; Canto et al., 2000; Peterson et al., 1997) or objective diagnostic information, and still find racial differences in receipt of care. Other studies find that overuse of cardiovascular services among whites does not explain racial differences in service use (Schneider et al., 2001).

Finally, some researchers have speculated that biologically based racial differences in clinical presentation or response to treatment may justify racial differences in the type and intensity of care provided. For example, racial and ethnic group differences are found in response to drug therapies such as enalapril, an angiotensin-converting–enzyme inhibitor used to reduce the risk of heart failure (Exner et al., 2001). These differences in response to drug therapy, however, are not due to "race" *per se* but can be traced to differences in the distribution of polymorphic traits between population groups (Wood, 2001), and are small in relation to the common benefits of most therapeutic interventions. Further, as noted above, the majority of studies document disparities in healthcare services and disease areas when interventions are equally effective across population groups—making the "racial differences" hypothesis an unlikely explanation for observed disparities in care.

>   **Finding 4-2: A small number of studies suggest that racial and ethnic minority patients are more likely than white patients to refuse treatment. These studies find that differences in refusal rates are generally small and that minority patient refusal does not fully explain healthcare disparities.**

Healthcare Systems-Level Factors

Aspects of health systems—such as the ways in which systems are organized and financed, and the availability of services—may exert different effects on patient care, particularly for racial and ethnic minorities. Language barriers, for example, pose a problem for many patients where health systems lack the resources, knowledge, or institutional priority to provide interpretation and translation services. Nearly 14 million Americans are not proficient in English, and as many as one in five Spanish-speaking Latinos reports not seeking medical care due to language barriers (The Robert Wood Johnson Foundation, 2001). Similarly, time pressures on physicians may hamper their ability to accurately assess presenting symptoms of minority patients, especially where cultural or linguistic barriers are present. Further, the geographic availability of healthcare institutions—while largely influenced by economic factors that are outside the charge of this study—may have a differential impact on racial and ethnic minorities, independent of insurance status (Kahn et al., 1994). A study of the availability of opioid supplies, for example, revealed that only one in four pharmacies located in predominantly non-white neighborhoods carried adequate supplies, compared with 72% of pharmacies in predominantly white neighborhoods (Morrison et al., 2000). Perhaps more significantly, changes in the financing and delivery of healthcare services—such as the shifts brought by cost-control efforts and the movement to managed care—may pose greater barriers to care for racial and ethnic minorities than for non-minorities (Rice, this volume). Increasing efforts by states to enroll Medicaid patients in managed care systems, for example, may disrupt traditional community-based care and displace providers who are familiar with the language, culture, and values of ethnic minority communities (Leigh, Lillie-Blanton, Martinez, and Collins, 1999). In addition, research indicates that minorities enrolled in publicly funded managed care plans are less likely to access services after mandatory enrollment in an HMO, compared with whites and other minorities enrolled in non-managed care plans (Tai-Seale et al., 2001).

Care Process-Level Variables:
The Role of Bias, Stereotyping, Uncertainty

Three mechanisms might be operative in healthcare disparities from the provider's side of the exchange: bias (or prejudice) against minorities; greater clinical uncertainty when interacting with minority patients; and beliefs (or stereotypes) held by the provider about the behavior or health of minorities (Balsa and McGuire, 2001). Patients might also react to providers' behavior associated with these practices in a way that also contributes to disparities. Unfortunately, little research has been conducted to elucidate how patient race or ethnicity may influence physician decision-making and how these influences affect the quality of care provided. In the absence of such research, the study committee drew upon a mix of theory and relevant research to understand how clinical uncertainty, biases or stereotypes, and prejudice might operate in the clinical encounter.

Clinical Uncertainty

Any degree of uncertainty a physician may have relative to the condition of a patient can contribute to disparities in treatment. Doctors must depend on inferences about severity based on what they can see about the illness and on what else they observe about the patient (e.g., race). The doctor can therefore be viewed as operating with prior beliefs about the likelihood of patients' conditions, "priors" that will be different according to age, gender, socioeconomic status, and race or ethnicity. When these priors—which are taught as a cognitive heuristic to medical students—are considered alongside the information gained in a clinical encounter, both influence medical decisions.

Doctors must balance new information gained from the patient (sometimes with varying levels of accuracy) and their prior expectations about the patient to determine the diagnosis and course of treatment. If the physician has difficulty accurately understanding the symptoms or is less sure of the "signal"—the set of clues and indications that physicians rely upon to make diagnostic decisions—then he or she is likely to place greater weight on the "priors." The consequence is that treatment decisions and patients' needs are potentially less well matched.

The Implicit Nature of Stereotypes

A large body of research in psychology has explored how stereotypes evolve, persist, shape expectations, and affect interpersonal interactions. Stereotyping can be defined as the process by which people use social categories (e.g., race, sex) in acquiring, processing, and recalling information about others. The beliefs (stereotypes) and general orientations (attitudes) that people bring to their interactions help to organize and simplify complex or uncertain situations and give perceivers greater confidence in their ability to understand a situation and respond in efficient and effective ways (Mackie, Hamilton, Susskind, and Rosselli, 1996). Although functional, social stereotypes and attitudes also tend to be systematically biased. These biases may exist in overt, explicit forms, as represented by traditional bigotry. However, because their origins arise from virtually universal social categorization processes, they may also exist, often unconsciously, among people who strongly endorse egalitarian principles and truly believe that they are not prejudiced (Dovidio and Gaertner, 1998). In the United States, because of shared socialization influences, there is considerable empirical evidence that even well-meaning whites who are not overtly biased and who do not believe that they are prejudiced typically demonstrate unconscious implicit negative racial attitudes and stereotypes (Dovidio, Brigham, Johnson, and Gaertner, 1996). Both implicit and explicit stereotypes significantly shape interpersonal interactions, influencing how information is recalled and guiding expectations and inferences in systematic ways. They can also produce self-fulfilling prophecies in social interaction, in that the stereotypes of the perceiver influence the interaction with others in ways that conform to stereotypical expectations (Jussim, 1991).

Healthcare Provider Prejudice or Bias

Prejudice is defined in psychology as an unjustified negative attitude based on a person's group membership (Dovidio et al., 1996). Survey research suggests that among white Americans, prejudicial attitudes toward minorities remain more common than not, as over half to three-quarters believe that relative to whites, minorities—particularly African Americans—are less intelligent, more prone to violence, and prefer to live off of welfare (Bobo, 2001). It is reasonable to assume, however, that the vast majority of healthcare providers find prejudice morally abhorrent and at odds with their professional values. But healthcare providers, like other members of society, may not recognize manifestations of prejudice in their own behavior.

While there is no direct evidence that provider biases affect the quality of care for minority patients, research suggests that healthcare providers' diagnostic and treatment decisions, as well as their feelings about patients, are influenced by patients' race or ethnicity. Schulman et al. (1999), for example, found that physicians referred white male, black male, and white female hypothetical "patients" (actually videotaped actors who displayed the same symptoms of cardiac disease) for cardiac catheterization at the same rates (approximately 90% for each group), but were significantly less likely to recommend catheterization procedures for black female patients exhibiting the same symptoms. Weisse et al. (2001), using a similar methodology as that of Schulman, found that male physicians prescribed twice the level of analgesic medication for white "patients" than for black "patients." Female physicians, in contrast, prescribed higher doses of analgesics for black than for white "patients," suggesting that male and female physicians may respond differently to gender and/or racial cues. In another experimental design, Abreu (1999) found that mental health professionals subliminally "primed" with African American stereotype-laden words were more likely to evaluate the same hypothetical patient (whose race was not identified) more negatively than when primed with neutral words. And in a study based on actual clinical encounters, van Ryn and Burke (2000) found that doctors rated black patients as less intelligent, less educated, more likely to abuse drugs and alcohol, more likely to fail to comply with medical advice, more likely to lack social support, and less likely to participate in cardiac rehabilitation than white patients, even after patients' income, education, and personality characteristics were taken into account. These findings suggest that while the relationship between race or ethnicity and treatment decisions is complex and may also be influenced by gender, providers' perceptions and attitudes toward patients are influenced by patient race or ethnicity, often in subtle ways.

Medical Decisions Under Time Pressure with Limited Information

Studies suggest that several characteristics of the clinical encounter increase the likelihood that stereotypes, prejudice, or uncertainly may influence the quality of care for minorities (van Ryn, 2002). In the process of care, health professionals must come to judgments about patients' conditions and make decisions about treatment, often without complete and accurate information. In most cases, they must do so under severe time pressure and resource constraints. The assembly and use of these data are affected by many influences, including various "gestalts" or cognitive shortcuts. In fact, physicians are commonly trained to rely on clusters of information that functionally resemble the application of "prototypic" or stereotypic constellations. These conditions of time pressure, resource constraints, and the need to rely on gestalts map closely onto those factors identified by social psychologists as likely to produce negative outcomes due to lack of information, to stereotypes, and to biases (van Ryn, 2002).

Patient Response: Mistrust and Refusal

As noted above, the responses of racial and ethnic minority patients to healthcare providers are also a potential source of disparities. Little research has been conducted as to how patients may influence the clinical encounter. It is reasonable to speculate, however, that if patients convey mistrust, refuse treatment, or comply poorly with treatment, providers may become less engaged in the treatment process, and patients are less likely to be provided with more vigorous treatments and services. But these kinds of reactions from minority patients may be understandable as a response to negative racial experiences in other contexts, or to real or perceived mistreatment by providers. Survey research, for example, indicates that minority patients perceive higher levels of racial discrimination in healthcare than non-minorities (LaVeist, Nickerson, and Bowie, 2000; Lillie-Blanton et al., 2000). Patients' and providers' behavior and attitudes may therefore influence each other reciprocally, but reflect the attitudes, expectations, and perceptions that each has developed in a context where race and ethnicity are often more salient than these participants are even aware of. In addition, it is clear that the healthcare provider, rather than the patient, is the more powerful actor in clinical encounters. Providers' expectations, beliefs, attitudes, and behaviors are therefore likely to be a more important target for intervention efforts.

> **Finding 3-1: Many sources—including health systems, healthcare providers, patients, and utilization managers—may contribute to racial and ethnic disparities in healthcare.**

> **Finding 4-1: Bias, stereotyping, prejudice, and clinical uncertainty on the part of healthcare providers may contribute to racial and ethnic disparities in healthcare. While indirect evidence from several lines of research supports this statement, a greater understanding of the prevalence and influence of these processes is needed and should be sought through research.**

INTERVENTIONS TO ELIMINATE RACIAL AND ETHNIC DISPARITIES IN HEALTHCARE

Legal, Regulatory, and Policy Interventions

"De-Fragmentation" of Healthcare Financing and Delivery

Racial and ethnic minorities are more likely than whites to be enrolled in "lower-end" health plans, which are characterized by higher per capita resource constraints and stricter limits on covered services (Phillips et al., 2000). The disproportionate presence of racial and ethnic minorities in lower-end health plans is a potential source of healthcare disparities, given that efforts to control for insurance status in studies of healthcare disparities have not taken detailed account of variations among health plans. Such socioeconomic fragmentation of health plans engenders different clinical cultures, with different practice norms, tied to varying per capita resource constraints (Bloche, 2001).

Equalizing access to high-quality plans can limit such fragmentation. Public healthcare payors such as Medicaid should strive to help beneficiaries access the same health products as privately-insured patients. This recommendation is also reflected in the IOM *Quality Chasm* report's strategies for focusing health systems on quality, in its call to "eliminate or modify payment practices that fragment the care system" (IOM, 2001, p. 13).

Recommendation 5-1: Avoid fragmentation of health plans along socioeconomic lines.

Strengthening Doctor-Patient Relationships

Several lines of research suggest that the consistency and stability of the doctor-patient relationship is an important determinant of patient satisfaction and access to care. Having a usual source of care is associated, for example, with use of preventive care services (Agency for Healthcare Research and Quality, 2001). In addition, having a consistent relationship with a primary care provider may help to address minority patient mistrust of healthcare systems and providers, particularly if the relationship is with a provider who is able to bridge cultural and linguistic gaps (LaViest, Nickerson, and Bowie, 2000). Minority patients, however, are less likely to enjoy a consistent relationship with a provider, even when insured at the same levels as white patients (Lillie-Blanton, Martinez, and Salganicoff, 2001). This is due in part to the types of health systems in which they are enrolled and the relative lack of providers located in minority communities.

Health systems should attempt to ensure that every patient, whether insured privately or publicly, has a sustained relationship with an attending physician able to help the patient effectively navigate the healthcare bureaucracy. Federal and state performance standards for Medicaid managed care plans, for example, should include guidelines to ensure the stability of patients' assignments to primary care providers (and these providers' accessibility), reasonable patient loads per primary care physician, and time allotments for patient visits.

Recommendation 5-2: Strengthen the stability of patient-provider relationships in publicly funded health plans.

Patient and provider relationships will also be strengthened by greater racial and ethnic diversity in the health professions. Racial concordance of patient and provider is associated with greater patient participation in care processes, higher patient satisfaction, and greater adherence to treatment (Cooper-Patrick et al., 1999). In addition, racial and ethnic minority providers are more likely than their non-minority colleagues to serve in minority and medically underserved communities (Komaromy et al., 1996). The benefits of diversity in health professions fields are significant, and illustrate that a continued commitment to affirmative action is necessary for graduate health professions education programs, residency recruitment, and other professional opportunities.

Recommendation 5-3: Increase the proportion of underrepresented U.S. racial and ethnic minorities among health professionals.

Patient Protections

Much of the political focus on Capitol Hill in the summer of 2001 was devoted to managed care regulation. To one extent or another, the various bills debated would all extend protections to enrollees in private managed care organizations, providing avenues for appeal of care denial decisions, improving access to specialty care, requiring health plans to disclose information about coverage, banning physician "gag" clauses, and providing other legal remedies to resolve disputes. Publicly funded health plans, however, are not addressed in these legislative proposals. Given that many minorities are disproportionately represented among the publicly insured who receive care within managed care organizations, the same patient protections that apply to the privately insured should apply to those in publicly funded plans (Hashimoto, 2001).

Recommendation 5-4: Apply the same managed care protections to publicly funded HMO enrollees that apply to private HMO enrollees.

Civil Rights Enforcement

Enforcement of regulation and statute is also an important component of a comprehensive strategy to address healthcare disparities, but unfortunately has been too often relegated to low-priority status. The U.S. DHHS Office of Civil Rights (OCR) is charged with enforcing several relevant federal statutes and regulations that prohibit discrimination in healthcare (principally Title VI of the 1964 Civil Rights Act). The agency, however, has suffered from insufficient resources to investigate complaints of possible violations, and has long abandoned proactive, investigative strategies (Smith, 1999). Complaints to the agency declined in the early 1990s, but have increased in recent years, while funding has remained level in terms of appropriated dollars but lower in terms of spending power after adjusting for inflation (U.S. Commission on Civil Rights, 2001). The agency should be equipped with sufficient resources to better address these complaints and carry out its oversight responsibilities.

Recommendation 5-5: Provide greater resources to the U.S. DHHS Office for Civil Rights to enforce civil rights laws.

Health Systems Interventions

A variety of interventions applied at the level of health systems may be effective as a part of a comprehensive, multi-level strategy to address racial and ethnic disparities in healthcare.

Evidence-Based Cost Control

In the current era of continually escalating healthcare costs, cost containment is an important goal of all health systems. To the extent possible, however, medical limit setting by health plans should be based on evidence of effectiveness. The application of evidence to healthcare delivery, such as through the use of evidence-based guidelines, can help to address the problem of potential underuse of services resulting from capitation or per case payment methods, as noted in the IOM *Quality Chasm* report (IOM, 2001). Evidence-based guidelines offer the advantages of consistency, predictability, and objectivity that general, discretionary advisory statements do not. In addition, because evidence-based guidelines and standards directly promote accountability, they also indirectly affect equity of care.

In actual practice, however, a pragmatic balance must be sought between the advantages and limitations of guidelines, such as the tension between the goal of standardization versus the need for clinical flexibility. Disclosing health plans' clinical protocols offers one means of achieving this balance, as it would aid both private sector and public efforts in balancing the virtues of rules and discretion. To achieve this, private accrediting entities and state regulatory bodies could require that health plans publish their clinical practice protocols, along with supporting evidence, thereby opening these protocols to professional and consumer review (Bloche, 2001).

Recommendation 5-6: Promote the consistency and equity of care through the use of evidence-based guidelines.

Financial Incentives in Healthcare

Financial factors, such as capitation and health plan incentives to providers to practice frugally, can pose greater barriers to racial and ethnic minority patients than to white patients, even among patients insured at the same level. Low payment rates limit the supply of physician (and other healthcare provider) services to low-income groups, disproportionately affecting ethnic minorities (Rice, this volume). Inadequate supply takes the form of too few providers participating in plans serving the poor, and provider unwillingness to spend adequate time with patients. This time pressure may contribute to poor information exchange between physicians and members of minority groups.

If appropriately crafted, however, financial incentives to physicians can serve a positive role in efforts to reduce disparities in care. Economic rewards for time spent engaging patients and their families can help physicians to overcome barriers of culture, communication, and empathy. In addition, incentives that encourage physicians to adhere to evidence-based protocols for frugal practice and to engage in age- and gender-appropriate disease screening can promote efficient, quality care and penalize deviations, regardless of race or ethnicity. Further, financial incentives linked to favorable clinical outcomes, where reasonably measurable (e.g. control of diabetes, asthma, and high blood pressure) can also promote equity of care (Bloche, 2001). Again, this recommendation is consistent with the IOM *Quality Chasm* report, which calls for healthcare organizations, clinicians, purchasers, and other stakeholders to "align the incentives inherent in payment and accountability processes with the goal of quality improvement" (IOM, 2001, p.10).

Recommendation 5-7: Structure payment systems to ensure an adequate supply of services to minority patients and limit provider incentives that may promote disparities.

Recommendation 5-8: Enhance patient-provider communication and trust by providing financial incentives for practices that reduce barriers and encourage evidence-based practice.

Interpretation Services

As noted above, many racial and ethnic minorities find that language barriers pose a significant problem in their efforts to access healthcare. Language barriers may affect the delivery of adequate care through poor exchange of information, loss of important cultural information, misunderstanding of physician instruction, poor shared decision making, or ethical compromises (e.g., difficulty obtaining informed consent; Woloshin et al., 1995). Linguistic difficulties may also result in decreased adherence with medication regimes, poor appointment attendance (Manson, 1988), and decreased satisfaction with services (Carrasquillo et al., 1999; David and Rhee, 1998; Derose and Baker, 2000).

Broader use of professional interpretation services has been hampered by a number of logistical and resource constraints. For example, in some regions of the country, few trained professional interpreters are available, and reimbursement for interpretation services via publicly funded insurance such as Medicaid is often inadequate. Greater resources are needed to support professional interpretation services, and more research and innovation should identify effective means to harness new technologies (e.g., simultaneous telephone interpretation) to aid interpretation.

Recommendation 5-9: Support the use of interpretation services where community need exists.

Community Health Workers

Community health workers—often termed lay health advisors, neighborhood workers, indigenous health workers, health aides, *consejera*, or *promotora*—fulfill multiple functions in helping to improve access to healthcare. Community health workers can serve as liaisons between patients and providers, educate providers about community needs and the culture of the community, provide patient education, contribute to continuity and coordination of care, assist in appointment attendance and adherence to medication regimens, and help to increase the use of preventive and primary care services (Brownstein et al., 1992; Earp and Flax,

1999; Jackson and Parks, 1997). In addition, some evidence suggests that lay health workers can help improve the quality of care and reduce costs (Witmer et al., 1995), and improve general wellness by facilitating community access to and negotiation for services (Rodney et al., 1998).

Recommendation 5-10: Support the use of community health workers.

Multidisciplinary Teams

Research demonstrates that multidisciplinary team approaches—including physicians, nurses, dietitians, and social workers, among others—can effectively optimize patient care. This effect is found in randomized controlled studies of patients with coronary heart disease, hypertension, and other diseases, and has extended to strategies for reducing risk behaviors and conditions such as smoking, sedentary lifestyle and obesity (Hill and Miller, 1996). Multidisciplinary teams coordinate and streamline care, enhance patient adherence through follow-up techniques, and address the multiple behavioral and social risks faced by patients. These teams may save costs and improve the efficiency of care by reducing the need for face-to-face physician visits and improve patients' day-to-day care between visits. Further, such strategies have proven effective in improving health outcomes of minorities previously viewed as "difficult to serve" (Hill and Miller, 1996). Multidisciplinary team approaches should be more widely instituted as strategy for improving care delivery, implementing secondary prevention strategies, and enhancing risk reduction.

Recommendation 5-11: Implement multidisciplinary treatment and preventive care teams.

Patient Education and Empowerment

Increasingly, researchers are recognizing the important role of patients as active participants in clinical encounters (Korsch, 1984). Patient education efforts have taken many forms, including the use of books and pamphlets, in-person instruction, CD-ROM-based educational materials, and internet-based information. These materials guide patients through typical office visits and provide information about asking appropriate questions and having their questions answered, communicating with the provider when instructions are not understood or cannot be followed, and being an active participant in decision-making. While evaluation data are limited, particularly with respect to racial and ethnic minority patients, preliminary evidence suggests that patient education can improve patients' skills and knowledge of clinical encounters and improve their participation in care decisions.

Recommendation 5-12: Implement patient education programs to increase patients' knowledge of how to best access care and participate in treatment decisions.

Cross-Cultural Education in the Health Professions

Given the increasing racial and ethnic diversity of the U.S. population, the development and implementation of training programs for healthcare providers offers promise as a key intervention strategy in reducing healthcare disparities. As a result, cross-cultural education programs have been developed to enhance health professionals' awareness of how cultural and social factors influence healthcare, while providing methods to obtain, negotiate and manage this information clinically once it is obtained. Cross-cultural education can be divided into three conceptual approaches focusing on *attitudes* (cultural sensitivity/awareness approach), *knowledge* (multicultural/categorical approach), and *skills* (cross-cultural approach), and has been taught using a variety of interactive and experiential methodologies. Research to date demonstrates that training

---

Summary of Findings

Finding 1-1: Racial and ethnic disparities in healthcare exist and, because they are associated with worse outcomes in many cases, are unacceptable.

Finding 2-1: Racial and ethnic disparities in healthcare occur in the context of broader historic and contemporary social and economic inequality, and evidence of persistent racial and ethnic discrimination in many sectors of American life.

Finding 3-1: Many sources—including health systems, healthcare providers, patients, and utilization managers—may contribute to racial and ethnic disparities in healthcare.

Finding 4-1: Bias, stereotyping, prejudice, and clinical uncertainty on the part of healthcare providers may contribute to racial and ethnic disparities in healthcare. While indirect evidence from several lines of research supports this statement, a greater understanding of the prevalence and influence of these processes is needed and should be sought through research.

Finding 4-2: A small number of studies suggest that racial and ethnic minority patients are more likely than white patients to refuse treatment. These studies find that differences in refusal rates are generally small and that minority patient refusal does not fully explain healthcare disparities.

Summary of Recommendations

General Recommendations
Recommendation 2-1: Increase awareness of racial and ethnic disparities in healthcare among the general public and key stakeholders.
Recommendation 2-2: Increase healthcare providers' awareness of disparities.

Legal, Regulatory, and Policy Interventions
Recommendation 5-1: Avoid fragmentation of health plans along socioeconomic lines.
Recommendation 5-2: Strengthen the stability of patient-provider relationships in publicly funded health plans.
Recommendation 5-3: Increase the proportion of underrepresented U.S. racial and ethnic minorities among health professionals.
Recommendation 5-4: Apply the same managed care protections to publicly funded HMO enrollees that apply to private HMO enrollees.
Recommendation 5-5: Provide greater resources to the U.S. DHHS Office for Civil Rights to enforce civil rights laws.

Health Systems Interventions
Recommendation 5-6: Promote the consistency and equity of care through the use of evidence-based guidelines.
Recommendation 5-7: Structure payment systems to ensure an adequate supply of services to minority patients, and limit provider incentives that may promote disparities.
Recommendation 5-8: Enhance patient-provided communication and trust by providing financial incentives for practices that reduce barriers and encourage evidence-based practice.
Recommendation 5-9: Support the use of interpretation services where community need exists.

is effective in improving provider knowledge of cultural and behavioral aspects of healthcare and building effective communication strategies. Despite progress in the field, however, several challenges exist, including the need to define educational core competencies, reach consensus on approaches and methodologies, determine methods of integration into the medical and nursing curriculum, and develop and implement appropriate evaluation strategies. These challenges should be addressed to realize the potential of cross-cultural education strategies.

Recommendation 6-1: Integrate cross-cultural education into the training of all current and future health professionals.

Recommendation 5-10: Support the use of community health workers.
Recommendation 5-11: Implement multidisciplinary treatment and preventive care teams.

Patient Education and Empowerment
Recommendation 5-12: Implement patient education programs to increase patients' knowledge of how to best access care and participate in treatment decisions.

Cross-Cultural Education in the Health Professions
Recommendation 6-1: Integrate cross-cultural education into the training of all current and future health professionals.

Data Collection and Monitoring
Recommendation 7-1: Collect and report data on health care access and utilization by patients' race, ethnicity, socioeconomic status, and where possible, primary language.
Recommendation 7-2: Include measures of racial and ethnic disparities in performance measurement.
Recommendation 7-3: Monitor progress toward the elimination of healthcare disparities.
Recommendation 7-4: Report racial and ethnic data by OMB categories, but use subpopulation groups where possible.

Research Needs
Recommendation 8-1: Conduct further research to identify sources of racial and ethnic disparities and assess promising intervention strategies.
Recommendation 8-2: Conduct research on ethical issues and other barriers to eliminating disparities.

DATA COLLECTION AND MONITORING

Standardized data collection is critically important in the effort to understand and eliminate racial and ethnic disparities in healthcare. Data on patient and provider race and ethnicity would allow researchers to better disentangle factors that are associated with healthcare disparities, help health plans to monitor performance, ensure accountability to enrolled members and payors, improve patient choice, allow for evaluation of intervention programs, and help identify discriminatory practices. Unfortunately, standardized data on racial and ethnic differences in care are generally unavailable. Federal and state-supported data collection efforts are scattered and unsystematic, and many health plans, with a few notable exceptions, do not collect data on enrollees' race, ethnicity, or primary language.

A number of ethical, logistical, and fiscal concerns present challenges to data collection and monitoring, including the need to protect patient privacy, the costs of data collection, and resistance from healthcare providers, institutions, plans and patients. In addition, health plans have raised significant concerns about how such data will be analyzed and reported. The challenges to data collection should be addressed, as the costs of failing to assess racial and ethnic disparities in care may outweigh new burdens imposed by data collection and analysis efforts.

Recommendation 7-1: Collect and report data on healthcare access and utilization by patients' race, ethnicity, socioeconomic status, and where possible, primary language.

Recommendation 7-2: Include measures of racial and ethnic disparities in performance measurement.

Recommendation 7-3: Monitor progress toward the elimination of healthcare disparities.

Recommendation 7-4: Report racial and ethnic data by federally defined categories, but use subpopulation groups where possible.

NEEDED RESEARCH

While the literature that the committee reviewed provides significant evidence of racial and ethnic disparities in care, the evidence base from which to better understand and eliminate disparities in care remains less than clear. Several broad areas of research are needed to clarify how race and ethnicity are associated with disparities in the process, structure, and outcomes of care. Research must provide a better understanding of the contribution of patient, provider, and institutional characteristics on the quality of care for minorities. Research has been notably absent in other areas. More research is needed, for example, to understand the extent of disparities in care faced by Asian-American, Pacific-Islander, American Indian and Alaska Native, and Hispanic populations, and to better understand and surmount barriers to research on healthcare disparities, including those related to ethical issues in data collection.

Recommendation 8-1: Conduct further research to identify sources of racial and ethnic disparities and assess promising intervention strategies.

Recommendation 8-2: Conduct research on ethical issues and other barriers to eliminating disparities.

References

Abreu JM. (1999). Conscious and nonconscious African American stereotypes: Impact on first impression and diagnostic ratings by therapists. *Journal of Consulting and Clinical Psychology* 67(3):387-93.

Agency for Healthcare Research and Quality. (2001). Addressing racial and ethnic disparities in healthcare. Fact sheet accessed from internet site www. ahrq.gov/research/ disparit.htm on December 18, 2001.

Allison JJ, Kiefe CI, Centor RM, Box JB, Farmer RM. (1996). Racial differences in the medical treatment of elderly Medicare patients with acute myocardial infarction. *Journal of General Internal Medicine* 11:736-43.

Ayanian JZ, Udvarhelyi IS, Gatsonis CA, Pasho, CL, Epstein AM. (1993). Racial differences in the use of revascularization procedures after coronary angiography. *Journal of the American Medical Association* 269:2642-6.

Ayanian JZ, Weissman JS, Chasan-Taber S, Epstein AM. (1999). Quality of care by race and gender for congestive heart failure and pneumonia. *Medical Care* 37:1260-9.

Bach PB, Cramer LD, Warren JL, Begg CB. (1999). Racial differences in the treatment of early-stage lung cancer. *New England Journal of Medicine* 341:1198-205.

Balsa A, McGuire TG. (2001). Prejudice, uncertainty and stereotypes as sources of health care disparities. Boston University, unpublished manuscript.

Barker-Cummings C, McClellan W, Soucie, JM, Krisher J. (1995). Ethnic differences in the use of peritoneal dialysis as initial treatment for end-stage renal disease. *Journal of the American Medical Association* 274(23):1858-1862.

Bennett CL, Horner RD, Weinstein RA, Dickinson GM, Dehovitz JA, Cohn SE, Kessler HA, Jacobson J, Goetz MB, Simberkoff M, Pitrak D, George WL, Gilman SC, Shapiro MF. (1995). Racial differences in care among hospitalized patients with pneumocystis carinii pneumonia in Chicago, New York, Los Angeles, Miami, and Raleigh-Durham. *Archives of Internal Medicine* 155(15):1586-92.

Bernabei R, Gambassi G, Lapane K, et al. (1998). Management of pain in elderly patients with cancer. *Journal of the American Medical Association* 279:1877-82.

Bloche MG. (2001). Race and discretion in American medicine. *Yale Journal of Health Policy, Law, and Ethics* 1:95-131.

Bobo LD. (2001). Racial attitudes and relations at the close of the twentieth century. In Smelser NJ, Wilson WJ, and Mitchell F (Eds.), *America Becoming: Racial Trends and Their Consequences*. Washington, DC: National Academy Press.

Brogan D, Tuttle EP. (1988). Transplantation and the Medicare end-stage renal disease program [Letter]. *New England Journal of Medicine* 319:55.

Brownstein JN, Cheal N, Ackermann SP, Bassford TL, Campos-Outcalt D. (1992). Breast and cervical cancer screening in minority populations: A model for using lay health educators. *Journal of Cancer Education* 7(4):321-326.

Canto JG, Allison JJ, Kiefe CI, Fincher C, Farmer R, Sekar P, Person S, Weissman NW. (2000). Relation of race and sex to the use of reperfusion therapy in Medicare beneficiaries with acute myocardial infarction. *New England Journal of Medicine* 342:1094-1100.

Carrasquillo O, Orav EJ, Brennan TA, Burstin HR. (1999). Impact of language barriers on patient satisfaction in an emergency department. *Journal of General Internal Medicine* 14(2):82-7.

Chin MH, Zhang JX, Merrell K. (1998). Diabetes in the African-American Medicare population: Morbidity, quality of care, and resource utilization. *Diabetes Care* 21(7):1090-1095.

Cooper-Patrick L, Gallo JJ, Gonzales JJ, Vu HT, Powe NR, Nelson C, Ford DE. (1999). Race, gender, and partnership in the patient-physician relationship. *Journal of the American Medical Association* 282(6):583-9.

Cunningham WE, Mosen DM, Morales LS. (2000). Ethnic and racial differences in long-term survival from hospitalization for HIV infection. *Journal of Health Care for the Poor and Underserved* 11(2):163-178.

David RA, Rhee M. (1998). The impact of language as a barrier to effective health care in an underserved urban Hispanic community. *Mount Sinai Journal of Medicine* 65(5-6):393-397.

Derose KP, Baker DW. (2000). Limited English proficiency and Latinos' use of physician services. *Medical Care Research and Review* 57(1):76-91.

Dovidio JF, Brigham JC, Johnson BT, Gaertner SL. (1996). Stereotyping, prejudice, and discrimination: Another look. In Macrae N, Stangor C, and Hewstone M (Eds.), *Stereotypes and Stereotyping* 276-319. New York: Guilford.

Dovidio JF, Gaertner SL. (1998). On the nature of contemporary prejudice: The causes, consequences, and challenges of aversive racism. In Eberhardt J and Fiske ST (Eds.), *Confronting Racism: The Problem and the Response* 3-32. Thousand Oaks, CA: Sage.

Earp JL, Flax VL. (1999). What lay health advisors do: An evaluation of advisors' activities. *Cancer Practice* 7(1):16-21.

Epstein AM, Ayanian JZ, Keogh JH, Noonan SJ, Armistead N, Cleary PD, Weissman JS, David-Kasdan JA, Carlson D, Fuller J, March D, Conti R. (2000). Racial disparities in access to renal transplantation. *New England Journal of Medicine* 343(21):1537-1544.

Exner DV, Dries DL, Domanski MJ, Cohn JN. (2001). Lesser response to angiotensin-converting–enzyme inhibitor therapy in black as compared with white patients with left ventricular dysfunction. *New England Journal of Medicine* 344:1351-1357.

Gaylin DS, Held PJ, Port FK, et al. (1993). The impact of comorbid and sociodemographic factors on access to renal transplantation. *Journal of the American Medical Association* 269:603-608.

Geiger J. (this volume). Racial and ethnic disparities in diagnosis and treatment: A review of the evidence and a consideration of causes.

Giles WH, Anda RF, Casper ML, Escobedo LG, Taylor HA. (1995). Race and sex differences in rates of invasive cardiac procedures in U.S. hospitals. *Archives of Internal Medicine* 155:318-24.

Gomes C, McGuire TG. (2001). Identifying the sources of racial and ethnic disparities in health care use. Unpublished manuscript.

Gornick ME, Egers PW, Reilly TW, Mentnech RM, Fitterman LK, Kucken LE, Vladeck BC. (1996). Effects of race and income on mortality and use of services among Medicare beneficiaries. *New England Journal of Medicine* 335(11):791-799.

Hannan EL, Van Ryn M, Burke J, et al. (1999). Access to coronary artery bypass surgery by race/ethnicity and gender among patients who are appropriate for surgery. *Medical Care* 37:68-77.

Hashimoto DM. (2001). The proposed Patients' Bill of Rights: The case of the missing equal protection clause. *Yale Journal of Health Policy, Law, and Ethics* 1:77-93.

Herholz H, Goff DC, Ramsey DJ, Chan FA, Ortiz C, Labarthe DR, Nichaman MZ. (1996). Women and Mexican Americans receive fewer cardiovascular drugs following myocardial infarction than men and non-Hispanic whites: The Corpus Christi Heart Project, 1988-1990. *Journal of Clinical Epidemiology* 49(3):279-87.

Hill MN, Miller NH. (1996). Compliance enhancement. A call for multidisciplinary team approaches. *Circulation* 93(1):4-6.

House JS, Williams D. (2000). Understanding and reducing socioeconomic and racial/ethnic disparities in health. In Smedley BD and Syme SL (Eds.), *Promoting Health: Intervention Strategies from Social and Behavioral Research*. Washington, DC: National Academy Press.

Imperato PJ, Nenner RP, Will TO. (1996). Radical prostatectomy: Lower rates among African American men. *Journal of the National Medical Association* 88(9):589-94.

Institute of Medicine. (2001). *Crossing the Quality Chasm*. Washington, DC: The National Academy Press.

Jackson EJ, Parks CP. (1997). Recruitment and training issues from selected lay health advisor programs among African Americans: A 20-year perspective. *Health Education & Behavior* 24(4):418-431.

Johnson, PA, Lee TH, Cook EF, Rouan GW, Goldman L. (1993). Effect of race on the presentation and management of patients with acute chest pain. *Annals of Internal Medicine* 118:593-601.

Jussim, L. (1991). Social perception and social reality: A reflection-construction model. *Psychological Review* 98:54-73.

Kahn KL, Pearson ML, Harrison ER, Desmond KA, Rogers WH, Rubenstein LV, Brook RH, Keeler EB. (1994). Health care for black and poor hospitalized Medicare patients. *Journal of the American Medical Association* 271(15):1169-1174.

Kaplan GA, Everson SA, Lynch JW. (2000). The contribution of social and behavioral research to an understanding of the distribution of disease: A multilevel approach. In Smedley BD and Syme SL (Eds.), *Promoting Health: Intervention Strategies from Social and Behavioral Research*. Washington, DC: National Academy Press.

Kasiske B, London W, Ellison MD. (1998). Race and socioeconomic factors influencing early placement on the kidney transplant waiting list. *Journal of the American Society of Nephrology* 9(11):2142-2147.

Kjellstrand CM. (1988). Age, sex, and race inequality in renal transplantation. *Archives of Internal Medicine* 148(6):1305-9.

Komaromy M, Grumbach K, Drake M, Vranizan K, Lurie N, Keane D, Bindman AB. (1996). The role of black and Hispanic physicians in providing health care for underserved populations. *New England Journal of Medicine* 334:1305-1310.

Korsch BM. (1984). What do patients and parents want to know? What do they need to know? *Pediatrics* 74(5 Pt 2):917-919.

Kressin NR, Petersen LA. (2001). Racial differences in the use of invasive cardiovascular procedures: Review of the literature and prescription for future research. *Annals of Internal Medicine* 135(5):352-366.

Laouri M, Kravitz RL, French WJ, Yang I, Milliken JC, Hilborne L, Wachsner R, Brook RH. (1997). Underuse of coronary revascularization procedures: Application of a clinical method. *Journal of the American College of Cardiology* 29:891-897.

LaVeist TA, Nickerson KJ, Bowie JV. (2000). Attitudes about racism, medical mistrust, and satisfaction with care among African American and white cardiac patients. *Medical Care Research and Review* 57(Supplement 1):146-61.

Leigh WA, Lillie-Blanton M, Martinez RM, Collins KS. (1999). Managed care in three states: Experiences of low-income African-Americans and Hispanics. *Inquiry* 36(3):318-31.

Lillie-Blanton M, Brodie M, Rowland D, Altman D, McIntosh, M. (2000). Race, ethnicity, and the health care system: Public perceptions and experiences. *Medical Care Research and Review* 57(1):218-235.

Lillie-Blanton M, Martinez RM, Salganicoff A. (2001). Site of medical care: Do racial and ethnic differences persist? *Yale Journal of Health Policy, Law, and Ethics* 1(1):1-17.

Lowe RA, Chhaya S, Nasci K, Gavin LJ, Shaw K, Zwanger ML, Zeccardi JA, Dalsey WC, Abbuhl SB, Feldman H, Berlin JA. (2001). Effect of ethnicity on denial of authorization for emergency department care by managed care gatekeepers. *Academic Emergency Medicine* 8(3):259-66.

Mackie DM, Hamilton DL, Susskind J, Rosselli F. (1996). Social psychological foundations of stereotype formation. In Macrae N, Stangor C, and Hewstone M (Eds.), *Stereotypes and stereotyping* (pp.41-78). New York: Guilford Press.

Manson A. (1988). Language concordance as a determinant of patient compliance and emergency room use in patients with asthma. *Medical Care* 26(12):1119-1128.

Mayberry RM, Mili F, Ofili E. (2000). Racial and ethnic differences in access to medical care. *Medical Care Research and Review* 57(1):108-45.

McMahon LF, Wolfe RA, Huang S, Tedeschi P, Manning W, Edlund MJ. (1999). Racial and gender variation in use of diagnostic colonic procedures in the Michigan Medicare population. *Medical Care* 37(7):712-7.

Mitchell JB, McCormack LA. (1997). Time trends in late-stage diagnosis of cervical cancer: Differences by race/ethnicity and income. *Medical Care* 35(12):1220-4.

Moore RD, Stanton D, Gopalan R, Chaisson RE. (1994). Racial differences in the use of drug therapy for HIV disease in an urban community. *New England Journal of Medicine* 330(11):763-8.

Morin R. (2001). Misperceptions cloud whites' view of blacks. *The Washington Post*, July 11, 2001.

Morrison RS, Wallenstein S, Natale DK, Senzel RS, Huang L. (2000). "We don't carry that"— Failure of pharmacies in predominantly nonwhite neighborhoods to stock opioid analgesics. *New England Journal of Medicine* 342(14):1023-1026.

Mukamel DB, Murthy AS, Weimer DL. (2000). Racial differences in access to high-quality cardiac surgeons. *American Journal of Public Health* 90:1774-1777.

Petersen LA, Wright SM, Peterson ED, Daley J. (2002). Impact of race on cardiac care and outcomes in veterans with acute myocardial infarction. *Medical Care* 40(1Suppl):I-86-96.

Peterson ED, Shaw LK, DeLong ER, Pryor DB, Califf RM, Mark DB. (1997). Racial variation in the use of coronary-vascularization procedures: Are the differences real? Do they matter? *New England Journal of Medicine* 336:480-6.

Phillips KA, Mayer ML, Aday LA. (2000). Barriers to care among racial/ethnic groups under managed care. *Health Affairs* 19:65-75.

Rice T. (this volume). The impact of cost-containment efforts on racial and ethnic disparities in health care: A conceptualization.

Robert Wood Johnson Foundation. (2001). New survey shows language barriers causing many Spanish-speaking Latinos to skip care. Fact sheet presented at press briefing, December 12, 2001. Washington, DC.

Rodney M, Clasen C, Goldman G, Markert R, Deane D. (1998). Three evaluation methods of a community health advocate program. *Journal of Community Health* 23(5):371-381.

Schneider EC, Leape LL, Weissman JS, Piana RN, Gatsonis C, Epstein AM. (2001). Racial differences in cardiac revascularization rates: Does "overuse" explain higher rates among white patients? *Annals of Internal Medicine* 135(5):328-37.

Schulman KA, Berlin JA, Harless W, et al. (1999). The effect of race and sex on physicians' recommendations for cardiac catheterization. *New England Journal of Medicine* 340:618-626.

Sedlis SP, Fisher VJ, Tice D, Esposito R, Madmon L, Steinberg EH. (1997). Racial differences in performance of invasive cardiac procedures in a Department of Veterans Affairs Medical Center. *Journal of Clinical Epidemiology* 50(8):899-901.

Shapiro MF, Morton SC, McCaffrey DF, Senterfitt JW, Fleishman JA, Perlman JF, Athey LA, Keesey JW, Goldman DP, Berry SH, Bozette SA. (1999). Variations in the care of HIV-infected adults in the United States: Results from the HIV Vost and Services Utilization Study. *Journal of the American Medical Association* 281:2305-75.

Smith DB. (1999). *Health Care Divided: Race and Healing a Nation.* Ann Arbor: The University of Michigan Press.

Tai-Seale M, Freund D, LoSasso A. (2001). Racial disparities in service use among Medicaid beneficiaries after mandatory enrollment in managed care: A difference-in-differences approach. *Inquiry* 38(1):49-59.

U.S. Commission on Civil Rights. (2001). *Funding Federal Civil Rights Enforcement: 2000 and Beyond.* Washington, DC: U.S. Commission on Civil Rights.

van Ryn M. (2002). Research on the provider contribution to race/ethnicity disparities in medical care. *Medical Care* 40(1): I-140-I-151.

van Ryn M, Burke J. (2000). The effect of patient race and socio-economic status on physician's perceptions of patients. *Social Science and Medicine* 50:813-828.

Weisse CS, Sorum PC, Sanders KN, Syat BL. (2001). Do gender and race affect decisions about pain management? *Journal of General Internal Medicine* 16(4)211-217.

Weitzman S, Cooper L, Chambless L, Rosamond W, Clegg L, Marcucci G, Romm F, White A. (1997). Gender, racial, and geographic differences in the performance of cardiac diagnostic and therapeutic procedures for hospitalized acute myocardial infarction in four states. *The American Journal of Cardiology* 79:722-6.

Wenneker MB, Epstein AM. (1989) Racial inequalities in the use of procedures for patients with ischemic heart disease in Massachusetts. *Journal of the American Medical Association* 261:253-7.

Williams DR. (1999). Race, socioeconomic status, and health: The added effects of racism and discrimination. *Annals of the New York Academy of Sciences* 896:173-88.

Williams DR, Rucker TD (2000). Understanding and addressing racial disparities in health care. *Health Care Financing Review* 21:75-90.

Williams JF, Zimmerman JW, Wagner DP, Hawkins M, Knaus WA. (1995). African-American and white patients admitted to the intensive care unit: Is there a difference in therapy and outcome? *Critical Care Medicine* 23(4):626-636.

Witmer A, Seifer SD, Finocchio L, Leslie J, O'Neil EH. (1995). Community health workers: Integral members of the health care work force. *American Journal of Public Health* 85(8): 1055-1058.

Woloshin S, Bickell NA, Schwartz LM, Gany F, Welch HG. (1995). Language barriers in medicine in the United States. *Journal of the American Medical Association* 273(9):724-728.

Wood AJJ. (2001). Racial differences in the response to drugs—pointers to genetic differences. *New England Journal of Medicine* 344:1393-1395.

Yergan J, Food AB, LoGerfo JP, Diher P. Relationship between patient race and the intensity of hospital services. *Medical Care* 25:592-603.

1

Introduction and Literature Review

Despite steady improvement in the overall health of the U.S. population, racial and ethnic minorities, with few exceptions, experience higher rates of morbidity and mortality than non-minorities. African Americans, for example, experience the highest rates of mortality from heart disease, cancer, cerebrovascular disease, and HIV/AIDS than any other U.S. racial or ethnic group. American Indians disproportionately die from diabetes, liver disease and cirrhosis, and unintentional injuries. Hispanic Americans are almost twice as likely as non-Hispanic whites to die from diabetes. In addition, some Asian-American subpopulations experience rates of stomach, liver, and cervical cancers that are well above national averages. The reasons for these health status disparities are complex and poorly understood, but may largely reflect socioeconomic differences, differences in health-related risk factors, environmental degradation, and direct and indirect consequences of discrimination (Williams, 1999).

Differences in access to healthcare are also likely to play a role in these health disparities. Hispanics, Asian Americans, American Indians and Alaska Natives, and African Americans are less likely than whites to have health insurance, have more difficulty getting healthcare, and have fewer choices in where to receive care. Hispanic and African-American patients are also more likely to receive care in hospital emergency rooms, and are less likely than whites to have a regular primary care provider (Collins, Hall, and Neuhaus, 1999).

Concern is growing, however, that even at equivalent levels of access to care, racial and ethnic minorities experience a lower quality of health services and are less likely to receive even routine medical procedures than white Americans. For example, relative to whites, African Americans and Hispanics are less likely to receive appropriate cardiac medication (e.g., thrombolytic therapy, aspirin and beta blockers) or to undergo coronary artery bypass surgery, even when variations in such factors as insurance status, income, age, co-morbid conditions, and symptom expression are taken into account (Ayanian et al., 1993; Hannan et al., 1999; Ramsey et al., 1997; Johnson et al., 1993; Canto et al., 2000). African Americans with end-stage renal disease are less likely to receive peritoneal dialysis and kidney transplantation (Kasiske, London, and Ellison, 1998; Barker-Cummings, McClellan, Soucie, and Krisher, 1995; Gaylin et al., 1993), and African-American and Hispanic patients with bone fractures seen in hospital emergency departments are less likely than whites to receive analgesia (Todd et al., 2000; Todd, Samaroo, and Hoffman, 1993). In terms of quality of care, a recent study of Medicare patients revealed that African-American patients with congestive heart failure or pneumonia received poorer quality care than whites, using explicit process criteria and implicit review by physicians (Ayanian, Weissman, Chasen-Taber, and Epstein, 1999). Further, these differences are associated with greater mortality among African-American patients (Peterson et al., 1997).

STUDY CHARGE AND COMMITTEE ASSUMPTIONS

These disparities prompted Congress in 1999 to request an Institute of Medicine (IOM) study to assess disparities in the kinds and quality of healthcare received by U.S. racial and ethnic minorities and non-minorities. Specifically, Congress requested that the IOM:

- Assess the extent of racial and ethnic differences in healthcare that are not otherwise attributable to known factors such as access to care (e.g., ability to pay or insurance coverage);
- Evaluate potential sources of racial and ethnic disparities in healthcare, including the role of bias, discrimination, and stereotyping at the individual (provider and patient), institutional, and health system levels; and
- Provide recommendations regarding interventions to eliminate healthcare disparities.

In its interpretation of the charge, the study committee assumes responsibility for assessing variation in the quality of healthcare services provided to individuals of different racial and ethnic backgrounds, independently of patients' insurance status, education, income, or other factors that are known to affect access to care. This is a somewhat artificial and difficult distinction, as many access-related factors, such as the type of health insurance coverage that healthcare consumers purchase or are provided, as well as their level of education and other unmeasured aspects of socioeconomic status (e.g., assertiveness in seeking care) significantly affect the quality and intensity of healthcare that they receive, and are highly correlated with race and ethnicity. The relationship of these variables to healthcare quality is therefore highlighted where appropriate in this report. For purposes of addressing the study charge, however, the committee's focus extends only to the direct and indirect effects of race and ethnicity in the process, structure, and outcomes of healthcare.

Further, the committee assumes that *healthcare* refers to the continuum of services provided in traditional healthcare settings—including public and private clinics, hospitals, community health centers, nursing homes, and other healthcare facilities—as well as home-based care. These include services provided by a range of healthcare professionals, including physicians, nurses, physician assistants, psychologists, and other licensed professionals. The term *healthcare services* refers to the provision of preventive, diagnostic, rehabilitative and/or therapeutic medical or health services to individuals or populations. *Quality of care* refers to the degree to which health services for individuals and populations increase the likelihood of desired health outcomes and are consistent with current professional knowledge. These definitions, and their interrelationship, are best summarized in the 1999 IOM report, *Measuring the Quality of Health Care*:

> The IOM stated . . . that "quality of care is the degree to which health services for individuals and populations increase the likelihood of desired health outcomes and are consistent with current professional knowledge" (IOM, 1990, p. 21). This definition has been widely accepted and has proven to be a robust and useful reference in the formulation of practical approaches to quality assessment and improvement (Blumenthal, 1996). Several ideas in this definition deserve elaboration.
>
> The term *health services* refers to a wide array of services that affect health, including those for physical and mental illnesses. Furthermore, the definition applies to many types of healthcare practitioners (physicians, nurses, and various other health professionals) and to all settings of care (from hospitals and nursing homes to physicians' offices, community sites, and even private homes). . . .
>
> The inclusion in the definition of both *populations* and *individuals* draws attention to the different perspectives that need to be addressed. On the one hand, there is concern with the quality of care that individual organizations, health plans, and clinicians deliver. On the other hand, attention must be paid to the quality of care across the entire system. In particular, one must ask whether all parts of the population have access to needed and appropriate services, whether services meet or exceed their expectations, and whether their health status is improving. That focus embraces all groups, whether or not they have access to care and whether they are

defined by cultural heritage, sociodemographic characteristics, geography (e.g., a state or a region), or diagnosis. It recognizes that such individuals will include the most vulnerable, whether the source of vulnerability is economic, the rarity or severity of the health problem, physical frailty, or physical or emotional impairment. (Institute of Medicine, 1999a; emphasis in text).

The study committee defines *disparities* in healthcare as racial or ethnic differences in the quality of healthcare that are not due to access-related factors or clinical needs, preferences,[1] and appropriateness of intervention (Figure 1-1). The committee's analysis is focused at two levels: 1) the operation of healthcare systems and the legal and regulatory climate in which health systems function; and 2) discrimination at the individual, patient-provider level. Discrimination, as the committee uses the term, refers to differences in care that result from biases, prejudices, stereotyping, and uncertainty in clinical communication and decision-making. It should be emphasized that these definitions are not legal definitions. Different sources of federal, state and international law define discrimination in varying ways, some focusing on intent and others emphasizing disparate impact.

Finally, in defining *racial and ethnic minority groups*, the committee uses the definitions provided by the federal Office of Management and Budget in its proposed Revisions to the Standards for the Classification of Federal Data on Race and Ethnicity (Office of Management and Budget, 2001). The revised standards (see Box 1-1) establish five categories for "racial" groups (American Indian or Alaska Native, Asian, Black or African American, Native Hawaiian or other Pacific Islander, and White), and two categories for "ethnic" groups (Hispanic or Latino and Not Hispanic or Latino).[2] It should be noted that these definitions have been subject to considerable criticism, including:

---

[1]The committee defines patient *preferences* as patients' choices regarding healthcare that are based on a full and accurate understanding of treatment options. As discussed in Chapter 3 of this report, patients' understanding of treatment options is often shaped by the quality and content of provider-patient communication, which in turn may be influenced by factors correlated with patients' and providers' race, ethnicity, and culture. Patient preferences that are not based on a full and accurate understanding of treatment options may therefore be a source of racial and ethnic disparities in care. The committee recognizes that patients' preferences and clinicians' presentation of clinical information and alternatives influence each other, but found separation of the two to be analytically useful.

[2]Consistent with the OMB classification scheme, the terms "African American" and "black" are used interchangeably throughout this report, as are the terms "Hispanic" and "Latino."

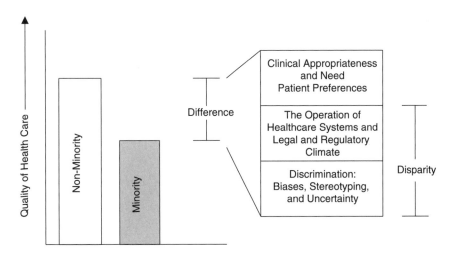

FIGURE 1-1 Differences, disparities, and discrimination: Populations with equal access to healthcare. SOURCE: Gomes and McGuire, 2001.

- reinforcement of the concept of "race" as reflecting genetic or biologic differences between population groups;
- failure to reflect the fluid and dynamic nature of sociopolitical identity, and
- failure to reflect the way many Americans choose to define themselves (Institute of Medicine, 1999b).

Nonetheless, the committee adopts these racial and ethnic definitions because they are commonly accepted among researchers, and most federally funded research utilizes these terms. Further, as will be noted below, access to and the allocation of healthcare resources differ with striking consistency across these population groups, making them useful in tracking disparities in care.

To summarize, racial and ethnic minorities are less likely than whites to posses health insurance (Collins, Hall, and Neuhaus, 1999), are more likely to be beneficiaries of publicly funded health insurance (e.g., Medicaid [The Henry J. Kaiser Family Foundation, 2000b]), and even when insured, may face additional barriers to care due to other socioeconomic factors, such as high co-payments, geographic factors (e.g., the relative scarcity of healthcare providers and healthcare facilities in minority communities), and insufficient transportation. These access-related factors are likely the most significant barriers to equitable care, and must be addressed as an important first step toward eliminating healthcare disparities. The

---

BOX 1-1
Revised Standards for the Classification of Federal Data on
Race and Ethnicity

Categories for Race:
American Indian or Alaska Native. A person having origins in any of the original peoples of North and South America (including Central America), and who maintains tribal affiliation or community attachment.
Asian. A person having origins in any of the original peoples of the Far East, Southeast Asia, or the Indian subcontinent including, for example, Cambodia, China, India, Japan, Korea, Malaysia, Pakistan, the Philippine Islands, Thailand, and Vietnam.
Black or African American. A person having origins in any of the black racial groups or Africa. Terms such as "Haitian" or "Negro" can be used in addition to "Black or African American."
Native Hawaiian or Other Pacific Islander. A person having origins in any of the original peoples of Hawaii, Guam, Samoa, or other Pacific Islands.
White. A person having origins in any of the original peoples of Europe, the Middle East, or North Africa.

Categories for Ethnicity:
Hispanic or Latino. A person of Cuban, Mexican, Puerto Rican, South or Central American, of other Spanish culture or origin, regardless of race. The term "Spanish origin" can be used in addition to "Hispanic or Latino."
Not Hispanic or Latino.

SOURCE: Office of Management and Budget, 2001.

---

committee is asked, however, to assess whether other factors may contribute to health-care disparities once these "threshold" factors (i.e., racial and ethnic differences in income, health insurance status, and geography) are held constant, and to specifically address whether bias, discrimination, or stereotyping at the individual, institutional, and health systems levels may explain some part of these disparities. To a great extent, attempts to separate the relative contribution of these factors risks presenting an incomplete picture of the complex interrelationship between racial and ethnic minority status, socioeconomic differences, and discrimination in the United States. For example, as will be discussed in Chapter 2, racial and ethnic housing segregation is a by-product of both historic and contemporary racism and discrimination, as well as socioeconomic differences (itself the legacy of poorer opportunities for many minority groups). The committee therefore stresses that attempts to "parcel out" access-related factors from the quality of healthcare for minorities remains an artificial exercise, and that policy solutions must consider the historic and contemporary forces that contribute to differences in access to and quality of healthcare.

THE RELATIONSHIP BETWEEN RACIAL AND ETHNIC DISPARITIES IN HEALTH STATUS AND HEALTHCARE

The health gap between minority and non-minority Americans has persisted, and in some cases, has increased in recent years. African-American men, for example, experienced an average life expectancy of 61 years in 1960, compared with 67 years for their white male peers; in 1996, this gap increased to 8 years, as white males enjoyed an average life expectancy of 74 years, relative to 66 years for African-American males. American-Indian men in some regions of the country can expect to live only into their mid-fifties. Further, African-American and American-Indian infant mortality rates remain approximately 2.5 and 1.5 times higher, respectively, than rates for whites (Collins, Hall, and Neuhaus, 1999).

As noted above, the reasons for these health status disparities are complex. Individual risk factors for poor health are pronounced among many racial and ethnic minorities, yet these risks are confounded by the disproportionate representation of minorities in the lower socioeconomic tiers. Moreover, socioeconomic position in and of itself is correlated with health status, independently of individual risk factors, as people in each ascending step along the socioeconomic gradient tend to have better health, even when individual health risk factors are accounted for (Kaplan, Everson, and Lynch, 2000). Cultural factors also play an important role in health disparities; among some immigrant Hispanic populations, for example, birth outcomes have been found to be better than among those of their U.S.-born peers, suggesting that sociocultural risk *increases* with subsequent generations living in the United States (Korenbrot and Moss, 2000). Further, environmental health risks, such as degradation, air, water, and soil pollution, and other physical health hazards are more prevalent in low-income racial and ethnic minority communities. These and other risk factors associated with health and poor health illustrate that racial and ethnic disparities in health status largely reflect differences in social, socioeconomic, and behavioral risk factors and environmental living conditions (House and Williams, 2000). Healthcare is therefore necessary but insufficient in and of itself to redress racial and ethnic disparities in health status (Williams, 1999). A broad and intensive strategy to address socioeconomic inequality, concentrated poverty in many racial and ethnic minority communities, inequitable and segregated housing and educational facilities, individual behavioral risk factors, as well as disparate access to and use of healthcare services is needed to seriously address racial and ethnic disparities in health status.

WHY ARE RACIAL AND ETHNIC DISPARITIES IN HEALTHCARE IMPORTANT?

The preceding discussion should not be interpreted as suggesting that racial and ethnic disparities in healthcare are unimportant, either to individuals in need of care or to a society that prides itself on equality of opportunity. To the contrary, disparities in healthcare are problems that have significant implications for health professionals, administrators and policymakers, and healthcare consumers of all backgrounds.

For the health professions, racial and ethnic disparities in healthcare pose moral and ethical dilemmas that will be among the most significant challenges of today's rapidly changing health systems. Increasingly, physicians and other health professionals are faced with a complex set of societal expectations. On one hand, they are expected to adhere to the highest ethical standards of service that mandate fairness and compassion. On the other hand, physicians are placed in the position of serving as managers of vital, yet limited healthcare resources. Their decisions may result in the allocation of more resources to some individuals than to others, resulting in the unequal distribution of healthcare across population groups. These challenges occur in the context of increasing financial and bureaucratic pressures on healthcare providers, which may exacerbate the problem of inequitable care. Yet the public's trust in the health professions may be irrevocably harmed should the healthcare industry be engaged, even inadvertently, in "social triaging." It is vitally important to preserve this trust, which is already fragile in many racial and ethnic minority communities, as it can significantly affect patients' willingness to seek care and adhere to treatment regimens.

Health professionals and policymakers must also be cognizant of the importance of healthcare as a resource that is tied to social justice, opportunity, and the quality of life for individuals and groups. The productivity of the workforce is closely linked with its health status, yet if some segments of the population, such as racial and ethnic minorities, receive a lower quality and intensity of healthcare, then these groups are further hindered in their efforts to advance economically and professionally. It is therefore important from an egalitarian perspective to expect equal performance in healthcare, especially for those disproportionately burdened with poor health.

From a public health standpoint, racial and ethnic disparities in healthcare threaten to hamper efforts to improve the nation's health. As will be discussed in Chapter 3, the United States is becoming increasingly diverse; while white Americans currently constitute 71% of the population, by the year 2050 nearly one in two Americans will be a person of color (U.S. Bureau of the Census, 2000). These groups, as noted earlier, experience a poorer overall health status and lower levels of access to heathcare than white Americans, and experience a disproportionate burden of chronic and infectious illness. This higher burden of disease and mortality among minorities has profound implications for all Americans, as it results in a less healthy nation and higher costs for health and rehabilitative care. All members of a community are affected by the poor health status of its least healthy members—infectious diseases, for example, know no racial/ethnic or socioeconomic boundaries. For this reason, the federal *Healthy People 2010* initiative has established an overarching goal of eliminating health disparities, noting that "the health of the individual is almost inseparable from the health of the larger community, and . . . the health of every community in every State and territory determines the overall health status of the Nation" (U.S. Department of Health and Human Services, 2000a, p. 15).

From an economic standpoint, the costs of inadequate care may have significant implications for overall healthcare expenditures. Poorly managed chronic conditions or missed diagnoses can result in avoidable, higher subsequent healthcare costs. For example, inadequately treated and managed diabetes can result in far more expensive complications, such as kidney disorder requiring dialysis or transplantation. To the extent that minority beneficiaries of publicly funded health programs are less likely to receive high quality care, these beneficiaries—as well as the taxpayers that support public healthcare programs—may face higher future healthcare costs.

Further, the problem of racial and ethnic disparities in healthcare poses a significant dilemma for a society that is still wrestling with a legacy of racial discrimination (Byrd and Clayton, this volume). Public opinion polls indicate that the vast majority of Americans abhor any form of racial discrimination and believe that all Americans should—and do—enjoy equal opportunities in accessing educational and job opportunities, as well as healthcare (Morin, 2001). Yet this ideal falls far from reality in many sectors of American life, including healthcare, as will be discussed in later sections of this report. The discrepancy between Americans' widely held values and beliefs regarding the importance of equality and the reality of persistent racial inequities tears at the social fabric of the nation and contributes to the gulf of understanding between racial, ethnic and socioeconomic groups.

Finally, for the population at large, racial and ethnic disparities in healthcare raise concerns about the overall quality of care in the United States. Given that racial and ethnic minority groups experience greater challenges and barriers to high quality care, their experiences expose healthcare systems' greatest weaknesses and problems—problems that any American may face in attempting to access healthcare. In this context, the extent to which minorities are well or poorly served provides an important indicator of the state of healthcare in the nation. The provision of equitable care that does not vary by patient race, ethnicity, gender, and age is therefore among one of the six overarching goals identified in the Institute of Medicine's *Crossing the Quality Chasm* report (IOM, 2001a). As the *Chasm* report suggests, evidence of unequal or substandard care for some segments of the population, particularly on the basis of group membership, should raise the concern that the provision of care may be inconsistently and subjectively administered. Inequities in care, therefore, expose a threat to quality care for all Americans.

For all of these reasons, should evidence be available to suggest that racial and ethnic disparities in care are widespread, these disparities would be unacceptable.

EVIDENCE OF RACIAL AND ETHNIC DISPARITIES IN HEALTHCARE

The literature review that follows summarizes articles published in peer-reviewed journals within the last 10 years, with an emphasis on the most recent publications. In selecting literature to review, the committee identified studies that assess racial and ethnic variation in healthcare while controlling for differences in access to healthcare (e.g., by studying similarly insured patients or by statistically adjusting for differences in insurance status) and/or socioeconomic status. To ensure that the committee's search was not limited to studies with "positive" findings of racial and ethnic differences in care, searches were conducted for studies that attempted to assess variations in care by patient socioeconomic status and geographic region. These studies were included if the researchers assessed racial or ethnic differences in care while controlling, as noted above, for patient access-related factors. In addition, the committee focused its review on those studies that attempt to assess the contribution of a range of other potential confounding variables, such as racial and ethnic differences in disease severity, stage of illness progression, patient preferences for non-invasive procedures or to avoid complex treatments, types of settings where care is received (e.g., public vs. private clinics, teaching vs. non-teaching hospitals), availability of procedures (e.g., whether catheterization is offered on-site), suitability of intervention (e.g., whether subtle racial differences in response to treatments may counter-indicate use), as well as other factors. Further, the committee paid particular attention to studies that assessed the appropriateness of services relative to established clinical guidelines. To the extent that these studies shed light on potential sources of disparities in care, they are summarized in this review. The committee's criteria for selecting literature to review are listed in Box 1-2.

Almost all of the studies reviewed by the committee contained one or more weaknesses of study design, methodology, or data analysis that limited the committee's ability to draw findings and conclusions. These weaknesses are noted below, where appropriate. The majority of studies of racial and ethnic disparities in care, for example, use odds ratios, which is a consequence of using logistic regression models, rather than risk ratios to assess the extent of disparities in care. Relative to risk ratios, odds ratios exaggerate the apparent effect of a co-variable when the prevalence of the dependent variable is above 5%-10%. The committee therefore cautions that in some instances, the magnitude of racial and ethnic disparities as reported in the literature may be exaggerated. In addition, as will be discussed below, no single study adequately controlled for all potential confounding factors (e.g., patient preferences, racial differences in disease severity or presentation, geographic availability of specific services or procedures) simultaneously. The committee therefore considered findings in light of the preponderance of evidence and the merits of each individual study. Noting the importance of assessing study strengths and limitations in context, Mayberry and colleagues (2000) write, "[t]he methodological inadequacy of an individual study may be a relatively moot point in the context of the body of literature that gives consistent findings and in which one study, often the more recent study, may overcome the specific failing of a previous investigation" (Mayberry, Mili, and Ofili, 2000, p. 116).

This review yielded over 100 studies (summarized in Appendix B) that assessed racial and ethnic variation in a range of clinical procedures, including the use of diagnostic and therapeutic technologies. This body of literature, however, represents only a fraction of the published studies that investigate racial and ethnic differences in access to and use of healthcare services. Geiger (this volume), for example, has identified over 600 such articles published over the last three decades. For a more comprehensive review of this literature, the reader is referred to Geiger (this volume) or the reviews of Mayberry and colleagues (Mayberry, Mili, and Ofili, 2000); Kressin and Petersen (2001); Sheifer, Escarce, and Schulman (2000); Ford and Cooper (1995); and the AMA Council on Ethical and Judicial Affairs (1990).

Cardiovascular Care

Some of the strongest and most consistent evidence for the existence of racial and ethnic disparities in care is found in studies of cardiovascu-

BOX 1-2
Criteria for Literature Review

To assess the evidence regarding racial and ethnic differences in healthcare, the committee conducted literature searches via PUBMED and MEDLINE databases to identify studies examining racial and ethnic differences in medical care for a variety of disease categories and clinical services. Searches were performed using combinations of following keywords:

• *Race, racial, ethnicity, ethnic, minority/ies, groups, African American, Black, American Indian, Alaska Native, Native American, Asian, Pacific Islander, Hispanic, Latino.*
• *Differences, disparities, care*
• *Cardiac, coronary, cancer, asthma, HIV, AIDS, pediatric, children, mental health, psychiatric, eye, ophthalmic, glaucoma, emergency, diabetes, renal, gall bladder, ICU, peripheral vascular, transplant, organ, cesarean, prenatal, hip, hypertension, injury, surgery/surgical, knee, pain, procedure, treatment, diagnostic.*

This search yielded over 600 citations. To further examine this evidence base and address the study charge that called for an analysis of "the extent of racial and ethnic differences in healthcare that are not otherwise attributable to known factors such as access to care," only studies that provided some measure of control or adjustment for racial and ethnic differences in insurance status (e.g., ability to pay/insurance coverage or co-morbidities) were included in the literature review. Other "threshold" criteria included:

• Publication in past 10 years (1992-2002; this criterion was established because more recent studies tend to employ more rigorous research methods and present a more accurate assessment of contemporary patterns of variation in care);
• Publication in peer-reviewed journals;
• Elimination of studies focused on racial and ethnic differences in health status (except as it is affected by the quality of healthcare) and healthcare access, as well as publications that were editorials, letters, published in a foreign language, were non-empirical, or studies that controlled for race or ethnicity; and
• Inclusion only of studies whose primary purpose was to examine variation in medical care by race and ethnicity, contained original findings, and met generally established principles of scientific research (e.g., studies that stated a clear research question, provided a detailed description of data sources, collection, and analysis methods, included samples large enough to permit statistical analysis, and employed appropriate statistical measures).

In addition, to ensure the comprehensiveness of the review, the committee examined the reference lists of major review papers that summarize this literature (e.g., Geiger, this volume; Kressin and Petersen, 2001; Bonham, 2001; Sheifer, Escarce, and Schulman, 2000; Mayberry, Mili, and Ofili, 2000; Ford and Cooper, 1995). Articles not originally identified in the initial search were retrieved and analyzed for appropriateness of inclusion in the committee's review. Finally, to ensure that the committee's search was not limited to studies with "positive" findings of racial and ethnic differences in care, searches were conducted for studies that attempted to assess variations in care by patient socioeconomic status and geographic region. These studies were included if the researchers assessed racial or ethnic differences in care while controlling, as noted above, for patient access-related factors.

To assess the quality of this evidence base, the committee ranked studies on several criteria:

- Adequacy of control for insurance status (studies of patients covered under the same health system or insurance plan were considered to be more rigorous than studies that merely assessed the availability of health insurance among the study population);
- Use of appropriate indicators for patient socioeconomic status (e.g., studies that measured patients' level of income, education, or other indicators of socioeconomic status);
- Analysis of clinical data, as opposed to administrative claims data (see limitations of administrative claims data noted below);
- Prospective or retrospective data collection (prospective studies were considered to be more rigorous than retrospective analyses);
- Appropriate control for patient co-morbid conditions;
- Appropriate control for racial differences in disease severity or stage of illness at presentation;
- Assessment of patients' appropriateness for procedures (e.g., studies that provide primary diagnosis and include well-defined measures of disease status, as in studies of cardiovascular care that assess racial differences in care following angiography) or that compare rates of service use relative to standardized, widely accepted clinical guidelines; and
- Assessment of racial differences in rates of refusal or patient preferences for non-invasive treatment.

Studies that met the committee's "threshold" criteria are summarized in Appendix B. Many of these studies are summarized in this chapter, with an emphasis on more rigorous studies, as defined by the committee's quality criteria, above.

lar care. The most rigorous studies in this area assess both potential underuse and overuse of services and appropriateness of care using well-established clinical and diagnostic criteria. Several studies, for example, have assessed racial and ethnic differences in cardiovascular care relative to RAND criteria for the necessity of revascularization procedures. These studies have therefore been able to demonstrate that differences in treatment are not due to factors such as racial differences in the severity of coronary disease.

No one study reviewed by the committee simultaneously controlled for all of the variables likely to confound the relationship between race/ethnicity and receipt of care. In addition, in almost all cases, studies that employ rigorous measures of potential confounding variables find that racial and ethnic disparities diminish once these variables are included in multivariate analysis. The preponderance of studies, however, find that even after adjustment for many potentially confounding factors—including racial differences in access to care, disease severity, site of care (e.g., geographic variation or type of hospital or clinic), disease prevalence, co-morbidities or clinical characteristics, refusal rates, and overuse of services by whites—racial and ethnic disparities in cardiovascular care remain. This conclusion was also reached by authors of all major review articles that the committee identified in its search, including Kressin and Petersen (2001); Mayberry, Mili, and Ofili (2000); Sheifer, Escarce, and Schulman, (2000); Ford and Cooper (1995); Gonzalez-Klayman and Barnhart (1998); the AMA Council on Ethical and Judicial Affairs (1990); and Geiger (this volume).

The preponderance of studies . . . find that even after adjustment for many potentially confounding factors—including racial differences in access to care, disease severity, site of care (e.g., geographic variation or type of hospital or clinic), disease prevalence, comorbidities or clinical characteristics, refusal rates, and overuse of services by whites—racial and ethnic disparities in cardiovascular care remain.

Studies Using Administrative Databases

Data from several large, national datasets have been analyzed and demonstrate both national and regional patterns of disparities in care. These datasets typically rely on administrative claims data to assess differences in receipt of services. A variety of limitations should be noted regarding administrative claims data. One, these data provide little or no information regarding co-morbid illnesses, the severity of disease, or the stage at which illness was detected. Findings of racial differences in these studies therefore cannot rule out the possibility that minority patients might be less appropriate for specific clinical services. Second, administrative data provide little indication as to whether patients were presented with all clinical options, whether patients accepted or refused recommendations, or whether the physician did not recommend clinical procedures. Third, these data typically provide no information regarding patients' education level or other socioeconomic background information. Given that whites generally enjoy higher socioeconomic and educational status, and given the correlation between these attributes and care-seeking behavior (e.g., greater assertiveness in seeking care), socioeconomic status is potentially a significant confounding factor. Fourth, administrative data typically provide no information regarding the appropriateness of services relative to patients' needs, and therefore overuse of services among whites and/or underuse among minorities cannot be ruled out.

Nonetheless, the consistency of findings from these studies, many using large sample sizes, is striking. Ford et al. (1989), for example, assessed rates of coronary arteriography and coronary artery bypass graft surgery (CABG) among nearly 4 million patients with acute myocardial infarction sampled in the National Hospital Discharge Survey (NHDS). The authors found that African-American men and women were significantly less likely to undergo CABG or angiography than whites. Escarce et al. (1993), McBean et al. (1994), and Gornick et al. (1996) found significant racial differences in rates of cardiovascular procedures among Medicare patients, with African-American patients approximately one-half to one-third less likely to receive services. Similarly, Goldberg et al. (1992), in an analysis of over 86,000 Medicare patients, found that whites were nearly four times more likely than African Americans to receive CABG, after adjusting for age- and gender-related differences in rates of myocardial infarction (MI). When data were analyzed by state, the authors found greater racial differences in CABG rates in the Southeast, particularly in non-metropolitan areas. For whites, CABG rates were significantly associated with the availability of thoracic surgeons and location in the Southeast, but physician availability and location were not correlated with CABG rates for African Americans.

To address some of the deficiencies of studies using administrative data, several studies have adjusted for the influence of variables such as site of care (e.g., geographic location or type of hospital or clinic) to assess racial differences in the receipt of coronary revascularization procedures. Ayanian et al. (1993) assessed racial differences in rates of revascularization following angiography and the relationship of these differences to hospital characteristics among more than 27,000 Medicare patients. Controlling for age, sex, region, Medicaid eligibility, and principal and secondary diagnoses, the authors found that whites were 78% more likely than African Americans to receive a revascularization procedure. These differences were apparent in public, private, teaching, non-teaching, and urban/suburban hospitals, as well as in hospitals where patients were referred to other facilities for revascularization procedures and those that offer such procedures in-house. Similarly, Weitzman et al. (1997) assessed rates of performance of cardiac procedures in relation to gender, race, and geographic location among 5,462 patients in four states (North Carolina, Mississippi, Maryland, and Minnesota) hospitalized for MI. After controlling for the severity of MI and co-morbid conditions, blacks admitted to teaching hospitals in this study were significantly less likely to receive percutaneous transluminal coronary angiography (PTCA), CABG, or thrombolytic therapy. Similarly, blacks admitted to non-teaching hospitals were significantly less likely to receive these procedures.

Giles et al. (1995) used data from NHDS to assess race and sex differences in the rate of receipt of catheterization, PTCA, or coronary artery bypass surgery (CABS), while adjusting for differences in the type of hospital admission, insurance status, and disease severity among 10,348 patients hospitalized with acute myocardial infarction (AMI). Significant differences by race and gender were found after statistical adjustment and a patient matching procedure, which matched individuals admitted to the same hospital and who underwent a cardiac procedure with individuals who did not undergo a procedure. With white males as the referent, black men were less likely to receive catheterization or CABS, while black women were less likely to receive catheterization, PTCA, or CABS. Among only those patients who underwent catheterization (and therefore had access to a cardiologist), black women were less likely to receive subsequent PTCA or CABS.

Similarly, Allison et al. (1996) assessed the rate of receipt of thrombolysis, beta-adrenergic blockade and aspirin in a retrospective medical record review of 4,052 patients hospitalized in all acute care hospitals in Alabama with principle discharge diagnosis of AMI. After controlling for patient age, gender, clinical factors, severity of illness, algorithm-determined candidacy for therapy, and hospital characteristics (e.g., rural vs. urban, teaching vs. non-teaching), the authors found that white patients were 50% more likely to receive thrombolytics than black patients. No differences were found in receipt of beta-blockers or aspirin by patient race.

In one of the few studies to assess rates of revascularization procedures among a multiethnic sample of patients, Carlisle et al. (1995) found that African Americans, Hispanics, and Asian Americans were significantly less likely than whites to receive coronary angiography, CABG, and/or angioplasty, controlling for primary diagnosis, age, gender, insurance type, income, and co-morbid factors. When differences in the volume of revascularization procedures among hospitals were controlled, however, Asian Americans did not differ from whites in the rates of cardiac procedures. African-American and Hispanic patients remained less likely than whites to receive angioplasty, and African Americans were less likely to receive CABG when hospital characteristics were controlled. Similarly, Herholz et al. (1996) analyzed discharge data for 982 Mexican-American and white patients hospitalized for definite or possible myocardial infarction. Mexican Americans received 38% fewer medications than whites, even after adjusting for clinical and demographic characteristics. Mexican Americans were less likely to receive almost all major medications, especially antiarrhythmics, anticoagulants, and lipid-lowering therapy. Using data from the same study as Herholz et al. (1996), Ramsey et al. (1997) found that after adjusting for age, sex, previous diagnosis of coronary heart disease, MI, diabetes mellitus, hypertension, occurrence of congestive heart failure during MI, and location and type of MI, Mexican Americans were less likely to receive PTCA, but not aortocoronary bypass surgery, than whites.

Other studies indicate that the likelihood of receiving revascularization procedures varies by the stage or typical sequence of events leading to care. Blustein, Arons, and Shea (1995), for example, found that among patients hospitalized for acute myocardial infarction, race and insurance status significantly predicted the likelihood of 1) gaining initial admittance to a hospital that offers revascularization services; 2) actually receiving revascularization following initial admission; or 3) receiving revascularization services following transfer or subsequent readmission. Whites, those with private insurance, and those with more severe heart disease were more likely to gain initial admittance to hospitals providing revascularization services. Once hospitalized, whites, males, those with private insurance, and those with more severe disease were more likely to actually receive revascularization. Racial disparities grew larger as patients "progressed" though the phases leading to revascularization.

Studies of the Role of Financial and Institutional Characteristics

Several studies suggest that financial and institutional characteristics may mediate the relationship between the use of cardiac procedures and patient race, in some cases significantly attenuating or eliminating racial and ethnic disparities. Leape et al. (1999) explored racial differences in revascularization procedures as a function of demographic characteristics and type of hospital among 631 patients at 13 New York City hospitals for whom revascularization procedures were deemed clinically necessary according to RAND criteria. The authors found no racial differences in rates of revascularization procedures among African-American patients (72%), Hispanic patients (67%) and white patients (75%). Rates of revascularization were significantly lower, however, among patients initially seen in hospitals that did not provide revascularization services (and therefore had to refer patients to other hospitals) than those treated in settings that did provide revascularization (59% to 76%, respectively). Subsequent criticism of the study noted that the limited sample and geographic setting, coupled with the fact that most of the facilities studied offered both angiography and revascularization on-site, may have limited the study's ability to detect group differences in procedure use (Kressin and Peterson, 2001).

Similarly, Gregory et al. (1999) studied the relationship between the availability of hospital-based invasive cardiac procedures and racial differences in the use of these services. The authors studied records of 13,690 black and white New Jersey residents hospitalized with a primary diagnosis of AMI. For all patients, the likelihood of receiving catheterization within 90 days of AMI was significantly greater among those hospitalized in facilities that provided cardiac services. Black patients in this sample were more likely to be admitted first to hospitals equipped to perform cardiac catheterization and/or PTCA or CABG. Despite this, blacks were less likely to receive catheterization than whites within 90 days of admission, even after controlling for age, sex, health insurance status (for those younger than age 65), anatomic location of primary infarct, co-morbidities, and the availability of cardiac services. Similarly, blacks were less likely than whites to receive revascularization procedures within 90 days of admission, again after controlling for patient demographic and clinical factors and availability of cardiac services.

Other researchers have assessed whether racial and ethnic disparities in healthcare are mediated by the type of health system in which care is delivered. Taylor et al. (1997), for example, abstracted chart reviews from 1,441 patients with principal or secondary diagnosis of AMI receiving care in one of 125 military hospitals. The authors found no differences in rates of catheterization procedures between white and "non-white" patients (all patients who described their race or ethnicity as other than white or Caucasian, including African Americans) during AMI admission or between white and black patients. Similarly, no differences were found in rates of revascularization (PTCA or CABG) between white and "non-white" patients or between white and black patients. No differences were found in mortality or rates of readmission within 180 days following initial discharge. However, white patients were significantly more likely than non-white patients to be considered for future catheterization. Among studies of disparities in Veterans Administration hospitals, which significantly reduce financial barriers to care, findings are mixed. Mickelson et al. (1997) found no differences between white and Hispanic VA patients in receipt of cardiovascular procedures following AMI. In contrast, Peterson et al. (1994), Mirvis et al. (1994), Whittle et al. (1993), and Mirvis and Graney (1998) all found that African-American VA patients were less likely to receive cardiovascular procedures. Sedlis et al. (1997) found that therapeutic cardiac procedures (surgery or PTCA) were offered more frequently for white VA patients (72.9%) than African-American VA patients (64.3%). This difference could not be explained by simple clinical differences between the two groups. Even though they were offered care at lower rates, however, African-American patients were more than twice as likely as whites to refuse invasive procedures. In contrast, Petersen et al. (2002) found significant differences in rates of thrombolytic therapy and bypass surgery among a sample of African-American and white VA patients with a confirmed diagnosis of acute myocardial infarction, with black patients receiving lower rates of these invasive procedures. Like Sedlis et al. (1997), Petersen et al. assess racial differences in rates of refusal for these procedures, but found no differences in rates of refusal when angiography, PTCA, or bypass surgery were offered.

Daumit et al. (1999), in one of the few studies to longitudinally assess receipt of cardiovascular procedures among a cohort of patients, followed nearly 5,000 African-American and white patients with end-stage renal disease (ESRD) to determine whether the acquisition of health insurance (ESRD patients are eligible for Medicare and generally enter a comprehensive system of care, if not already enrolled in one, upon diagnosis) could reduce racial and ethnic disparities in receipt of cardiovascular procedures (ESRD patients are at high risk for cardiovascular disease). Prior to development of ESRD, white patients were nearly three times more likely than African-American patients to receive catheterization, angioplasty, or CABG, even after controlling for clinical and socioeconomic variables. At follow-up, this disparity diminished to the point where whites were only 40% more likely to receive a cardiovascular procedure. Significantly, among patients who were already enrolled in Medicare at baseline, racial disparities in cardiovascular procedures disappeared at follow-up. Daumit et al. caution, however, that "a substantial baseline disparity between black and white patients . . . exists in the privately insured and Medicare subgroups, providing evidence against acquisition of health insurance as the only factor in narrowing the ethnic gap" (Daumit et al., 1999, p. 179). As with many of the studies reviewed above, however, this study did not obtain detailed clinical data or information on patient preferences, which could explain some of the observed differences (Kravitz, 1999).

These studies strongly suggest that addressing racial and ethnic gaps in insurance coverage is one of the most important factors in narrowing the racial and ethnic gap in cardiovascular services. Health insurance alone does not completely eliminate disparities, however, as the studies above illustrate. This finding is confirmed in a study of cardiovascular care in the United Kingdom, which offers universal access and free care at the point of use. In a prospective study of 2,552 patients seen in London hospitals who were deemed "appropriate" for cardiovascular procedures according to standardized criteria, Hemingway et al. (2001) found that "non-white" patients were more likely to receive only medical treatment (received by 20% of these patients), rather than CABG (received by 14% of these patients), after controlling for demographic and clinical variables. These differences were not found among white patients similarly deemed appropriate for invasive treatment.

Studies to Assess Appropriateness of Services

Critics of many of the studies reviewed above charge that comparisons of minority patients' receipt of revascularization procedures with that of whites' may identify differences caused by overuse of procedures by whites, rather than clinical necessity. To address this concern, several studies have examined use of coronary procedures relative to established criteria for necessity. Hannan et al. (1999) assessed rates of CABG among 1,261 post-angiography patients who would benefit from CABG according to RAND appropriateness and necessity criteria. Controlling for age, gender, severity of disease, patient risk status, type of insurance, and other clinical characteristics, the authors found that African-American and Hispanic patients were significantly less likely than whites to undergo CABG. Similarly, Laouri et al. (1997), using RAND/UCLA criteria for necessity of revascularization procedures, found that African Americans were half as likely as whites to undergo necessary CABG and one-fifth as likely to undergo PTCA. In this study, patients at public hospitals were less likely to undergo PTCA than those at private hospitals. Conigliaro et al. (2000) also assessed racial variation in coronary revascularization relative to RAND appropriateness criteria at six hospital sites that offered CABG on site or at an adjacent university hospital. This was a VA patient population with few financial barriers to care. Further, all patients had unstable angina or acute myocardial infarction and had undergone coronary angiography. Overall, African-American patients were found to be less likely then whites to undergo CABG and PTCA, but when RAND appropriateness criteria were considered, African Americans were still less likely to receive CABG when deemed "necessary."

In a larger study, Canto et al. (2000) studied the use of reperfusion therapy among more than 26,000 patients meeting eligibility criteria as a result of acute myocardial infarction. After controlling for clinical and demographic characteristics, the authors found that African Americans were slightly less likely than whites to undergo reperfusion therapy. Further, Schneider et al. (2001) used RAND criteria to assess whether overuse of PTCA or CABG by whites explained racial differences in revascularization rates among 3,960 African-American and white Medicare patients. As with other studies cited above, Schneider et al. found that whites were more likely than African Americans to receive PTCA and CABG. When assessed relative to RAND appropriateness criteria, white males were found to be nearly 2.5 times more likely to receive PTCA than African Americans when the procedure was judged to be "inappropriate;" no other racial or gender differences were found in rates of inappropriate CABG. The authors conclude, however, that the racial difference in rates of inappropriate PTCA "was not sufficiently large to account for more than a small fraction of the substantial disparities in rates of revascularization between white patients and African-American patients" (Schneider et al., 2001b, p. 334).

These studies of disparities in cardiovascular care relative to appropriateness criteria offer an important means of assessing whether observed racial and ethnic differences in care may be "explained" by differences in clinical necessity. It should be noted, however, that even among studies employing objective criteria to assess racial and ethnic differences in care relative to clinical necessity, "there may not always be a perfect fit between the clinical indications considered by the [panel evaluating appropriateness] and the characteristics of real patients" (Kravitz, 1999).

In a more comprehensive study of whether racial disparities in receipt of revascularization procedures reflect clinical necessity or merely overuse among whites, Peterson et al. (1997) assessed racial differences in receipt of coronary angioplasty and CABG among patients with documented coronary disease, and assessed whether differences were associated with survival. Peterson et al. followed 12,402 patients seen annually at Duke University Medical Center for an average of five and a half years, and found that African Americans were 13% less likely than whites to undergo angioplasty and 32% less likely to undergo CABG during the study period. Racial differences in procedure rates were more marked among patients with severe disease. Analysis of survival benefit of surgery also revealed racial differences; among patients expected to survive more than one year, 42% of African Americans underwent surgery, compared with 61% of whites. Finally, analysis of the adjusted five-year mortality rate among patients revealed that African-American patients were 18% more likely than whites to die. The Peterson et al. study can be criticized on the grounds that the findings may not generalize beyond the single study setting. Nevertheless, the study provides strong evidence that lower rates of intervention among this sample of African-American patients were associated with lower rates of survival.

Summary of Literature on Racial and Ethnic Disparities in Cardiovascular Care

The literature reviewed above illustrates that racial and ethnic disparities in cardiovascular care are robust and consistent across a range of studies conducted in different geographic regions with diverse patient populations seen in a range of clinical settings. This literature does not, however, provide a clear account of the sources of these disparities; rather, these studies provide clues regarding the types of factors that are *not* likely to fully explain disparities in cardiovascular care. Racial differences in clinical presentation or disease severity do not fully explain differences in receipt of services (Hannan et al., 1999; Lauori et al., 1997; Conigliaro et al., 2000; Canto et al., 2000), although minority and non-minority patients may not respond equally well to some therapeutic interventions, as will be discussed in Chapter 3. White patients have been found to use some clinical services at higher rates than minorities, even when not necessarily indicated. Therefore, when minority patients' use of services is compared with that of whites, differences may be observed. But this "overuse" of cardiovascular procedures by whites does not fully explain disparities in care (Schneider et al., 2001), and studies that assess racial differences in care relative to established clinical criteria still find significant differences (Conigliaro et al., 2000b; Hannan et al., 1999; Laouri et al, 1997). Racial and ethnic disparities in cardiovascular services are found among patients insured by Medicare (Gornick et al., 1996; McBean et al., 1994; Escarce et al., 1993), and among patients in VA settings (Peterson et al., 1994; Mirvis et al., 1994; Whittle et al., 1993; Mirvis and Graney, 1998; Sedlis et al., 1997; Petersen et al., 2002), although these findings are not consistent (Mickelson et al., 1997). Significantly, however, even among patients whose care is covered by nationalized health plans (e.g., Great Britain), minority racial and ethnic groups are found to receive fewer clinical services (Hemingway et al., 2001).

Several studies find that African-American patients are more likely than whites to refuse invasive procedures (e.g., Hannan et al., 1999; Oddone et al., 1998; Sedlis et al., 1997), but when the relative contribution of patient refusal to racial differences in care is assessed, this factor is not found to account completely for these disparities. Further, physician recommendation appears to be the major factor in determining whether patients receive invasive cardiac procedures (Hannan et al., 1999). These factors as potential sources of disparities will be assessed in greater detail in Chapter 3.

Almost all of the studies reviewed here find that as more potentially confounding variables are controlled, the magnitude of racial and ethnic disparities in care decreases. In a few studies, disparities disappeared entirely when appropriate confounding variables were included in multivariate analysis. In general, these findings are limited to studies of patients seen in universally accessible care settings, such as the U.S. Department of Defense healthcare systems (e.g., Taylor et al., 1997), or studies employing small samples in one or a handful of clinical settings (e.g., Leape et al., 1999). These findings strongly suggest that access-related factors, such as insurance status, ability to pay, and characteristics of institutional and clinical settings are the largest contributors to observed racial and ethnic disparities in cardiovascular care. The vast majority of studies assessing disparities in cardiac care, however, find that racial and ethnic disparities persist even after variations in insurance status are controlled.

As a "second level" analysis of the quality of evidence regarding racial and ethnic disparities in cardiovascular care, the committee identified a subset of studies that permit a more detailed analysis of the relationship between patient race or ethnicity and quality of care, while considering potential confounding variables such as clinical differences in presentation and disease severity. Several criteria were established to identify these studies, using generally accepted criteria of research rigor and quality. To begin, the committee identified only studies using clinical, as opposed to administrative data, for the reasons cited above. Secondly, the committee identified studies that provided appropriate controls for likely confounding variables, and/or employed other rigorous research methods. These criteria included the use of adequate control or adjustment for racial and ethnic differences in insurance status; prospective, rather than retrospective data collection; adjustment for racial and ethnic differences in co-morbid conditions; adjustment for racial and ethnic differences in disease severity; comparison of rates of cardiovascular services relative to measures of appropriateness; and assessment of patient outcomes.

Several caveats should be noted in undertaking this approach. One, studies using clinical data allow researchers to better assess whether disparities in care exist and are significant after potential confounding factors such as clinical variation and the appropriateness of intervention are taken into account. However, these studies often are limited to small patient samples in one or only a few clinical settings, therefore sacrificing statistical power and potentially underestimating the role of institutional variables as contributing to healthcare disparities. Second, assessments of racial and ethnic differences in patients' clinical outcomes following intervention must be made with caution. Patients' outcomes following medical intervention reflect a wide range of factors, some of which are unrelated to the intervention itself (e.g., the degree of social support available to patients following treatment) and may vary systematically by race or ethnicity. In addition, a finding of no racial or ethnic differences in patient outcomes (e.g., survival) despite disparate rates of treatment should not be interpreted as demonstrating that disparities in the use of medical intervention are inconsequential. In such instances, researchers should ask whether equivalent rates of intervention might be associated with *better* patient outcomes among minorities. Finally, this second level of analysis should not be interpreted as suggesting that the larger literature presented above is insufficient to draw conclusions regarding disparities in healthcare. Almost all of the individual studies reviewed earlier possess limitations, but the collective body of this evidence is robust. Despite these caveats, this second review afforded an opportunity to assess whether racial and ethnic disparities in care remain when racial differences in clinical presentation and other potentially confounding variables are controlled. Studies were considered in this second review only if they met four of six criteria noted above, in addition to the "threshold" criteria that studies employ clinical databases. Thirteen studies were identified through this process (see Table B-2 in Appendix B). Of these, only two (Leape et al., 1999; Carlisle et al., 1999) found no evidence of racial and ethnic disparities in care after adjustment for racial and ethnic differences in insurance status, co-morbid factors, disease severity, and other potential confounders as noted above. The remaining studies found racial and ethnic disparities in one or more cardiac procedures, following multivariate analysis. Almost all studies found that adjustment for one or more confounding factors reduced the magnitude of unadjusted racial and ethnic differences in care. Among the five studies that collected data prospectively, however, all found racial and ethnic disparities remained after adjustment for confounding factors.

Cancer

Studies of racial disparities in cancer diagnosis and treatment are less clear and consistent than studies of cardiac care, in part because many studies rely on data that use crude or incomplete indicators of the type of treatment provided and/or do not control for co-morbid factors. Variations in the extent of disease among patients are rarely well controlled, and the comprehensiveness of treatment cannot be evaluated. In addition, many studies indicate that ethnic minorities are diagnosed at later stages of cancer progression, further confounding efforts to assess the quality of treatment. Nonetheless, several studies demonstrate significant racial differences in the receipt of appropriate cancer treatments and analgesics.

Studies of racial disparities in cancer diagnosis and treatment are less clear and consistent than studies of cardiac care, in part because many studies rely on data that use crude or incomplete indicators of the type of treatment provided and/or do not control for co-morbid factors. Variations in the extent of disease among patients are rarely well controlled, and the comprehensiveness of treatment cannot be evaluated. In addition, many studies indicate that racial and ethnic minorities are diagnosed at later stages of cancer progression (for example, Mitchell and McCormack, 1997), further confounding efforts to assess the quality of treatment. Nonetheless, several studies demonstrate significant racial differences in the receipt of appropriate cancer treatments and analgesics.

In one of the largest early studies of racial disparities in cancer care, Diehr et al. (1989) assessed the quality of care for 7,781 women treated for breast cancer in 107 hospitals relative to 10 dimensions of breast cancer care established by a panel of experts convened by the National Cancer Institute (NCI). While African Americans were less likely than whites to have health insurance, were less likely to be treated by an experienced, board-certified physician, and were more likely to be treated in large, public hospitals, racial differences in care persisted when these and other clinical and demographic factors were controlled. African-American women were less likely than white women to receive progesterone receptor assays (a prognostic test), were less likely to receive radiation therapy in combination with radical/modified mastectomy, and were less likely to receive rehabilitation support services following mastectomy.

Similarly, Harlan et al. (1995) assessed variations in the use of radical prostatectomy and radiation to treat prostate cancer by geographic area, age, and race. Data for 67,693 men with localized and regional cancer, obtained from Surveillance, Epidemiology, and End Results (SEER) program database, revealed that black men aged 50 to 69 years were less likely than similarly aged white men to undergo prostatectomy. For black and white men aged 70 to 79 years, rates of prostatectomy were similar in 1984, but became significantly divergent by 1991, as a larger proportion of white men underwent the procedure. In 1991, a significantly higher proportion of black men aged 50 to 59 years received radiation. For all age groups in 1991, twice as many blacks as whites (12.5% vs. 6.6%) received no treatment. In a similar analysis of 4,154 Medicare claims for radical prostatectomy to treat prostate cancer, Imperato et al. (1996), found that rates of prostatectomy were lower among African Americans than among whites, with the black/white ratio ranging from 0.59 in 1991 to 0.86 in 1993.

McMahon et al. (1999) assessed the contribution of patient age, sex, race, urbanicity, per capita income, and education level of patients' community, and availability of physicians, internists, and gastroenterologists per 100,000 population to predict use of diagnostic procedures for colon cancer among all Medicare Part B transactions in the state of Michigan from 1986 to 1989. African Americans were more likely than whites to receive a barium enema only, were less likely to receive a combination of barium enema and sigmoidoscopy, and were less likely to undergo colonoscopy. While this study could not control for stage of disease and the reason for performing diagnostic procedures, it suggests that African Americans received less effective diagnostic evaluations. Relative to whites, African Americans in this study received 28% fewer sigmoidoscopic examinations—which are generally considered to be more technically advanced diagnostic procedures than barium enema— despite a 20% higher incidence of colon cancer.

African-American cancer patients are also less likely to receive post-treatment surveillance care. Elston Lafata et al. (2001) assessed colorectal cancer surveillance care among 251 patients enrolled in a managed care organization at diagnosis, and found that within 18 months of treatment, over half of the total cohort received a colon examination (55%), nearly three-fourths had received carcinoembryonic antigen (CEA) testing, and nearly six in ten (59%) received metastatic disease testing. Whites were more likely than African Americans, however, to receive CEA testing and displayed a slight but non-significant trend toward higher rates of colonic examination. The small sample size and single setting of this study, however, may limit these findings.

In one of the few studies to analyze the effect of both stage of illness at the time of diagnosis and reasons for no receipt of treatment, Merrill, Merrill, and Mayer (2000) assessed the receipt of surgery or radiation therapy among 8,119 white and African-American women with invasive cervical cancer. Overall, 8.03% of whites and 11.64% of blacks did not receive either radiation therapy or surgery. For both blacks and whites, the odds of not receiving treatment increased with older age, distant and unstaged disease (vs. localized disease), unknown grade (vs. well-differentiated disease), and unknown lymph node (vs. no lymph node) status. Blacks were more likely to be diagnosed unstaged and were less likely to have localized disease; once stage was accounted for, racial differences in treatment status became insignificant. However, among those not treated, blacks were more likely than whites to have treatment not recommended (53.68% vs. 40.32%). Of those cases not receiving therapy, few were due to patient refusal (3.76% among whites, 5.88% among blacks).

Similarly, Howard, Penchansky, and Brown (1998) assessed racial differences in of breast cancer survival among 246 black and white women who sought care for breast cancer in one of three health maintenance organizations (HMOs). No significant racial differences were found in stage of disease, utilization of health services before diagnosis of breast cancer, or receipt of breast examination. However, African-American patients were more likely to die than whites (30% vs. 18%, respectively) and experienced shorter average survival (1.63 years vs. 2.77 years, respectively). Two percent of whites and eight percent of African Americans missed two or more appointments following diagnosis; after adjusting for the number of appointments made, African Americans were more likely than whites to miss appointments. Missed appointments and stage of diagnosis were strongly associated with survival, and reduced the impact of race on survival. As with the study by Elston Lafata et al. (2001), however, findings of this study are limited by the small sample size and study setting.

In a larger study, Ball and Elixhauser (1996) assessed racial differences in treatment for colorectal cancer among over 20,000 patients in a national sample. Among patients with primary tumor and no metastasis, African Americans were 41% less likely than whites to receive a major procedure for treatment of colorectal cancer (i.e., colon resection, total cholecystectomy, colonoscopy, or bronchoscopy), after controlling for patient demographic characteristics, comorbidities, therapeutic complications, and hospital characteristics. Among patients with metastasis, African-American patients were 27% less likely to receive a major treatment. Bach et al. (1999) found similar results in a study of nearly 11,000 Medicare patients with a diagnosis of resectable non-small-cell lung cancer. The authors found that African-American and white patients who underwent surgery had similar rates of survival at five years (39.1% and 42.9%, respectively). No racial differences were found in survival rates at five years for those patients who did not undergo surgery (4% among African Americans and 5% among whites). African Americans, however, were 12.7% less likely to undergo resection, a difference that was not due to comorbid factors, age, gender, income, geographic region, or type of Medicare insurance. Further, using survival analysis, the authors estimate that 308 African-American patients would have been alive at five years if black patients had undergone surgery at a rate similar to that of white patients.

Racial and ethnic differences are also found in the use of analgesics to manage pain due to cancer. Bernabei et al. (1998) assessed the adequacy of pain management among 13,625 elderly and minority cancer patients admitted to nursing homes following treatment. More than a quarter of patients who experienced daily pain (26%), as assessed by self-report and independent raters, received no pain medication. After adjusting for gender, cognitive status, communication skills, and indicators of disease severity (e.g., explicit terminal prognosis), being bedridden, number of diagnoses, and use of other medications, the authors found that African Americans had a 63% greater probability of being untreated for pain relative to whites. Older age, low cognitive performance, and increased number of other medications were also associated with failure to receive any analgesic agent. Similarly, Cleeland et al. (1997) assessed the adequacy of pain management among minority patients receiving care in settings that primarily serve minorities vs. patients who receive care in settings where few minority patients are treated. In addition, the authors compared the adequacy of analgesia received by minority patients vs. that received by non-minority patients, as determined by independent, widely accepted pain assessment criteria. Sixty-five percent of patients in this study who reported pain received inadequate pain medication. Patients treated in settings where the patient population was primarily black or Hispanic and those who were treated at university medical centers were more likely to receive inadequate analgesia (77%) than those who received treatment in settings where the patient population was primarily white (52%). In addition, minority patients were more likely to be undermedicated for pain than white patients (65% vs. 50%, respectively), and were more likely to have the severity of their pain underestimated by physicians.

As is the case with some studies of cardiovascular care, the type of health system in which minority patients access care may influence the quality of cancer care received. Optenberg and colleagues, for example (Optenberg et al., 1995), assessed the long-term survival of 1,606 black and white prostate cancer patients who were active duty personnel, dependents, or retirees eligible for care in the military medical system. Black patients in this study presented at a significantly higher stage of cancer development than whites (26.4% of blacks presenting with distant metastases compared to 12.3% of whites), and demonstrated a greater percentage of recurrence (30.6% vs. 21.4%, respectively). There were no significant racial differences in wait time to receive treatment, and no significant differences were found in the type of treatment when stratified by stage of presentation. Overall, stage, grade, and age were found to affect survival, but not race. When analyzed by stage, blacks demonstrated longer survival for distant metastatic disease. Similarly, Dominitz et al. (1998) assessed racial differences in receipt of treatment and survival among 3,176 patients with colorectal cancer treated in the "equal access" Veterans Administration (VA) health system. After adjusting for patient demographic characteristics, co-morbidities, distant metastases, and tumor location, no significant racial differences were found in rates of receipt of surgical resection (70% among blacks, 73% among whites), chemotherapy (23% for both black and whites), or radiation therapy (17% among blacks, 16% among whites). Five-year relative survival rates were similar for black and white patients (42% vs. 39% respectively). These findings are not consistent, however; Dominitz et al. (2002), for example, assessed rates of surgical intervention versus chemotherapy and radiation therapy among a sample of African-American and white male veterans diagnosed with esophageal cancer and treated at VA hospitals. The authors found that after controlling for a variety of patient demographic and clinical characteristics, African-American patients with esophageal adenocarcinoma were less likely to undergo surgery than whites, but had similar rates of chemotherapy and radiation therapy. Similarly, black patients with squamous cell carcinoma were less likely than whites to undergo surgical resection, but were more likely to receive radiation therapy and chemotherapy. Further, in contrast to Optenberg et al. (1995) and his earlier study (Dominitz et al., 1998), in this study Dominitz and colleagues (2002) found that post-treatment mortality was higher for African-American than white patients with squamous cell carcinoma.

Cerebrovascular Disease

Racial and ethnic variation in the rates of diagnostic tests and clinical procedures for cerebrovascular disease have not been studied as extensively as variation in cardiac procedures, despite the relatively higher risk among African Americans for stroke (Mitchell et al., 2000). Moreover, few studies have compared rates of procedures conditional upon angiography or other diagnostic testing. The preponderance of studies, however, finds generally lower rates of diagnostic and therapeutic procedures among African Americans with cerebrovascular disease.

Oddone et al. (1999) studied racial differences in rates of carotid artery imaging among patients diagnosed with transient ischemic attack, ischemic stroke, or amaurosis fugax seen at one of four VA Medical Centers. After controlling for patients' age, co-morbid factors, clinical presentation, anticipated operative risk, and hospital, African-American patients were found to be half as likely as whites to receive carotid imaging. White patients in this study, however, were more likely to be assessed as appropriate candidates for surgery using RAND criteria because of a higher prevalence of significant carotid artery stenosis among blacks.

Mitchell and colleagues (Mitchell et al., 2000) assessed rates of tests and treatment (including noninvasive cerebrovascular tests, cerebral angiography, carotid endarterectomy, and anticoagulant therapy) for cerebrovascular disease among a sample of Medicare patients admitted to hospitals with a principal diagnosis of transient ischemic attack (TIA). Further, they assessed the relative probability of receiving care from a neurologist. After adjusting for comorbid illness (including hypertension and prior history of stroke), ability to pay (using a proxy based on dual Medicaid-Medicare eligibility and area of residence), and other clinical and demographic variables, the authors found that African Americans were 83% less likely than whites to receive noninvasive cerebrovascular testing. Among those receiving noninvasive testing, African Americans were 54% as likely to receive cerebral angiography, and among those receiving angiography, the odds of African Americans receiving carotid endarterectomy was 0.27. African Americans were 62% less likely than whites to receive anticoagulant therapy, but this difference was not statistically significant given the small number of African-American subjects. African-American patients were 21% less likely than whites to receive care from a neurologist. Overall, patients who received care from a neurologist were more likely to receive both noninvasive and invasive cerebrovascular testing, but were significantly less likely to undergo surgery. The authors note that while the findings could have been affected by unmeasured differences in the severity of carotid artery stenosis that could explain the lower rates of carotid endarterectomy among African Americans (African Americans are less likely to have extracranial disease that is most amenable to carotid endarterectomy), this difference would not explain the disparity in rates of testing (Mitchell et al., 2000).

Renal Transplantation

African Americans are at greater risk for end-stage renal disease (ESRD) than white Americans. Although African Americans constitute 12% of the U.S. population, they represent almost one-third of those with ESRD. Kidney dialysis was once considered the optimal treatment for ESRD, but recent advancements in kidney transplantation techniques have made transplantation more cost-effective than dialysis. African-American patients with ESRD, however, are less likely than similar white patients to receive a kidney transplant (Epstein et al., 2000). African-American patients are also less likely than white patients to be referred for transplantation and to appear on waiting lists within the first year of Medicare eligibility (Kasiske, London, and Ellison, 1998). In addition, average waiting time for African-American patients awaiting kidney transplantation is almost twice as long as that for white patients, a difference that is not apparent for transplantation of other solid organs (Young and Gaston, 2000). These findings, however, must be interpreted with caution, as many clinical considerations complicate interpretation of these data. For example, in general, fewer African Americans than whites desire or are appropriate for transplantation, and immunologic matching criteria result in fewer donor matches for African Americans than whites.

Several studies are consistent in finding that African-American patients (and in some instances, other ethnic minority patients) are less likely to be judged as appropriate for transplantation, are less likely to appear on transplantation waiting lists, and are less likely to undergo transplantation procedures, even after patients' insurance status and other factors are considered. Garg, Diener-West, and Powe (2001) longitudinally followed adult ESRD patients to assess racial differences in rates of placement on transplantation waiting lists over time. The authors found that lower rates of placement on the waiting list for blacks than whites persisted after adjustment for differences in both sociodemographic characteristics and health status, and that the gap between blacks and whites did not narrow over time. Epstein and colleagues (2000), in a study of patients with end-stage renal disease from four regional networks in geographically diverse areas, found that African-American patients were less likely than white patients to be rated as appropriate candidates for transplantation, according to expert-identified criteria (9.0% vs. 20.9%, respectively). Among patients considered appropriate for transplantation, however, African-American patients were less likely than whites to be referred for evaluation (90.1% vs. 98.0% respectively), were less likely to be placed on a waiting list (71.0% vs. 86.7% respectively), and were less likely to ultimately undergo transplantation (16.9% vs. 52.0%, respectively). Similarly, in a study of over 41,000 patients awaiting transplantation, Kasiske, London, and Ellison (1998) found that white patients were more likely to be placed on waiting lists before initiating maintenance dialysis than African-American, Hispanic, or "Asian/other" patients. Other factors predicting being placed on waiting lists before dialysis included patients' age, receipt of a prior transplant, level of education, employment status, insurance status, receiving insulin, listing for kidney and pancreas transplant vs. kidney only, and listing through a center that performs a high volume of procedures.

Several studies are consistent in finding that African-American patients (and in some instances, other ethnic minority patients) are less likely to be judged as appropriate for transplantation, are less likely to appear on transplantation waiting lists, and are less likely to undergo transplantation procedures, even after patients' insurance status and other factors are considered.

African-American patients are also found to be less likely to receive dialysis as an initial treatment for ESRD. Barker-Cummings, McClellan, Soucie, and Krisher (1995) found that after controlling for patients' sociodemographic and clinical characteristics (including age, education, social support, home ownership, functional status, albumin level, presence of hypertension, history of MI, peripheral neuropathy, and comorbid diabetes), African Americans were half as likely as white patients to be initially treated with peritoneal dialysis.

Some evidence suggests that African-American patients are less likely than whites to desire kidney transplantation. Ayanian, Cleary, Weissman, and Epstein (1999) found that African-American male patients were significantly less likely than white males to report wanting a transplant. This difference was not significant among female patients. However, even when differences in preference were taken into account, African-American patients were much less likely than white patients to have been referred to a transplant center for evaluation (50.5% of African-American women vs. 70.7% of white women, and 53.9% of African-American men vs. 76.2% of white men), and to have been placed on a waiting list or to have received a transplant within 18 months after initiating dialysis (31.9% of African-American women vs. 56.5% of white women, and 35.3% for African-American men vs. 60.6% of white men). Similarly, Alexander and Sehgal (1998) found that African-American patients were less likely than white patients to be "definitely interested" in receiving a transplant, to complete pre-transplant workup, and finally, to progress on waiting lists to receive a transplant. These analyses controlled for patient age, gender, cause of renal failure, years receiving dialysis, and median income of patients' zip code area. Ozminkowski et al. (1997) surveyed 456 ESRD patients to assess the effects of patient sociodemographic characteristics, health and functional status, and attitudes about dialysis or transplantation on waiting list entry and receipt of a cadaver kidney transplant. The authors found that approximately 60% of the differences between African-American and white waiting list entry rates and 52% of the black-white differences in transplantation rates were due to race-related differences in socioeconomic status, health and functional status, severity of illness, biological factors, the existence of contraindications to transplantation, transplant center characteristics, and patients' attitudes about dialysis and transplantation.

At least one study has assessed the influence of patients' clinical and non-clinical factors, including race, on physicians' recommendations for renal transplantation. Thamer et al. (2001) surveyed 271 nephrologists who were presented with scenarios that varied the age, race, gender, living situation (alone or with family), history of compliance with treatment, diabetic status, residual renal function status, HIV status, weight, and cardiac ejection fraction of hypothetical patients. Asian-American males were less likely than white males to be recommended for transplantation, as were women, those with a history of non-compliance, low cardiac ejection fraction, overweight, or positive HIV status. The fact that African-American and white "patients" were recommended for transplantation at similar rates suggests that the observed black-white differences may emerge at other steps in the transplantation process, according to the authors. The low rate of recommendation for Asian-American males, however, is inconsistent with the fact that Asians have the highest cadaveric allograft survival rates of all racial and ethnic groups, the authors note.

HIV/AIDS

HIV infection continues to spread more rapidly among African-American and Hispanic populations than any other racial/ethnic group in the United States. While federal programs have been expanded in recent years to increase the availability of antiretroviral therapies, especially among low-income and ethnic minority populations, minorities face greater barriers than whites to appropriate care. African Americans with HIV infection are less likely to receive antiretroviral therapy, less likely to receive prophylaxis for pneumocystic pneumonia, and less likely to receive protease inhibitors than non-minorities with HIV. These disparities remain even after adjusting for age, gender, education, and insurance coverage (Shapiro et al., 1999). Differences in the quality of HIV care may be related to survival rates, even at equivalent levels of access to care. Cunningham et al. (2000), for example, in a study of relative risk of six-year mortality for Hispanic, African-American, and white patients hospitalized as a result of HIV-related illness, found that Hispanics experience twice the risk of dying as whites, after controlling for sociodemographic characteristics, (e.g., access to care and insurance) and clinical characteristics (e.g., severity of illness and disease stage). Use of antiretroviral drugs prior to hospitalization did not diminish the impact of ethnicity on survival.

African Americans with HIV infection are less likely to receive antiretroviral therapy, less likely to receive prophylaxis for pneumocystic pneumonia, and less likely to receive protease inhibitors than non-minorities with HIV. These disparities remain even after adjusting for age, gender, education, and insurance coverage.

Shapiro et al. (1999) assessed racial/ethnic, gender, and other socio-demographic variations in care (number of care-seeking visits and use of protease inhibitors [PI] or nonnucleoside reverse transcriptase inhibitors [NNRTI]) for persons infected with HIV. Adjusting for insurance status, CD4 cell count, sex, age, method of exposure to HIV, and region of country, African-American and Hispanic patients were 24% less likely than whites to receive PI or NNRTI at initial assessment. This disparity declined to 8% at the final assessment stage, a difference that remained statistically significant. On average, blacks waited 13.5 months to receive these medications, compared with 10.6 months for whites.

Moore et al. (1994) assessed use of anti-retroviral drugs and prophylactic therapy to treat Pneumocystis carinii pneumonia (PCP) in an urban population infected with HIV. No racial differences were found in the stage of HIV disease at the time of presentation. However, 63% of eligible whites, but only 48% of eligible blacks received antiretroviral therapy, and PCP prophylaxis was received by 82% of eligible whites and only 58% of eligible blacks. African-American patients were significantly less likely than whites to receive antiretroviral therapy or PCP prophylaxis. Noting that whites were more likely to report a usual source of care (59%) than African Americans (34%), the authors suggested that increased access to regular healthcare providers among minorities might reduce disparities in HIV treatment.

Bennett et al. (1995) assessed quality of care for Pneumocystis carinii pneumonia (PCP) among white, Hispanic and African-American patients with HIV receiving care in either Veterans Administration (VA) hospitals or non-VA systems. For all patients, regardless of the type of hospital in which they were treated, anti-PCP medications were initiated within two days of admission for 70% to 77% of patients. Approximately 60% of patients underwent a bronchoscopy at some point during hospitalization. Black and Hispanic patients at non-VA hospitals, however, were more likely to die during hospitalization, and were less likely to undergo bronchoscopy in the first two days of admission. No racial differences were found in use of bronchoscopy, receipt of anti-PCP medications within two days of admission, or mortality in VA hospitals.

Asthma

African Americans, particularly those living in urban areas characterized by concentrated poverty, are at greater risk of morbidity and mortality due to asthma. It is unclear if the greater prevalence of asthma among African Americans is due to biologic or genetic predisposition, socioeconomic factors, or environmental living conditions, although high rates of air pollutants in urban communities is likely a key factor (Institute of Medicine, 1999c). Management and control of the disease is affected by socioeconomic as well as cultural considerations; African Americans are more likely to receive treatment for asthma in emergency rooms, and are more likely to use inhaled bronchodilator medications than inhaled corticosteroids, suggesting that management of the disease in this population has been focused more on acute symptom control as opposed to suppression of chronic airway inflammation. These patterns are not fully explained by socioeconomic differences between blacks and whites (Zoratti et al., 1998).

Zoratti and colleagues (Zoratti et al., 1998), in a study of African-American and white patients enrolled in a managed care system, found that after controlling for income, marital status, gender, and age, African-American patients were more likely than whites to access care in emergency rooms, were hospitalized more often, and were less likely to be seen by an asthma specialist. African Americans were also more likely to use oral corticosteroids and were less likely to be prescribed inhaled anticholinergic medications. The authors note that the population at highest risk for the most severe asthma and the poorest management of the disease had the least access to specialists and the appropriate medications to manage chronic symptoms. While this study was unable to assess the severity of disease in the patient population and could not assess long-term follow-up, African Americans seen in emergency rooms appeared not to receive appropriate rates of referral to specialty care. The authors speculate that several barriers to referral may exist, particularly for low-income African Americans, including geographic distance from specialists (who are primarily located in suburban and higher-income communities), the presence of other life demands and challenges, and assumptions on the part of primary care physicians that low-income patients would be unable to maintain compliance with treatment regimens.

A combination of poor patient understanding of asthma management and inadequate physician monitoring may contribute to disparities in asthma care. Blixen et al. (1997) surveyed 24 African-American patients with asthma who were treated in an emergency department for acute asthma symptoms, and found that despite having relatively high levels of access to care (half reported belonging to an HMO, 54% lived within 10 minutes away from a regular source of healthcare, and 70.8% reported having a regular physician to treat their asthma), the disease was typically poorly managed. Overall disease-related quality of life scores suggested that these respondents experienced poorer quality of life related to asthma than white patients assessed with the same instrument in prior studies. Fewer than half (45.8%) used NIH-recommended prophylactic anti-inflammatory medication, and a majority (70.8%) managed symptoms with an inhaled beta agonist inhaler. Over half (58.3%) knew what a home peak flow meter was, but fewer than half reported that their doctor had recommended its use and only 29.2% had one in the home. A majority (62.5%) made one to three visits to the emergency departments within the past three months, and fewer than half reported speaking with their physician or nurse about asthma-related problems.

In contrast, in a study of over 5,000 patients to assess the consistency of asthma care in relation to national guidelines, Krishnan et al. (2001) found that after controlling for patient age, education, employment, and symptom frequency, no significant differences existed between African-American and white patients in use of medication regimens and asthma specialty care. Findings of racial or ethnic differences in asthma care are therefore somewhat mixed, and may vary as a function of the educational level of patient populations studied.

Diabetes

African Americans, Hispanics, and Native Americans experience a 50%-100% higher burden of illness and mortality due to diabetes than white Americans, yet the disease appears to be more poorly managed among minority patients. In a study of nearly 1,400 Medicare beneficiaries with a diagnosis of diabetes, Chin, Zhang, and Merrell (1998) found that even after controlling for patients' gender, education, and age, African-American patients were less likely to undergo a measurement of glycosylated hemoglobin, lipid testing, ophthalmologic visits, and influenza vaccinations than white patients. African-American patients with diabetes were also more likely to use hospital emergency departments and had fewer physician visits. Similarly, Cowie and Harris (1997) found that African-American non-insulin dependent diabetes patients were more likely to be treated with insulin than whites and Mexican Americans. No significant differences were found among the racial and ethnic groups, however, in rates of visits to specialists for diabetes complications, physician testing of blood glucose, and screening for hypertension, retinopathy, and foot problems. In addition, a higher proportion of African-American patients than non-Hispanic whites and Mexican Americans were found to receive patient education, but the median number of hours of instruction was lower for African Americans. Harris et al. (1999) found that while the majority of subjects in a nationwide study of adults with type 2 diabetes used pharmacologic treatment to manage the disease, a higher proportion of African-American patients were treated with insulin and a higher proportion of Mexican-American patients were treated with oral agents when compared with non-Hispanic whites. Multiple daily insulin injections were also more common among whites. Further, a larger percentage of African-American women and Mexican-American men were found to have poor glycemic control (HbA1c > 8%) when compared with other groups. There was no relationship between glycemic control and patient socioeconomic status or access to care for any racial or ethnic group.

Analgesia

Given the role of cultural and linguistic factors in both patients' perceptions of pain and in physicians' ability to accurately assess patients' pain (to be discussed in greater detail in Chapter 3), it is reasonable to suspect that healthcare disparities might be greater in pain treatment and other aspects of symptom management than in treatment of objectively verifiable disease. Several studies have documented underuse of analgesics among minority patients, both in in-patient and outpatient settings.

Todd, Samaroo, and Hoffman (1993), for example, found that among Hispanic and non-Hispanic white patients with long-bone fracture treated at the UCLA Medical Center emergency department, Hispanic patients were twice as likely as white patients to receive no pain medication, even after controlling for patient, injury, and physician characteristics. A follow-up study (Todd, Lee, and Hoffman, 1994) revealed that physicians' assessments of pain severity did not differ among Hispanic and non-Hispanic white patients presenting to the emergency department with extremity trauma, ruling out physicians' ability to assess pain as a possible explanation for disparities in analgesic use. Todd and colleagues (Todd et al., 2000) also found that after controlling for time since injury, time in the emergency department, need for fracture reduction, and payer status, African-American patients with long-bone fractures seen in emergency rooms were less likely than whites to receive analgesia. Similarly, as noted above, Bernabei et al. (1998), in a study of elderly nursing home residents with cancer, found that African Americans were 63% more likely than whites to receive no pain medication, after accounting for patients' gender, marital status, severity of illness, and cognitive status. Cleeland et al. (1997) found that minority cancer patients were more likely than whites to receive inadequate pain medication.

Study findings regarding use of analgesia, however, are not entirely consistent. Ng et al. (1996), for example, found that white and African-American post-operative patients were prescribed more narcotics than Asian-American and Hispanic patients. This difference persisted after adjustment for age, gender, preoperative use of narcotics, health insurance, and pain site. These findings suggest that cultural and linguistic barriers, which may have been more pronounced among Hispanic and Asian-American patients, may indeed play a significant role in physicians' ability to detect pain symptoms. These findings are in contrast to that of Todd and colleagues (Todd, Lee, and Hoffman, 1994; Todd, Samaroo, and Hoffman, 1993), who controlled for patient characteristics such as language in finding that Hispanic patients seen in emergency care settings were less likely to receive analgesia. In addition, Weisse et al. (2001) used an experimental design to assess primary care physicians' recommendations regarding treatment of hypothetical patients presenting with pain (kidney stone pain or lower back pain) or a control condition (sinusitis). Symptom presentation and severity were held constant, but the investigators varied the "patients'" race (African American or white) and gender. No overall racial or gender differences were found in treatment recommendations. However, when the physicians' recommendations were analyzed by gender, a significant interaction was observed. Male physicians prescribed higher doses of pain treatment to white than African-American patients and to male than female patients. Female physicians, on the other hand, prescribed higher doses to African Americans than whites and females than males. Among "patients" presenting with sinusitis, no overall differences were observed in physicians' decisions to treat patients with antibiotics, but white patients were prescribed a longer course of antibiotics and were prescribed refills more often than African-American patients. These findings lead the authors to conclude that male and female physicians respond differently to patients' gender and race.

Rehabilitative Services

Studies of racial differences in the use of rehabilitative services, such as occupational or physical therapy, yield mixed results. Hoenig, Rubenstein, and Kahn (1996) assessed racial and other sociodemographic and geographic differences in the use of physical and occupational therapy among elderly Medicare patients with acute hip fracture. Assessing records of 2,762 Medicare patients treated in 297 randomly selected hospitals from five states, the authors found that after controlling for patient clinical characteristics, African-American patients (63%) were more likely to receive a lower intensity of physical or occupational therapy than non-African Americans (43%). Similarly, Harada et al. (2000) assessed use of physical therapy among patients hospitalized in acute and/or postacute settings following hip fracture, and found that African-American patients were less likely than whites to receive acute physical therapy only, were less likely to receive therapy in both acute care and skilled nursing facilities, and were more likely to receive no physical therapy at all.

In contrast, Horner et al. (1997), in a study of inpatient utilization of physical and occupational therapy following stroke, found that a larger proportion of African American patients received physical or occupational therapy during hospitalization. After adjusting for clinical and socioeconomic factors associated with the use of physical and occupational therapy, however, no racial differences were found in the likelihood of use of therapy or time to initiate therapy (African Americans = 6.6 days, whites = 7.4). Similarly, no racial differences were found in length of physical or occupational therapy in days or as a proportion of hospital stay.

Maternal and Child Health

In recent years, several federal and state initiatives have been implemented to promote access to appropriate prenatal, perinatal and postnatal care for pregnant women and their children. Despite these efforts, many of which have been directed at low-income and uninsured women, racial and ethnic disparities have been found with modest consistency in a range of maternal and child health services.

Aron et al. (2000) assessed differences in rates of cesarean delivery by patient race and insurance status among over 25,000 women seen in 21 hospitals in northeastern Ohio. While the unadjusted overall rate of cesarean delivery was similar in white and non-white (over 90% African-American and other racial and ethnic groups) patients, adjusted analyses that controlled for clinical risk factors revealed that non-white patients were more likely to receive cesarean delivery. In contrast, Braveman et al. (1995) found that after adjusting for insurance status and personal, community, medical, and hospital characteristics, black women were 24% more likely to undergo cesarean than whites. Latino women were also at a slightly elevated risk for cesarean delivery compared with whites. Among women who delivered high-birth-weight babies, gave birth at for-profit hospitals, or resided in communities where 25% or more of the population were non-English speaking, cesarean delivery was more likely among non-whites and was more than 40% more likely among black women than white women.

Brett, Schoendorf, and Kiely (1994) assessed use of prenatal care technologies (i.e., ultrasonography, tocolysis, amniocentesis) among African-American, Hispanic, and white women, and found inconsistent racial differences in these services, after controlling for maternal age, education, marital status, location of residence, birth order, timing of first prenatal care visit, and plural births. Amniocentesis was used substantially less frequently by black women, while black women underwent ultrasonography slightly less frequently than white women. Black women with singleton births were slightly more likely to receive tocolysis than white women, although the risk of idiopathic pre-term delivery is estimated to be three times higher in black women. Black women with plural births received tocolysis two-thirds as often as white women.

In a study of civilian vs. military outcomes in prenatal care utilization, birth weight distribution, and fetal and neonatal mortality rates, Barfield et al. (1996) found that prenatal care utilization was lower for black patients than white patients in both military and civilian populations. The magnitude of the disparity was lower, however, in the military population. Similarly, Kogan et al. (1994) assessed self-reported receipt of prenatal care advice from providers among over 8,300 white and African-American women. After adjusting for age, marital status, education, income, site of prenatal care, type of payment, maternal health behaviors, when trimester care began, and prior adverse pregnancy outcomes, the authors found that white women were more likely to report receiving advice for alcohol and smoking cessation than African-American women.

Breast-feeding promotion narrowly missed significance with a trend toward more advice for white women. A significant interaction between race and marital status emerged, such that black single women were 1.4 times more likely than single white women to not receive advice on drug cessation, while there were no racial differences among married women.

Childrens' Health Services

As is the case with maternal and infant health services, several federal and state initiatives have been initiated to improve access to healthcare among low-income children and adolescents (most notably, the federal State Child Health Insurance Program [SCHIP]). Several studies note racial and ethnic disparities in hospital-based and outpatient child health services. However, no studies to date have assessed the effectiveness of SCHIP in reducing racial and ethnic disparities in care.

Furth et al. (2000) assessed access to kidney transplantation among over 3,000 African-American and white youth under age 20 with ESRD. Controlling for factors such as age, gender, cause of ESRD, family socioeconomic status (SES), incident year of ESRD, ESRD network, and facility characteristics, the authors found that African-American youth were 12% less likely than white patients to be activated on the kidney transplant wait list. Family socioeconomic characteristics, however, reduced this disparity; the relative hazard for black patients in the lowest SES quartile being activated on the wait list was .84, compared with relative hazard of 1.0 for black patients in the highest SES quartile.

Hahn (1995) assessed use of prescription medications between two samples of children (ages 1 to 5 and ages 6 to 17) who had at least one ambulatory care visit in 1987. Among children aged one to five, African-American children were half as likely to receive prescription medication compared with white children. Adding health factors to the model did not change this relationship. However, the addition of numbers of physician visits reduced these differences, such that they were no longer significant. There was no difference in the probability of receiving medication for Hispanic children compared with white children. After controlling for age, maternal education, insurance, poverty status, source of care, geographic location, health status, number of bed days, number of reduced activity days, and physician visits, black children received the fewest number of medications. The average number of medications for black children was 86.5% compared to that of white children, while Hispanic children averaged 94.1% of medications compared to that of white children. Among children aged 6 to 17 years, African-American and Hispanic children were 46% and 38% less likely, respectively, to receive any prescription medication compared with white children. The addition of health factors and numbers of physician visits did not change these relationships, and they remained after controlling for age, maternal education, insurance, poverty status, source of care, geographic location, health status, number of bed days, number of reduced activity days, and physician visits. Similarly, Zito et al. (1998) found that white children were twice as likely to receive psychotropic prescriptions compared with African-American children.

A study examining parents' perceptions of pediatric care found striking racial and ethnic differences. Weech-Maldonado et al. (2001) used data from the National Consumer Assessment of Health Plans (CAHPS) Benchmarking database and found that minority parents, particularly non-English speakers, were less satisfied than white parents with pediatric services, after controlling for parents' gender, age, education, and their children's health status. African-American and American-Indian parents were found to be less satisfied than whites in getting needed care, the timeliness of care, provider communication, and health plan services. Among Asian-American and Hispanic parents, parental satisfaction was lower than for whites only among those who were non-English speakers. Asian-American and Hispanic non-English speakers rated staff helpfulness, timeliness of care, provider communication, health plan services, and getting needed care lower than did white parents, while Asian-American and Hispanic parents who were proficient in English did not differ significantly from whites on any reports of care.

Mental Health Services

Several studies document racial and ethnic variation in receipt of mental health services. Significantly, the U.S. Surgeon General recently completed a major report assessing racial and ethnic disparities in mental health and mental healthcare that reviews much of the available literature. That report finds that more so than in other areas of health and medicine, mental health services are "plagued by disparities in the availability of and access to its services," and that "these disparities are viewed readily through the lenses of racial and cultural diversity, age, and gender" (U.S. DHHS, 2001a, p. vi). Major findings of the report include that: mental illnesses are real and disabling conditions that affect all populations (regardless of race/ethnicity); striking disparities are found for racial and ethnic minorities; and these disparities impose a greater disability burden on racial and ethnic minorities. In addition to universal barriers to quality care (e.g., cost, fragmentation of services), the report notes that other barriers, such as mistrust, fear, discrimination, and language differences carry special significance for minorities in mental health treatment, as these barriers affect patients' thoughts, moods, and behavior. Communication and trust are particularly critical in treatment, the report notes, and differences in the cultural perspectives of the patient and clinician/healthcare system must be acknowledged and addressed (U.S. DHHS, 2001a).

The U.S. Surgeon General . . . finds that more so than in other areas of health and medicine, mental health services are "plagued by disparities in the availability of and access to its services," and that "these disparities are viewed readily through the lenses of racial and cultural diversity, age, and gender."

Several studies have examined disparate use of psychotropic medications and mental health services and find disparities, with minorities in some cases receiving *higher* quantities of medications. For example, in a study examining prescriptions of antipsychotic medications by physicians in psychiatric emergency services, Segal, Bola, and Watson (1996) found that African-American patients received more oral doses and injections of antipsychotic medications. The 24-hour dosage of antipsychotic medication given to African Americans was also significantly higher that for other patients. Analyses controlled for several clinical factors including presence of psychotic disorder, severity of disturbance, dangerousness, psychiatric history, if physical restraints were used, hours spent in the emergency service, clinician's efforts to engage patient in treatment, and whether optimum time was spend on the evaluation. The study also found that the tendency to overmedicate African-American patients was lower when a clinician's efforts to engage the patients in treatment were rated as being higher. Models predicting number of medications, number of oral and injected antipsychotic and 24-hour dosage became non-significant.

In contrast, a study examining medication prescribed for depression yielded different results. Melfi and colleagues (2000) assessed antidepressant treatment in a population of Medicaid beneficiaries diagnosed with depression. Analyses controlled for age, gender, Medicaid eligibility status, and several clinical factors. Forty-four percent of whites and 27.8% of blacks received antidepressant treatment within 30 days of the first indicator of depression. White patients were more likely to receive antidepressants than black patients and patients in the other/unknown racial category.

An examination of privately insured federal employees, conducted by Padgett and colleagues (1994), assessed racial and ethnic differences in use of inpatient psychiatric services. Analyses controlled for a variety of predisposing factors (e.g., education, family size, racial/ethnic composition of residing county), enabling factors (region of country, salary, high or low option selected for insurance coverage), and need factors (annual medical expenses, family's annual medical expenses, other family member receipt of inpatient psychiatric care, sum of outpatient mental heath visits by other family members). No significant differences were found among blacks, whites and Hispanics as to the probability of a psychiatric hospitalization or in number of inpatient psychiatric days.

Racial and Ethnic Differences in Other Clinical and Hospital-Based Services

Several studies document racial and ethnic disparities in other clinical and hospital-based services. Ebell et al. (1995) assessed the rate of survival by patient race following in-hospital cardiopulmonary resuscitation (CPR) of 656 patients at one of three teaching hospitals. Black patients in this study were less likely than non-black patients to have an admitting diagnosis of myocardial infarction (MI), were less likely to have a history of coronary artery disease, but had a higher severity of illness according to a standard screening instrument. Controlling for these variables, black patients were found to have poorer survival to discharge than non-black patients. Because resuscitation was provided in-hospital, differences in ambulance response time, access to telephones, or other community factors could not account for this difference. Further, because there were no significant racial differences in the success of the resuscitation effort, the difference in survival appears to be related to the quality of care after resuscitation, or to other unmeasured factors.

Devgan et al. (2000) assessed surgical treatment for glaucoma among large samples of African-American and white Medicare patients, and found that African-American patients received argon laser trabeculoplasty or trabeculectomy surgery at nearly half of expected rates, once the age-race prevalence of glaucoma was considered. Arozullah et al. (1999) assessed rates of laparoscopic cholecystectomy among more than 16,000 Veterans Administration (VA) patients diagnosed with gall bladder or biliary disease. After controlling for patient age, marital status, co-morbid illness, year of surgery, and hospital geographic location, the investigators found that African-American patients who underwent cholecystectomy were less likely than white patients to undergo the laparoscopic procedure. In contrast, another study of VA patients (Selim et al., 2001) found that among patients presenting with low-back pain, "non-white" patients in higher levels of pain were more likely to receive lumbar spine radiographs than white patients experiencing similar pain levels, although this racial difference disappeared after controlling for clinical characteristics.

Fewer studies have assessed the quality of basic healthcare services.

In one such study, Ayanian et al. (1999) utilized explicit process criteria and implicit review by physicians to assess the quality of care for patients hospitalized with congestive heart failure and pneumonia. Using records from a stratified random sample of over 2,000 Medicare beneficiaries, the authors found that among patients with congestive heart failure, African Americans received a lower overall quality of care than other patients by implicit review, but not explicit review. Among patients with pneumonia, African-American patients received a lower quality of care by explicit criteria, but not explicit review. These differences persisted in analyses adjusting for patient and hospital characteristics. Adjusted analyses also revealed no significant differences in quality of care for patients from poor communities, as compared with other patients. Similarly, in a review of discharge data from over 1.7 million patients assessed via the Hospital Cost and Utilization Project (HCUP-2), Harris, Andrews, and Elixhauser (1997) found that African Americans were less likely than whites to receive major therapeutic procedures for 37 of 77 conditions, and more likely than whites to receive a major therapeutic procedure in 9.1% of conditions studied. These differences persisted even after controlling for patients' age, expected pay source, indicators of clinical condition, and hospital-level characteristics (e.g., bed size, public ownership, teaching status, and urban location).

In a study of racial differences in mortality and resource use among patients admitted to intensive care units, Williams et al. (1995) found no significant differences in risk-adjusted in-hospital mortality. The authors did find, however, that African-American patients had a shorter length of stay and lower resource use in the first seven days compared with white patients. For example, whites received more technological monitoring (arterial and pulmonary artery catheters, pulse oximetry), more laboratory testing, and a greater proportion of life-saving treatments. These differences persisted after adjusting for patient characteristics and insurance status, leading the researchers to conclude that these differences could reflect undertreatment for African Americans or overutilization of services by whites.

In another study of Medicare patients, Wilson, May, and Kelly (1994) assessed racial differences in receipt of total knee arthroplasty among older adults with osteoarthritis. The authors found that while osteoarthritis was slightly, but not significantly, more common among African Americans, whites were more likely to receive total knee arthroplasty. This relationship held true at all income levels and could not be explained by prior procedures or the use of alternative procedures.

White-Means (2000) assessed the use of long-term care services (paid caregiver, therapist, mental health, dentist, foot doctor, optometrist, chiropractor, ER visit, doctor visits, prescription medications) by disabled elderly Medicare patients, as a function of medical conditions and disabilities, income, insurance status, regional and rural residence, whether unpaid caregivers provide in-home services, and sociodemographic characteristics (e.g., gender, education). Given similar medical conditions, African-American patients were found to be less likely to use long-term care services, particularly prescription medications and physician services. African-American patients who lived in rural areas, small cities, and western states or who had more joint and breathing problems were more likely to use services. Differences in personal attributes (e.g., income, health) did not fully explain racial differences in use of prescriptions and physician services. Similarly, Khandker and Simoni-Wastila (1998) assessed racial differences in use and level of use of prescription drugs among a sample of Medicaid patients, controlling for age, sex, and Medicaid eligibility characteristics. African-American children were found to use 2.7 fewer prescriptions compared with white children. African-American adults used 4.9 fewer prescriptions, and African-American elders used 6.3 fewer prescriptions than white elders. White Medicaid enrollees had higher use and spending than black enrollees across most high-volume therapeutic drug categories.

In a study of primary care, Shi (1999) assessed patients' perceptions of intake, service delivery, referral, and follow-up among nearly 15,000 white, African-American, Hispanic, and Asian respondents to the Medical Expenditure Panel Survey (MEPS). Controlling for patients' perceived need for care, ability to obtain services, and frequency of use of care, Shi found that African-American, Hispanic, and Asian-American patients tended to experience greater barriers to receiving primary care. Hispanic patients were over 40% less likely to have a usual source of care, while those African-American and Hispanic patients who did report a regular primary care provider tended to reference a facility (hospital or clinic) rather than an individual provider. African Americans were less likely to have a primary care specialist as a regular provider. All three minority groups were 39% to 48% more likely than whites to report long waiting periods before seeing their care provider, but Asian-American patients were more likely than any racial/ethnic groups to report that getting an appointment was "very difficult." On an encouraging note, this study also found that overwhelming numbers of whites and minority patients reported confidence in their provider and that their usual care provider "listened to them"—over 90% agreement for all groups.

A small number of studies have assessed racial and ethnic differences in preventable hospitalizations. Preventable hospitalizations are those that might not have occurred had patients received timely and appropriate preventive care in the case of acute conditions, as well as effective and continuous care for chronic conditions. Gaskin and Hoffman (2000) assessed rates of preventable hospitalizations among children, working-age adults, and the elderly, while adjusting for a range of sociodemographic (e.g., age, income, insurance status), community-level (e.g., neighborhood characteristics, physicians, and hospital beds per capita), and health status (e.g., co-morbidities) variables. Results indicated that African Americans and Hispanics were significantly more likely to be hospitalized for preventable conditions than whites, even after adjusting for patient differences in healthcare needs, socioeconomic status, insurance coverage, and the availability of primary care providers. Subsequent analyses of individuals within similar health insurance plans confirmed that these differences exist independently of insurance status. The findings were limited by the lack of information on the competency of providers seen by minority patients, the adequacy of insurance plans, and personal health-seeking behavior.

Minority patients are more likely to undergo amputation than white patients. Such is the case with limb amputation, where more than 50,000 procedures are performed each year among patients with diabetes. Guadagnoli et al. (1995) assessed racial differences in the use of amputation and leg-sparing surgery among a random sample of Medicare patients. The authors found that African-American patients were nearly twice as likely as whites to undergo above-knee amputation, and were slightly more likely than whites to undergo toe and/or foot amputation, controlling for co-morbid disease, prior hospitalizations, geographic region, hospital teaching status, and other factors. Whites, on the other hand, were more likely to undergo lower-extremity arterial revascularization and percutaneous transluminal angioplasty than African-American patients. The study did not, however, control for disease severity, although the authors note that controls for co-morbid disease and prior hospitalizations may attenuate this potential confounding factor. Similarly, Gornick et al. (1996), in a study of 26.3 million Medicare beneficiaries, found that African Americans were more likely than whites to undergo bilateral orchiectomy or amputation of the lower limbs, even after controlling for income differences. Finally, Collins et al. (2002) assessed racial and ethnic differences in rates of lower extremity amputation versus lower extremity bypass revascularization among a sample of VA patients with peripheral arterial disease. In this prospective study, the authors statistically adjusted for a range of factors that may be associated with the use of amputation versus revascularization (e.g., presence of diabetes, hypertension, heart disease, or other co-morbid conditions, behavioral risk factors such as smoking or alcohol use, geographic location of the VA hospital), and found that African-American and Hispanic patients were 1.5 and 1.4 times, respectively, more likely than white patients to undergo amputation than revascularization (Collins et al., 2002).

Gaps in Existing Research

While the research reviewed here points to significant variation in access to and use of services by race and ethnicity, several gaps exist that must be addressed to develop a more comprehensive understanding of racial and ethnic disparities in healthcare. The most significant gap in this research is the failure to identify mechanisms by which these disparities occur. A robust research agenda is needed to better understand how the process and structure of care may vary by patient race (see chapter on "Needed Research"). Such research must consider the range of influences on patients' and providers' attitudes and expectations in the clinical encounter, clinical decision-making processes employed by healthcare providers and the influence of patient race in these processes, the nature and quality of communication between patients and providers (particularly as it occurs across cultural and/or linguistic lines), the environments and settings in which care is delivered, and other factors that will be discussed later in this report. In addition, as noted below, no research has yet illuminated the relative contribution of these factors to the healthcare disparities observed in the literature.

Assessing sources of disparities in care in the current literature is also complicated by many methodological considerations. Attempts to control for SES differences are inconsistent, with some researchers employing patient income or education as sole indicators of SES, and others using proxy variables such as estimates of income on the basis of patients' zip code information. Most studies control for insurance status, but some combine data from patients insured via different types of health systems (e.g., HMO or fee-for-service) or different sources of insurance coverage (e.g., public vs. private).

Some studies have explicitly examined differences in where racial and ethnic groups receive care (e.g., public vs. private healthcare settings), and clinical factors such as stage of illness progression at presentation (e.g., on average, ethnic minority cancer patients present at later stages of disease progression, thereby limiting treatment options) or other co-morbid factors that may limit treatment options. Other studies have attempted to control for the quality of diagnostic evaluation and disease severity. Adequate assessment of these factors, however, is often limited by a lack of sufficient information in administrative claims data upon which many studies are based. These datasets often rely on crude or incomplete measures of disease severity and the types of treatment provided, and contain limited information on prior diagnoses or treatments. Further, most studies (with the exception of several studies of cardiovascular care) lack comparison to standards for the appropriateness of care, leaving open the question of whether care received was sufficient given the type and severity of disease.

Finally, one of the most significant limitations of existing research is the failure to analyze differences in care beyond comparisons of African-American and white patients. With the exception of a few large studies conducted in ethnically diverse regions of the United States such as California and New York, few studies have assessed whether disparities in care exist for Hispanic and Asian-American populations. Further, few studies have examined subgroup differences within these populations. These issues are particularly salient for Hispanic and Asian-American subgroups, whose healthcare may be complicated by linguistic and cultural differences, immigration status, and other access-related issues.

The Extent of Racial and Ethnic Disparities in Healthcare

As the discussion above suggests, many factors influence the provision and receipt of diagnostic and therapeutic healthcare services. Further, healthcare outcomes are influenced by a wide variety of factors, many of which are beyond the scope of clinical factors such as the efficacy of treatment protocols. Assessing the relative contribution of the many patient, provider, and system-level influences on care is therefore an imprecise exercise. Similarly, assessing the extent of racial and ethnic differences in healthcare that are not otherwise attributable to known factors such as access to care is not likely to yield reliable estimates.

Some studies have attempted to assess the extent of racial and ethnic disparities in a small number of key indicators of healthcare use. Weinick, Zuvekas, and Cohen (2000) assessed racial and ethnic differences in access to and use of healthcare services (i.e., having a usual source of care and the use of ambulatory care services), and evaluated the magnitude of these differences above and beyond access-related factors such as insurance status, income, and other socioeconomic characteristics. The authors found that after adjusting for health insurance, income, age, sex, marital status, education, health status, region of the country, and residence in a metropolitan area, Hispanics and African Americans were significantly more likely to lack a usual source of care and were less likely to use any ambulatory care services than white Americans. Hispanics were nearly 10% more likely to lack a usual source of care, and African Americans and Hispanics were nearly 9% and over 10% less likely, respectively, to have made any ambulatory care visits. The authors performed additional analyses to assess the extent of these disparities, simulating conditions in which all racial and ethnic groups earned equivalent income and were insured at the same level. For all groups, 55% to 77% of the observed differences remained, demonstrating that "health insurance coverage and income typically each account for only about one fifth, and never even as much as one half, of the disparities . . . observed" (Weinick, Zuvekas, and Cohen, 2000, p.43). The authors acknowledge, however, that these racial and ethnic disparities in the use of services could be related to unmeasured factors, such as job-related and non-financial barriers, poor cultural and linguistic access, an inadequate geographic distribution of healthcare providers in racial and ethnic minority communities, and other factors.

More such studies are needed to assess the relative contribution of access-related factors (e.g., insurance status), other socioeconomic and geographic variables (e.g., patients' education, income, and the availability of healthcare providers in a community), and racial and ethnic differences in healthcare preferences and attitudes to determine the extent of disparities in care. This research is needed across a range of health conditions. Currently, however, this research does not present a sufficient empirical foundation to assess the extent of racial and ethnic healthcare disparities. The committee therefore concludes that while evidence of racial and ethnic disparities in care appears consistently across a range of health conditions and medical procedures, attempts to assess or quantify the extent of these disparities, based on evidence currently available, are not likely to prove to be reliable or valid.

SUMMARY

Racial and ethnic minority patients are found to receive a lower quality and intensity of healthcare and diagnostic services across a wide range of procedures and disease areas. This finding is remarkably consistent and robust, as only a handful of the several hundred studies reviewed here and by others (e.g., Geiger, this volume; Kressin and Peterson, 2001; Mayberry et al., 2000) find no racial and ethnic differences in care. In studies where patients' sociodemographic characteristics (e.g., education level, income), insurance status (e.g., public or privately funded insurance) and clinical factors (e.g., co-morbid illness, severity of disease) are controlled, these racial and ethnic differences are generally attenuated, but rarely disappear completely. Further, in a few well-designed, prospective studies, these disparities in care have been linked to poorer clinical outcomes and higher mortality among minorities (Peterson et al., 1997; Bach et al., 1999).

Insurance status, in particular, emerges in several studies as a key predictor of the quality of care that patients receive. The privately insured generally receive a higher quality of care than those who are insured through publicly funded sources (e.g., Medicaid), or those who have no health insurance. Racial and ethnic minorities are disproportionately represented between the latter two categories, yet when sources of insurance are controlled statistically or by study design, race and ethnicity remain as significant predictors of the quality of care. This disparity is best illustrated in studies of care among Medicare populations (Gornick et al., 1996), which reveal lower rates of use of effective, higher technology diagnostic and therapeutic procedures among minorities for illnesses such as heart disease, cancer, and other chronic illnesses, and higher rates of less desirable procedures, such as amputation and bilateral orchiectomy.

The quality of care that minority and non-minority patients receive is also partly a function of where these populations tend to receive care. Several studies note that patient care is of lower quality in non-teaching hospitals, public hospitals and clinics than in teaching hospitals or private settings. While some minorities are more likely to receive care in the former settings, they are more likely to access care in emergency departments, and are less likely to have a regular source of care (Collins, Hall, and Neuhaus, 1999). Further, minorities tend to have lower access than whites to specialty care, and are less likely to be treated in settings that offer higher-technology procedures—all factors related to the quality of care in the studies reviewed here. Again, however, when these variables are controlled statistically or by study design, racial and ethnic minorities tend to receive a lower quality of care.

Most studies have compared the quality of care received by minority patients relative to that of whites as the standard of comparison. This type of analysis, however, fails to provide a complete picture of the appropriateness of care, as whites may over-utilize some services, and racial differences in the severity of disease at presentation or treatment response may contraindicate the use of similar therapeutic interventions. Some of the best-designed studies reviewed here, however, assessed the quality of care provided relative to well-established clinical criteria, and use objective diagnostic measures to assess the extent and severity of disease. In these studies, race and ethnicity again typically emerge as significant predictors of the quality of care received, indicating that disparities in care are not simply a function of disproportionate use by whites or greater disease severity among minorities.

These findings appear consistently in studies of differences in care received by African-American and white populations, and increasingly, in studies involving Hispanic patients. A few studies suggest that Asian Americans also are less likely to receive the same quality of care as whites (e.g., Carlisle et al., 1995). This review produced no studies where the quality of care for American Indian, Alaska Native, or Pacific Islander populations were explicitly studied, or where the sample size of these populations permitted analysis. Further, in few instances were subgroups of these populations explicitly studied. As will be discussed in a later chapter, research is urgently needed to assess the quality of care for these populations relative to the burden of illness.

A few of the studies that find no racial and ethnic differences in care indicate that characteristics of health systems may serve an important role in mediating these disparities. Studies of patients in military healthcare systems reviewed here indicate a lower prevalence of racial or ethnic differences in the quality of healthcare that active-duty personnel or their families receive. Similarly, some studies of patients in VA systems demonstrate reductions in racial and ethnic differences in care, although these studies are less consistent. Future research must assess the range of factors that distinguish these heath systems from other private or publicly funded systems to better understand how patient race and ethnicity are related to care and care outcomes. For example, the impact of differences in provider profiles should be investigated, as VA hospitals commonly are staffed by a larger percentage of trainees than other systems. Nonetheless, these studies suggest that characteristics of these health systems, perhaps related to universal or equal access to care, may attenuate disparities that are typically found in other systems.

Collectively, these findings support the hypothesis that patients' race and ethnicity significantly predict the quality and intensity of care that they receive. Succeeding chapters of this report will review the historical context in which these disparities occur, and examine the types of settings in which minorities typically receive care, as well as the characteristics of healthcare providers that serve them. Potential sources of healthcare disparities will be closely examined, including patient preferences; provider biases, stereotyping, and clinical decision-making; and the impact of financial and institutional characteristics of health systems on the quality of care for minority patients. Finally, several strategies to eliminate these disparities are proposed, and future research directions are outlined.

Finding 1-1: Racial and ethnic disparities in healthcare exist and, because they are associated with worse outcomes in many cases, are unacceptable.

Racial and ethnic disparities in healthcare exist. These disparities are consistent and extensive across a range of medical conditions and healthcare services, are associated with worse health outcomes, and occur independently of insurance status, income, and education, among other factors that influence access to healthcare. These disparities are unacceptable.

2

The Healthcare Environment and Its Relation to Disparities

Many aspects of the healthcare environment influence the quality of care received by U.S. racial and ethnic minority groups. The historical evolution of healthcare for persons of color, the current financial and organizational structures of health systems, the settings in which care is delivered, and the nature of the workforce providing care may, both independently and jointly, influence the quality of care that minorities receive. This chapter describes some of these environmental factors and the influences they may have on healthcare for racial and ethnic minorities.

The first two sections of this chapter describe aspects of the social and economic contexts in which racial and ethnic minority groups live in the United States. These sections review: a) the health, health insurance, and linguistic status of these groups, and b) racial attitudes and patterns of segregation and discrimination in various sectors of American life. The third section reviews the history of segregated healthcare and contemporary settings in which racial and ethnic minorities receive healthcare, including the influence and importance of community health centers. The last section focuses on the healthcare workforce in minority communities—how this workforce originated, where individuals practice, who they serve, and the influence of international medical graduates on healthcare in minority communities. The chapter concludes with a discussion of medical education, how affirmative action has served to increase the presence of underrepresented minorities in the health professions workforce, and how recent legal challenges to affirmative action have affected and may have a future impact on the healthcare workforce.

Much of the data presented in this chapter are drawn from available literature and large national data sources, such as the U.S. Census and the National Center for Vital and Health Statistics. Where possible, data on subpopulations of racial and ethnic groups (e.g., Cuban American, Puerto Rican, Mexican American, and other subgroups of the Hispanic population) are presented. This information is supplemented, where appropriate, by qualitative data regarding the experiences of racial and ethnic minority patients and healthcare professionals. These data, presented in individuals' own words, are offered as a means of understanding some of patients' and providers' experiences and perceptions of how race or ethnicity may affect both care processes and the systems and settings in which care takes place. As such, these data are not intended to substitute for empirical findings. Rather, they serve to "give voice" to the experiences of key actors in healthcare disparities, and illuminate how healthcare disparities are perceived by patients and their providers. Qualitative data were gathered via three mechanisms:

• Roundtable discussions with minority healthcare consumers, professionals and advocates at one of two large national conferences (the Asian American and Pacific Islander Health Forum conference and the Indian Health Service Research Conference, both held in April, 2001);
• Liaison panel discussions with consumer and professional groups, federal agency representatives, and minority health advocates held in the spring and summer, 2001;
• Focus group sessions conducted during this same time period; and interviews with American Indian and Alaska Native tribal leaders and a cadre of healthcare providers serving American Indian and Alaska Native communities (Joe, this volume).

For more information on these data collection activities and a summary of focus group and liaison panel findings, please see Appendixes A and D.

THE HEALTH, HEALTH INSURANCE, AND LANGUAGE STATUS OF RACIAL AND ETHNIC MINORITY POPULATIONS

This section provides an overview of factors that influence healthcare and healthcare needs of minority populations—including their health and insurance status, and linguistic barriers to care.

Health Status

Some racial and ethnic minorities experience higher rates of chronic and disabling illnesses, infectious diseases, and mortality than white

Americans. As depicted in Figure 2-1, African Americans have the highest rates of morbidity and mortality of any U.S. racial and ethnic group. The mortality rate for African Americans is approximately 1.6 times higher than that for whites—a ratio that is identical to the black/white mortality ratio in 1950 (Williams and Rucker, 2000). American Indians and Alaska Natives also experience higher mortality rates than whites, accompanied by low life expectancy. And while other racial and ethnic minorities experience lower overall mortality rates than whites, these data mask both inter-group variation (e.g., among Hispanics, Puerto Ricans experience higher infant mortality rates than whites [National Center for Health Statistics, 2000]), and an elevated burden of disease among some groups for specific causes of mortality. As depicted in Figure 2-2, some causes of mortality, such as diabetes, disproportionately affect African-American, Hispanic, and American Indian/Alaska Native populations. In addition, some subpopulations of racial and ethnic groups experience an elevated incidence and mortality due to specific diseases. Alaska Natives experience the highest rates of colon and rectal cancers of any racial or ethnic group in the United States (Institute of Medicine, 1999b). Korean Americans have the highest rates of stomach cancer (48.9 per 100,000 population) among U.S. males, followed by Japanese Americans (30.5 per 100,000 population; Institute of Medicine, 1999b). Similarly, Vietnamese-American women experience the highest incidence of cervical cancer in the United States, at rates nearly six times higher than that of white women (Institute of Medicine, 1999b).

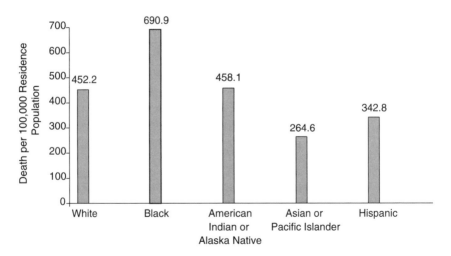

FIGURE 2-1 Age-adjusted death rates for all causes of death by race and Hispanic origin: United States, 1950-1998. SOURCE: Health, United States, 2000 (2001).

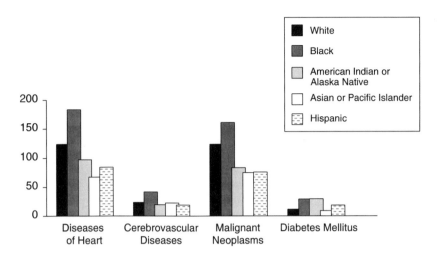

FIGURE 2-2 Age-adjusted death rates for selected causes of death by race and Hispanic origin: United States, 1950-1998. SOURCE: Health, United States 2000 (2001).

Insurance Status

Racial and ethnic minority Americans are significantly less likely than white Americans to possess health insurance (see Figures 2-3 and 2-4). The problem is particularly acute among the working poor and individuals who have no employment-based insurance, and among whom minori-

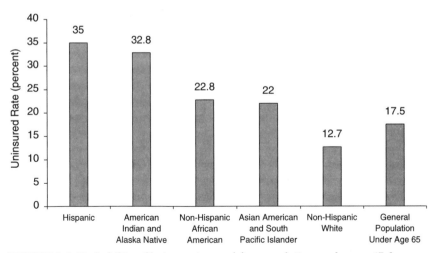

FIGURE 2-3 Probability of being uninsured for population under age 65, by race and ethnicity. SOURCE: Hoffman and Pohl, 2000.

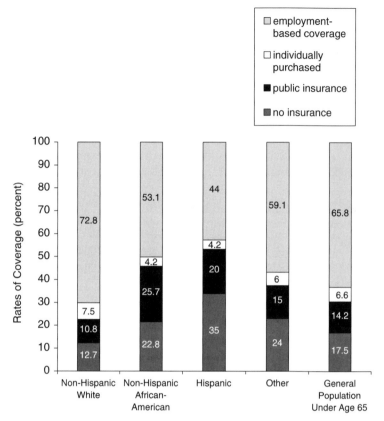

FIGURE 2-4 Sources of health insurance for population under age 65, by race and ethnicity, 1999. NOTE: Numbers may not add to 100 percent due to respondents reporting more than one source of coverage and due to rounding. SOURCE: Fronstin, 2000.

ties, particularly Hispanic Americans, are over-represented. Lack of insurance poses the most significant barrier to care. Insurance status, perhaps more than any other demographic or economic factor, determines the timeliness and quality of healthcare, if it is received at all (Institute of Medicine, 2001b).

African Americans

African Americans are less likely to possess private or employment-based health insurance relative to white Americans, and are more likely to be covered via Medicaid or other publicly funded insurance (see Figure

2-4). In addition, African Americans are almost twice as likely as non-Hispanic whites to be uninsured. High rates of uninsurance among this population occur despite the fact that over 8 in 10 African Americans are in working families, as a disproportionate percentage of African Americans work in jobs that provide no heath insurance (The Henry J. Kaiser Family Foundation, 2000a). As illustrated in Figure 2-3, the probability of being without health insurance coverage for African Americans is 22.8 percent, compared with 17.5 percent in the general population.

American Indians and Alaska Natives

The U.S. government is obligated through treaty and federal statutes to provide healthcare to members of federally recognized American Indian tribes. This trust, however, has not been fully met, for several reasons. The federal Indian Health Service (IHS) provides healthcare services primarily on Indian reservations, which are home to only a minority of American Indians (as few as 30%), as the majority of the population currently lives in urban or other non-reservation areas (Brown et al., 2000). To obtain IHS care, Indians must travel to their home reservation. Not surprisingly, a large majority (80%) of American Indians and Alaska Natives report no access to IHS facilities (The Henry J. Kaiser Family Foundation, 2000a). Although the federal government contracts with a number of urban Indian health organizations to provide services, such federal support is often limited. In general, the agency's resources (slightly over $2 billion was appropriated to the agency in fiscal year 1998) are far below needs. In fiscal year 1997, for example, the agency reported $1,430 in per capita expenditures, a figure that is 1.4 to 2.8 times below the per capita spending of other federal health programs and agencies such as Medicaid ($3,369) and the Veterans Administration ($5,458) (National Indian Health Board, 2001).

Figure 2-3 indicates that nearly one-third of American Indians and Alaska Natives (32.8%) lack health insurance, compared with 17.5% in the general population. Slightly less than half of American Indians and Alaska Natives have job-based health insurance, while one quarter receive Medicaid insurance and a similar proportion are uninsured or report only IHS coverage (The Henry J. Kaiser Family Foundation, 2000).

Asian Americans and Pacific Islanders

Some of the ethnic subgroups among Asian Americans and Pacific Islanders (API) have disproportionately high rates of uninsurance (Brown et al., 2000; Hoffman and Pohl, 2000). Rates vary considerably, although generally, only 64% of API populations have job-based health insurance, compared with nearly three-fourths of whites (73%). Nearly one-fourth of API populations are uninsured (see Figure 2-3). Generally, rates of public insurance are lower for Asian Americans and Pacific Islanders, except for some Southeast-Asian subpopulations (Brown et al., 2000).

Within API subgroups, Korean Americans are least likely to have health insurance. Less than half have job-based insurance (49%), while over one-third (34%) are uninsured and 14% receive Medicaid or other publicly funded insurance. Similarly, South East-Asian (e.g., Vietnamese, Cambodian, Laotian) and South-Asian (e.g. Indian, Pakistani, Bangladeshi) populations are disproportionately uninsured (27% and 22%, respectively). Less than half (49%) of South East-Asians have job-based insurance, while nearly seven in ten South-Asians (69%) have job-based insurance. Two in ten Chinese-American and Filipino-American families are uninsured (The Henry J. Kaiser Family Foundation, 2000b). These data are depicted in Figure 2-5.

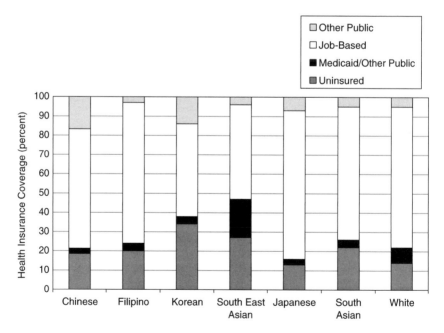

FIGURE 2-5 Health insurance coverage by Asian-American and Pacific-Islander subgroups vs. whites (Ages 0-64), 1997. SOURCE: The Henry J. Kaiser Family Foundation, 2000b.

Hispanic Americans

Hispanic Americans face greater barriers to health insurance than all other U.S. racial and ethnic groups. The probability of being uninsured among Hispanic Americans is 35 percent, compared with 17.5 percent for the general population (Hoffman and Pohl, 2000). This disparity, depicted in Figures 2-3 and 2-4, largely results from the lack of job-based insurance provided to Hispanic Americans, who disproportionately work in blue-collar and service-oriented jobs. The vast majority (87%) of uninsured Hispanics are in working families, yet only 43% of Hispanics receive health insurance through work. Further, nearly one-third of Hispanics (30%) work for an employer who does not offer health insurance to workers (The Henry J. Kaiser Family Foundation, 2000b). The high rate of uninsurance among Hispanics is also a reflection of a lower-than-average rate of participation in publicly funded health plans. In families with incomes less than the federal poverty level, 45 percent of all Hispanics are uninsured, compared with 32 percent of non-Hispanic whites (Fronstin, 2000). Differing eligibility standards may play a significant role in the lower rates of coverage for Hispanics under some publicly funded insurance plans, as many state and federal guidelines do not permit coverage for extended family members or families where married spouses live in the same household.

Hispanic subgroups vary in rates and sources of insurance coverage. Cuban Americans experience the highest rates of job-based or other private insurance (65%), and along with Puerto Ricans, are least likely to be uninsured (21%). Less than half of Puerto Rican, Central and South American-descendent, and Mexican Americans have job-based or other private insurance (45%, 46% and 44%, respectively), and over one-third of Puerto Rican Americans (34%) are insured by Medicaid or other publicly funded programs. More than 4 in 10 Central and South American descendent-Americans are uninsured (42%), as are 38% of Mexican Americans. These data are displayed in Figure 2-6.

Linguistic Barriers

Many racial and ethnic minority Americans experience language barriers. These barriers range from low or no English proficiency to limited proficiency in speaking, reading or comprehending English. In healthcare settings, these linguistic barriers can present significant challenges to both patients and providers, despite federal regulations that encourage and support the use of interpreters (Office of Civil Rights, U.S. Department of Health and Human Services, 2000). According to the 1990 U.S. Census, 14 million people living in the United States have no or limited English-language skills

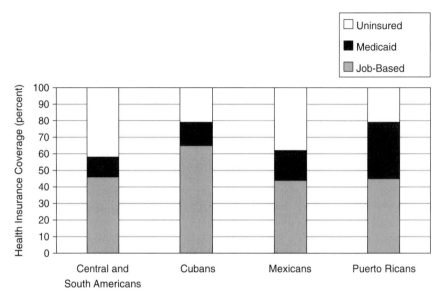

FIGURE 2-6 Health insurance coverage among Latino subgroups (Ages 0-64), 1997. SOURCE: The Henry J. Kaiser Family Foundation, 2000b.

(data from the 2000 Census are not available as of this writing). These populations can be found throughout the United States, although they are disproportionately represented in large urban centers and in five states (more than 10% of the population in California, New York, Texas, New Mexico, and Hawaii have limited English-language skills [Woloshin et al., 1995]). Nearly 8 million individuals (7,741,259) live in linguistically isolated households, e.g., households in which no person over age 14 speaks English "very well" (U.S. Bureau of the Census, 1993). The percentage of individuals living in linguistically isolated households for each racial and ethnic group is depicted in Figure 2-7.

Hispanic or Latino

More than 1 in 4 (25.3%) Hispanic individuals in the United States live in a linguistically isolated household. These include 4,560,000 individuals in over 1.5 million households. In addition, nearly 8 million Hispanic Americans (7,716,000) do not speak English "very well" (U.S. Bureau of the Census, 1993). Given recent population shifts (e.g., an increase in foreign-born Hispanic immigrants), it is likely that these figures grossly underestimate the number of Hispanic Americans with limited or low English proficiency.

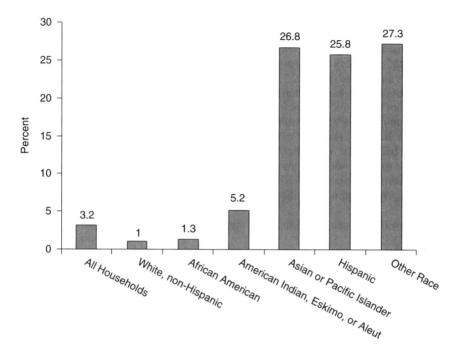

FIGURE 2-7 Percentage linguistically isolated households, by race and ethnicity, United States, 1990. SOURCE: U.S. Bureau of the Census, 1993.

American Indian and Alaska Native

More than one in 20 American Indians or Alaska Natives lives in a household in which no adolescent or adult speaks English "very well." According to the 1990 U.S. Census, 281,990 persons aged five years or older speak one of the American Indian languages at home; half of these (142,886) speak Navajo. Nearly 170,000 American Indians or Alaska Natives do not speak English "very well," and over 32,000 American Indian or Alaska Native households are linguistically isolated (U.S. Bureau of the Census, 1993).

Asian Americans and Pacific Islanders

Large segments of Asian-American and Pacific Islander communities face linguistic isolation. According to 1990 U.S. Census estimates, more than 1.5 million Asian or Pacific Islander Americans live in linguistically isolated households. Over half of Laotian, Cambodian, and Hmong families are linguistically isolated, while between 26%-42% of Thai, Chinese,

Korean, and Vietnamese families live in similar conditions. Figure 2-8 displays the percentage of Asian American households that are linguistically isolated.

Healthcare Providers

Many healthcare providers are acutely aware of the impact of language barriers and other cultural differences and how these factors affect their healthcare practice. In a recent survey of physicians who participate in the "Healthy Families" programs, L.A. Care (the local health authority of Los Angeles County) found that 71% of providers believe that language and culture are important in the delivery of care to patients. Slightly over half (51%) believe that their patients did not adhere to medical treatments as a result of cultural or linguistic barriers. Yet, over half of these providers (56%) report not having had any form of cultural competency training (Cho and Solis, 2001).

RACIAL ATTITUDES AND DISCRIMINATION IN THE UNITED STATES

"There are those that don't get promoted because of their race or whatever. The reason [may be because] they're not well liked by administration or it may be just that they [administrators] don't want that person in that setting because of their race—that is out there. Racism is alive and well, and those of us who think that it's not are living in some kind of dream world." (African-American nurse)

"I've had both positive and negative experiences. I know the negative one was based on race. It was [with] a previous primary care physician when I discovered I had diabetes. He said, 'I need to write this prescription for these pills, but

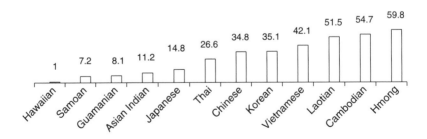

FIGURE 2-8 Percentage of Asian Americans that are linguistically isolated, by subgroup. SOURCE: U.S. Bureau of the Census, 1990 General Population Characteristics.

you'll never take them and you'll come back and tell me you're still eating pig's feet and everything...then why do I still need to write this prescription.' And I'm like 'I don't eat pig's feet.'" (African-American patient)

"My name is . . . [a common Hispanic surname] and when they see that name, I think there is some kind of prejudice [against] the name . . . we're talking about on the phone, there's a lack of respect. There's a lack of acknowledging the person and making one feel welcome. All of the courtesies that go with the profession that they are paid to do are kind of put aside. They think they can get away with a lot because 'Here's another dumb Mexican.'" (Hispanic patient)

"If you speak English well, then an American doctor, they will treat you better. If you speak Chinese and your English is not that good, they would also kind of look down on you. They would [be] kind of prejudiced." (Chinese patient)

The first chapter reviewed evidence of disparities in the process, structure, and outcomes of healthcare. This information alone presents an incomplete picture of the social, political, and economic contexts in which racial and ethnic disparities occur. In particular, to understand the question of whether discrimination occurs in healthcare, it is necessary to review what is known about racial attitudes and racial discrimination in other aspects of American life. This section reviews this evidence, with the goals of:

• illuminating trends in racial attitudes that may be assumed to carry over into healthcare settings; and

• understanding the persistence and pervasive quality of discrimination that has characterized the American racial and ethnic minority experience.

Indeed, towards this latter goal, it is useful to consider that the concept of "race" depends fundamentally on the existence of social hegemony. As Michael Omi (2001) notes, "[t]he idea of race and its persistence as a social category is only given meaning in a social order structured by forms of inequality—economic, political, and cultural—that are organized, to a significant degree, by race" (Omi, 2001, p. 254).

Racial Attitudes and Relations

"Often times, the system gets the concept of black people off the 6 o'clock news, and they treat us all the same way. Here's a guy coming in here with no insurance. He's low breed." (African-American patient)

Racial attitudes and relations in recent decades have been characterized by both progress and strife. Sociologist Lawrence Bobo (2001) notes
five trends regarding racial attitudes and race relations in this period that
offer, at times, a conflicting picture of race in America. The first, more
positive trend is that Americans' attitudes toward the goals of integration
and equality have improved steadily over the past three decades. Second,
this trend has not resulted in increasing public support for policies or
other significant efforts to improve educational, employment, housing,
and other opportunities for U.S. racial and ethnic minorities. Third, white
Americans continue to express support for negative stereotypes of minority groups in surprisingly large numbers, even though few of these individuals would identify themselves as bigoted or racist. Fourth, white and
non-white Americans differ significantly in their perception of the prevalence of racial discrimination in the United States. Finally, minorities'
attitudes regarding race relations suggest a deepening level of alienation
from U.S. society.

Regarding the first trend, Bobo notes that racial attitudes in America
have improved significantly over the past 50 years. In the 1940s, for example, opinion surveys indicated that over two-thirds of white Americans endorsed the view that African-American and white children should
attend separate schools, a view that was reflected in both formal policy
and practice. Over half of respondents felt that public transportation
should be segregated by race, and that whites should receive preference
over minorities in access to jobs. By 1995, 96% of white Americans expressed the view that black and white children should be allowed to attend the same schools. Similarly, by the 1970s, few whites endorsed the
view that public transportation should be segregated, or that whites
should receive preferential treatment in hiring. In 1965, slightly more
than 60% of whites stated that they would not move if a black family
moved next door; by 1995, well over 90% shared this belief. Bobo concludes that over time, "support for principles of racial equality and integration has been sweeping and robust. So much so, that it is reasonable to
describe it as a change in fundamental norms with regard to race" (Bobo,
2001, p. 273).

Despite these positive overall trends, Americans' attitudes cannot be
characterized as wholly egalitarian with regard to racial minorities, particularly when asked about policies and practices that might increase their
direct contact with minority groups. For example, while the vast majority
of Americans support school integration in principle, when asked whether
they would send their own children to integrated schools, support declines as the degree of contact with minorities increases. When asked if
they would object to sending their children to a school with a "few" black
children, over 90% of whites report no objection. If black children consti-

tuted half of the school enrollment, support dips to approximately three-quarters of respondents. If the school is presented as "mostly black," support falls to below 50%. While these trends have remained fairly stable since the mid-1970s, white support for sending their children to "mostly black" schools has fallen to below 40% at various points, particularly in the early and mid-1980s. Similarly, the percentage of white respondents who report that they would move should their neighborhood become integrated increases linearly with the proportion of blacks as residents (Bobo, 2001).

In addition, a substantial proportion of white Americans continue to endorse negative stereotypes about minorities. The 1990 General Social Survey (GSS) revealed that whites viewed blacks more negatively relative to whites on a number of dimensions, including intelligence (54% rated blacks as less intelligent in relation to whites), industriousness (62% rated blacks as lazier than whites), propensity towards violence (56% rated blacks as more prone to violence), and preference for living on public assistance (78% rated blacks as preferring to live off of welfare as compared with whites). Whites also rated Hispanics more negatively in relation to whites along the same dimensions, as 31% of whites gave Hispanics a low rating relative to whites in intelligence, 47% rated Hispanics as "lazier" than whites, 54% rated Hispanics as more prone to violence, and 59% believed that Hispanics are more likely than whites to prefer to live off of welfare (Bobo, 2001). It should be noted, however, that these percentages may be conservative due to tendencies among the general public to respond in a socially desirable, non-racist manner.

Negative stereotyping of minorities is not limited to African Americans and Hispanics. A recent survey commissioned by the Committee of 100 to study Americans' attitudes toward Asian Americans found that at least 1 in 4 Americans holds decidedly negative attitudes toward Chinese Americans, and an additional 43% hold "somewhat negative" attitudes. Many responses suggested that a significant segment of Americans fear Chinese Americans' influence and power; over one-third (34%) of respondents believe that Chinese Americans have "too much influence in the U.S. high technology sector," while 23% believe that Chinese Americans have "too much power in the business world." Nearly one in three (32%) respondents believe that Chinese Americans "always like to be at the head of things," and nearly 1 in 4 believes that Americans are losing jobs at the hands of Chinese Americans. Nearly 1 in 3 believe that Chinese Americans are more loyal to China than to the United States, and 46% of those surveyed believe that "Chinese Americans passing on information to the Chinese government is a big problem." Respondents who endorsed 5 or more of the 12 negative stereotypes posed about Chinese Americans—25% of the sample—were found to hold overwhelmingly negative attitudes toward Chinese Americans. These respondents, who tended to have lower levels of education, lower incomes, and were more likely from the South, believe in large majorities—ranging from 68% to 73%—that Chinese Americans "don't care what happens to anyone but their own kind," and are "taking away too many jobs from Americans" (Edsall, 2001).

Not surprisingly, white and non-white Americans hold widely diverging views of the prevalence of racial discrimination. A 1995 poll, for example, found that nearly nine in ten African Americans (88%) felt that police treat blacks unfairly, compared with 47% of whites (Schuman et al., 1997). In another poll, slightly over one in five whites (22%) but 57% of African Americans endorsed the view that blacks are discriminated against "a lot" (ABC News/Lifetime Television, 1999). Bobo (2001) cites a survey that finds African Americans to be three times as likely as whites to feel that there is "a lot" of discrimination against blacks in attaining "good-paying" jobs. Nearly 70% of African Americans endorsed this view, compared with slightly more than 20% of whites. Interestingly, 40% of Hispanics and slightly over 10% of Asian Americans supported this view. When asked whether Hispanics face "a lot" of discrimination in getting good-paying jobs, Hispanics (60%) were three times as likely as whites (20%) and one and a half times as likely as African Americans to endorse this view. Bobo (2001) summarizes these data, stating, "[minorities] not only perceive more discrimination, they also see it as more 'institutional' in character . . . [whereas] many whites tend to think of discrimination as either mainly a historical legacy of the past or as the idiosyncratic behavior of the isolated bigot" (Bobo, 2001, p. 281).

Strikingly, white Americans' perceptions of minorities appear to be based on inaccurate notions of racial progress. A national survey conducted by the Washington Post, The Henry J. Kaiser Family Foundation, and Harvard University revealed that "whether out of hostility, indifference or simple lack of knowledge, large numbers of white Americans incorrectly believe that blacks are as well off as whites in terms of their jobs, incomes, schooling, and healthcare" (Morin, 2001, p. 1). Over seven in ten (71%) white Americans surveyed expressed the view that African Americans enjoy the same or greater opportunities than whites; 65% of whites endorse this view with respect to Hispanics. In terms of income, 42% of whites surveyed believe that African Americans are better off or about the same as the "average white person," and nearly half (49%) believe that African Americans have similar or higher levels of education. Half of surveyed whites endorsed the view that African Americans hold similar or better jobs than whites. More than six in ten (61%) whites believe that African Americans have equal or better access to healthcare as whites, and nearly half (48%) of these respondents believe than Hispanics have equal or better access to healthcare (Morin, 2001). All of these responses are inaccurate with respect to major demographic data collected by the U.S. Bureau of the Census and other data sources, as outlined in this chapter. The following sections illustrate that despite the more optimistic view of some that unfair treatment on the basis of race is rare, racial discrimination persists in a wide range of important aspects of American life.

Racial Discrimination

"I felt that because of my race that I wasn't serviced as well as a Caucasian person was. The attitude that you would get. Information wasn't given to me as it would have [been given to] a Caucasian. The attitude made me feel like I was less important. I could come to the desk and they would be real nonchalant and someone of Caucasian color would come behind me and they'd be like 'Hi, how was your day?'" (African-American participant)

What Is Discrimination?

Discrimination, the differential and negative treatment of individuals on the basis of their race, ethnicity, gender, or other group membership, has been the source of significant policy debate over the past several decades. Federal and state laws adapted since the landmark 1964 Civil Rights Act outlaw most forms of discrimination in public accommodations, access to resources and services, and other areas. While this legislation appears to have spurred significant change in some segments of American society, such as in the overt behavior of lenders and real estate agents, debate continues regarding whether and how discrimination persists today. Conservative legal scholars and social scientists argue that discrimination has largely been eliminated from the American landscape (Thernstrom and Thernstrom, 1997; D'Souza, 1996), while others argue that discrimination has simply taken on subtler forms that make it difficult to define and identify. Complicating this assessment is the fact that while individual discrimination is often easier to identify, *institutional discrimination*—the uneven access by group membership to resources, status, and power that stems from facially neutral policies and practices of organizations and institutions—is harder to identify. Further, it is difficult to distinguish the extent to which many racial and ethnic disparities are the result of discrimination or other social and economic forces.

There is little doubt among researchers who study discrimination, however, that the United States' history of racial discrimination has left a lasting residue, even in a society that overtly abhors discrimination. "Deliberate discrimination by many institutions in American society in the past had left a legacy of [social and] economic inequality between whites and minorities that exists today . . . [but] legal evidence of discrimination in specific cases is not the same as statistical measures of the overall level at which discrimination exists" (Turner and Skidmore, 1999, p. 5-6).

Mortgage Lending

African-American and Hispanic applicants for conventional home mortgages are rejected at rates greater than twice that of white applicants (U.S. Department of Housing and Urban Development, 1999). But are these disparities due to minorities' generally lower credit ratings and lower income—important predictors of loan outcomes that are themselves by-products of past discrimination?

After controlling for measures of creditworthiness, such as loan type, property and credit, data compiled by the Federal Reserve Bank of Boston revealed large differences in loan denial rates between minority and white applicants. Hispanic and African-American applicants faced an 80% greater likelihood of loan denial. The Urban Institute reanalyzed these data and replicated the finding that creditworthiness or technical factors could not explain the disparity. These researchers concluded that "the Boston Fed Study results provide such strong evidence of differential denial rates (other things being equal) that they establish a presumption that discrimination exists, effectively shifting the 'burden of proof' to lenders" (Turner and Skidmore, 1999, p. 12).

A 1999 Urban Institute study of mortgage lending practices found that minorities face discrimination in several stages of the mortgage lending process. Paired testers sought loans using similar credit histories, incomes and financial histories, and presented the same mortgage needs. Overall, minorities received less information about loan products and were accorded less time with lending officers. Further, they were quoted higher lending rates than whites in most of the cities where tests were conducted. Potentially discriminatory practices began at early stages of the loan process, such as pre-application inquiries, and persisted through to the loan approval stage (Turner and Skidmore, 1999).

Housing Discrimination

Despite the presence of fair housing and anti-discrimination laws, American cities remain starkly segregated by race. Massey (2001), in an analysis of the largest 30 U.S. cities, finds that residential segregation is most profound and consistent over time among African Americans, and is less prominent, but still significant among Hispanic and Asian-American families. Using the indices of dissimilarity (the relative number of minorities who would have to change geographic locations so that an even racial distribution could be achieved) and isolation (the percentage of minorities residing in the geographic unit of the average minority individual), Massey found that, on average, African Americans live in communities that are overwhelmingly African American, with dissimilarity indices averaging 77.8 in northern cities and 66.5 in southern cities (indices above 60 are considered high). In six metropolitan areas (Chicago, Cleveland, Detroit, Gary, New York, and Newark), isolation indices for African Americans are 80 or more, indicating that in these cities, the average African American lives in a neighborhood that is more than 80% black. Further, other measures indicate that many African-American communities are characterized by "hypersegregation;" that is, African Americans tend to be concentrated in compact, densely packed, contiguous tracks in central cities. Black residents in these areas are unlikely to ever come into contact with non-blacks in their neighborhoods or in adjoining neighborhoods, and would have "little direct experience with the culture, norms, and behaviors of the rest of American society, and have few social contacts with members of other racial groups" (Massey, 2001, p. 410).

Patterns of segregation among Hispanic and Asian-American populations, in contrast, are less stark than that of African Americans. The dramatic increase of both Asian and Hispanic immigrants to the United States has led to large concentrations of these populations in some urban areas, but other segments of these populations have achieved remarkable levels of integration with whites. In several cities with large Hispanic populations, such as Brownsville and McAllen (Texas) and Miami (Florida), Hispanic segregation is high, with isolation indices averaging 77.2. This suggests that more than 3 of 4 Hispanics lacks regular neighborhood contact with individuals from other racial and ethnic backgrounds. In cities that are not majority Hispanic, concentration of Hispanics is less likely, with dissimilarity indices averaging 49.6 (suggesting that about half of communities in these cities are segregated by race and ethnicity) and isolation indices averaging 45.1 (both are in the moderate range). Asian-American segregation indices are quite moderate, with dissimilarity indices averaging 40.6 and isolation indices averaging 20.6 (Massey, 2001).

These patterns of segregation are not merely the product of socioeconomic differences, Massey notes. Segregation of African Americans, for example, occurs independently of social class. African-American families earning at least $50,000 annually are as likely to live in neighborhoods as segregated as those in which African-American families earning less than $2,500 per year reside. Further, the most affluent African Americans are even more segregated than lower-income Asian-American and Hispanic families; blacks earning more than $50,000 annually live in more segregated conditions than Asian-American or Hispanic families earning less than $2,500 annually (Massey, 2001).

Importantly, segregation does not appear to result merely from the choices of African-American and other minority groups to live apart from white Americans. Polling data indicate that African Americans strongly endorse the idea of residential integration, and would prefer to live in racially mixed neighborhoods. Virtually all African Americans endorse the statement that "black people should have a right to live wherever they can afford to," and over 70% would vote for a community law to enforce this right (Bobo, Schuman, and Steeh, 1986). Nearly 90% of African Americans state that they would be willing to live in any racially mixed area (Farley et al., 1994).

Similarly, most white Americans endorse the view that housing opportunities should be open to all and that housing discrimination should be abolished. In practice, however, white Americans' attitudes shift significantly with increasing residential segregation, as measured by polling data and patterns of movement after previously all-white neighborhoods become integrated. Farley et al. (1994) asked white residents in the Detroit metro area if they would feel uncomfortable in a neighborhood where 7% of the residents were black; 13% of respondents reported that they would be unwilling to enter such a neighborhood. When the percentage of black residents is presented as one-fifth of the total, one-third of whites reported that they would be unwilling to enter. If 30% of residents are African American, 59% of whites reported that they would be unwilling to move in, 44% reported that they would feel uncomfortable, and 29% reported that they would try to leave if they lived in such a neighborhood. If 50% of residents are African American, 73% of whites report that they would not want to live in the neighborhood, 65% reported that they would feel uncomfortable, and 53% would try to leave. In actual practice, the presence of smaller percentages of African Americans in previously all-white neighborhoods initiates a pattern of destabilization whereby whites tend to leave in large numbers. Summarizing studies of neighborhood racial transformation, Massey (2001) notes that the presence of one African-American family among every five white families tends to fuel a process of neighborhood turnover; in some cases, this turnover has accelerated when African Americans have numbered as few as three percent of a neighborhood (Massey, 2001).

Despite the existence of federal laws barring discrimination in housing, racial discrimination appears to be a key mechanism preventing neighborhood integration. Prior to passage of the 1968 Fair Housing Act, racial discrimination was institutionalized in the real estate industry and was widely practiced. Today, Massey (2001) states, minority home seekers, particularly African Americans, are more likely than not to face discrimination when attempting to purchase or rent a home. This discrimination occurs largely in the form of subtle, covert barriers. Housing audit studies, for example, provide a powerful means of assessing the likelihood of discriminatory practices. Auditors are trained to present comparable needs and desires in home purchases or rental properties, and are provided with similar socioeconomic traits. These studies, according to Massey, consistently indicate that housing discrimination has persisted in the years following passage of the Fair Housing Act. The U.S. Department of Housing and Urban Development's (HUD) Housing Discrimination Study, for example, was conducted in 20 audit sites around the United States and revealed that white auditors were, on average, provided with 45% more housing options in the rental market and 34% more options in the sales market than black auditors. In addition, whites were shown additional units 65% more often than blacks. Subtle "steering" of minority auditors away from predominantly white neighborhoods increased the likelihood of discrimination to 60%; in total, between 60% and 90% of the housing shown to white auditors were not shown to comparable black auditors (Yinger, 1995). For Hispanics, the likelihood of discriminatory treatment was equally high, as Hispanic auditors faced unfavorable treatment 43% of the time when seeking rental units, and 45% of the time when seeking to purchase a home (Fix, Galster, and Struyk, 1993).

White auditors also received greater assistance in obtaining credit; in 46% of encounters, whites received more favorable credit assistance in sales transactions and were offered more favorable terms in 17% of rental transactions. In addition, greater credit assistance was provided to whites; of all instances in which agents discussed a fixed-rate mortgage, 89% were with white auditors, as were 91% of instances in which adjustable-rate loans were discussed (Yinger, 1995).

These findings have been replicated in several other housing audit studies conducted in different locations in the United States. Galster (1990) found that racial steering occurred in approximately 50% of transactions, and that "selective commentary" from agents was common (including positive comments provided to white auditors regarding predominantly white neighborhoods that are not provided to African-American auditors). While housing audits have largely focused on the possibility of discrimination against African Americans, a few studies suggest that Hispanics face similar discrimination, particularly among darker-skinned Hispanics or those who identify themselves as mixed European and Indian ancestry (Massey, 2001). The consistency of these findings, coupled with data noting persistent racial segregation in the vast majority of American communities, prompts Massey to conclude, "rather than declining in significance, race remains the dominant organizing principle of U.S. urban housing markets" (2001, p. 420).

The consequences of such segregation for individual health status are significant (Williams, 2001; Massey, 2001). Many community resources that affect health, including access to employment and educational opportunities, are inequitably distributed; a close association exists between a group's spatial position in society and its socioeconomic opportunities. For example, some communities are characterized by better schools, safer streets, better public services, fewer environmentally based health hazards, and better access to quality healthcare. African Americans, regardless of income, tend to be segregated in neighborhoods characterized by fewer of these resources and higher levels of health risks. "Compared with whites of similar socioeconomic status," Massey (2001) notes, "blacks tend to live in systematically disadvantaged neighborhoods, even within suburbs" (2001, p. 392).

Employment

Audit studies using matched pairs of minority and non-minority auditors have also revealed consistent patterns of discrimination in hiring. As in housing audit studies, these studies carefully match testers on such attributes as educational level and personality characteristics, and carefully coach testers to ensure consistent responses to typical job interview questions. Fix, Galster, and Struyk (1993), for example, report findings from two studies of housing discrimination that assessed unfavorable treatment encountered by qualified job applicants responding to advertisements in major newspapers for entry-level positions. The first, conducted in San Diego and Chicago, assessed unfavorable treatment of Hispanics compared with white applicants. Because this study was part of a larger project assessing the potential adverse impact of new immigration legislation that banned the hiring of undocumented aliens, Hispanic testers were selected who "looked Hispanic and had definite accents" (Fix, Galster, and Struyk, 1993, p. 19). The second study, conducted in Chicago and Washington, D.C., assessed potential discriminatory treatment of African-American applicants relative to whites. Findings revealed that opportunity denial (defined as the denial of opportunity to obtain an application, obtain an interview, or receive an offer of employment) occurred 20% of the time in black-white audits and 31% of the time in Hispanic-Anglo audits, across all study sites. In other words, in nearly one-third of instances Hispanic applicants were denied an application, denied an interview, or did not receive an offer of employment while the matched white auditor received the opposite outcome.

Criminal Justice

Minority Youth in the Juvenile Justice System

Minority youth are overrepresented in the juvenile justice system in the United States. While minorities (African Americans, Hispanics, Asian

Americans, and American Indians) constituted only about one-third of juveniles in the United States in 1997, they represent two-thirds of detained and committed youth in juvenile facilities. These disparities are most pronounced among African-American youth; while they comprise 15% of the juvenile population, they account for more than one in every four juvenile arrests and 45% of delinquent cases involving detention. Further, nearly half (46%) of juvenile cases waived to criminal courts in 1996/7 involved African American youth (Office of Juvenile Justice and Delinquency Prevention, 1999).

Overrepresentation of minority youth in juvenile justice systems occurs in all 50 states and the District of Columbia. According to data collected by the U.S. Office of Juvenile Justice and Delinquency Prevention (OJJDP), minority youth face a higher probability than white youth of being arrested, referred to court intake, held in short-term detention, petitioned for formal processing, adjudicated delinquent, and confined in a secure juvenile facility. While these disparities may reflect a greater level of involvement in crimes (e.g., African-American youth are involved in 39% of violent crimes, as reported by victims), African-American youth disproportionately account for juvenile arrests for violent crime (44%) and confinement (45%), suggesting differential treatment by race (U.S. Office of Juvenile Justice and Delinquency Prevention, 1999).

A growing number of well-controlled studies demonstrate that minority youth are treated differently in the juvenile justice system than white youth, even considering the severity of crime and differences in rates of offenses. Minority youth, for example, are more likely than whites to be placed in public secure facilities, while white youth are more likely to be housed in private facilities or diverted from the juvenile justice system (U.S. Office of Juvenile Justice and Delinquency Prevention, 1999). These disparities are most pronounced at the beginning stages of processing within the juvenile justice system, but tend to accumulate as juveniles move through stages of the juvenile justice system. OJJDP researchers note that approximately two-thirds of studies of racial differences in processing demonstrate that race influences decision-making in the juvenile justice system, leading researchers to conclude that "there is substantial evidence that minority youth are treated differently from majority youth within the juvenile justice system" (U.S. Office of Juvenile Justice and Delinquency Prevention, 1999, p. 3).

What Is the Relationship Between Racial and Ethnic Disparities in Healthcare and Broader Racial Attitudes and Discrimination?

The study committee considered studies of racial and ethnic discrimination in sectors outside of healthcare as an important aspect of the evidence base to better understand the contexts in which care is delivered to racial and ethnic minority patients. These data are not meant to imply that inferences can be drawn from this literature regarding possible discrimination in healthcare settings. To the contrary, most social scientists agree that individuals with higher levels of education (such as healthcare professionals) generally hold more egalitarian attitudes than less educated individuals and abhor racial or ethnic prejudice and discrimination. In addition, as will be noted in later sections of this report, healthcare professionals are sworn to beneficence, and the vast majority are drawn to their disciplines out of feelings of compassion and a strong desire to heal. Data on the persistence of racial and ethnic discrimination in other sectors of American life are important, however, because they are likely to affect the clinical encounter and process of healthcare delivery in at least three ways:

- experiences of discrimination, whether real or perceived, are experiences that minority patients are likely to bring to the clinical encounter, and are thereby likely to shape their expectations, attitudes and behaviors toward providers and health systems;
- minority patients encountering health systems are likely to interact with many individuals in addition to healthcare providers, such as administrative and clerical staff, who may be expected to mirror social attitudes and trends regarding race and ethnicity; and
- healthcare providers, like all other individuals, are likely influenced in their racial and ethnic attitudes by broader social trends.

THE CONTEXT OF HEALTHCARE DELIVERY FOR RACIAL AND ETHNIC MINORITY PATIENTS—AN HISTORICAL OVERVIEW

"What would you recommend (to the IOM) to better understand what minorities experience in getting healthcare?" (Focus Group Moderator)

"Understand what the past healthcare history has been to Native Americans. Maybe just having an understanding of how Native American healthcare has been across the U.S., not just here in the Southwest, but everywhere. I think that would make [healthcare providers] effective because they would know what's happened in the past and not repeat the same mistakes." (American Indian healthcare consumer)

This section presents a discussion of the history of healthcare service delivery for racial and ethnic minority populations in the United States. The discussion is focused on the experience of African Americans only because historical documentation of healthcare for this group is more extensive than for other racial and ethnic minorities. It is not meant to exemplify other groups' healthcare experiences and histories (for a discussion of aspects of the history of U.S. healthcare for American Indians and Alaska Natives, see Joe, this volume). An historical account of the healthcare experience of African Americans is illustrative, however, of how the historic context shapes the contemporary structure of and access to care for racial and ethnic minorities. This section will discuss how the legacy of segregated and inferior healthcare for African Americans continues to reverberate in today's healthcare settings. Important factors such as the makeup of the healthcare workforce, primary settings in which racial and ethnic minorities receive care, opportunities for training of minority healthcare providers, and other aspects of the structure and delivery for healthcare for many African Americans are shaped by these historical trends.

A BRIEF HISTORY OF LEGALLY SEGREGATED HEALTHCARE FACILITIES AND CONTEMPORARY *DE FACTO* SEGREGATION

From the earliest periods in America's history, sharp divisions across racial and ethnic lines were customary in virtually all sectors of society, including healthcare. The origins of racially segregated healthcare systems can be traced back to slavery. While these systems were loosely organized, plantation health services were the earliest and one of the only systems comparable to today's managed-care plans (Smith, 1999). Plantation owners, as employers, had a significant financial interest in preserving the health of their employees (Byrd and Clayton, this volume). Slaves received care in hospitals-of-sorts on plantations. In some states, white physicians organized hospitals for slaves, or contracted with plantation owners to provide care to their slaves (Smith, 1999).

The early and mid 1800s also saw the emergence in America of scientific theories about race. Polygenism, and movements such as anthropometry, phrenology, and craniometry (theories that human races were distinct and hierarchical biological species) were at the forefront of scientific inquiry. Black soldiers during the Civil War were often used as subjects in studies comparing races to demonstrate black inferiority (Byrd and Clayton, this volume).

After emancipation, the plantation system of medical care ended and the Freedmen's Bureau was established by the federal government to provide assistance to former slaves. The medical department of the Bureau established nearly 100 hospitals for freed slaves, However, by 1868 only one (Howard University Medical Center) remained (Smith, 1999). After this point, African Americans received healthcare in segregated facilities in northern hospitals created by local governments. In the south, where most African Americans resided, local municipalities and states began to provide payments to hospitals to subsidize care for the underserved, which included segregated care for the poor (Smith, 1999). American Indians, who experienced displacement and high mortality, had little contact with health systems until the second half of the 19th century. This healthcare, administered by the government, was also poor, inadequately funded, and not sensitive to culture (Byrd and Clayton, this volume).

As the country approached the 20th century, two major social transformations converged to sharpen the racial divisions in healthcare services (Smith, 1999). First, with the development of surgical and other medical advances, both public and voluntary hospitals became important practice sites. Middle- and upper middle-class citizens began paying for services at these facilities, shifting power away from hospital boards to medical staff, who decided who received what kind of care. Second, the passage of Jim Crow laws solidified racial divides by legally separating facilities that provided care to black and white communities. In the scientific community, theories such as Darwinism, eugenics, and later, psychometric testing were developed to explain and predict the inferiority of certain groups, such as immigrants, African Americans, the poor, and the mentally retarded (Byrd and Clayton, this volume).

As hospital facilities became more important to the practice of medicine, organizations such as the American College of Surgeons sought to standardize hospital practices, which enabled medical staffs at hospitals to become more organized and exercise control over practices in their facilities (Smith, 1999). This essentially resulted in the exclusion of minority physicians from practicing in these institutions. Marginalized groups, including African Americans, American Indians, Hispanic Americans, and others from racial or religious minority groups were isolated, excluded from training, and professionally segregated (Byrd and Clayton, this volume). The response by minority physicians was to create their own facilities. American Indians and Alaska Natives, by treaty agreements, in large part received their healthcare through the Federal government. However, the diversity and dispersion within the Native American community made it difficult to provide consistent and reliable care (Byrd and Clayton, this volume). In a parallel movement, issues of payment for medical care became prominent as these services became increasingly important in peoples' lives. Questions about whether care should be based on need or ability to pay became influenced, in part, by race (Byrd and Clayton, this volume).

The passage of civil rights legislation in 1964 and Medicare and Medicaid legislation in 1965 stimulated profound changes in the structure of healthcare. With mandated integration, one of the most significant changes was the closing of black hospitals (Smith, 1999). Between 1961 and 1988, 70 black hospitals either closed or merged with white facilities. This transformation was taking place while white hospitals were experiencing growth and financial prosperity. While on the surface these closings may have seemed like a mere shifting of service sites, they had quite profound and devastating effects in minority communities. These closings meant a loss of geographic convenience and accessibility to care, a sense of safety with known institutions, and a loss of a major source of employment in the community (Smith, 1999). In addition to the loss of these facilities, a similar fate was befalling many public facilities that had provided access to many minority patients.

Another major, and more recent, shift in healthcare structure began in the late 1980s with the rise of managed care. This movement was initiated as both private and public payers were overwhelmed by rising costs and were searching for alternative ways to control their expenditures. By 1996, two-thirds of African Americans and Latinos with private insurance were enrolled in managed care plans. The transformation of Medicare programs to managed care formats led to further downsizing of large urban hospitals (Smith, 1999).

Historical Determinants of the Contemporary Minority Health Professions Workforce

During the post-Reconstruction period, several "Negro" medical schools and hospitals emerged. Eight medical schools for African Americans were established between 1865 and 1910 [Howard University Medical School, Washington, D.C. (1868); Meharry Medical College, Nashville, Tennessee (1876); Leonard (Shaw) Medical School, Raleigh, North Carolina (1882-1915); Louisville National Medical College, Louisville, Kentucky (1887-1911); Flint Medical College, New Orleans, Louisiana (1889-1911); Knoxville Medical College, Knoxville, Tennessee (1895-1910); the Medical Department of the University of West Tennessee (1900-1923); and Chattanooga National Medical College, Chattanooga, Tennessee (ca. 1902)] (Cobb, 1981). At least nine northern medical schools had admitted blacks by 1860. As a result, by 1895 there were approximately 385 black doctors, 7% of whom had been trained in white medical schools. Numbers of African Americans graduating from white institutions gradually increased, and in 1905, 14.5% of the country's 1,465 black physicians were from white medical schools (Duke University Medical Center, 1999).

Training black health professionals was essential to African-American communities during the prolonged post-Reconstruction period of crushing poverty, poor health status and inadequate or absent healthcare (Byrd and Clayton, this volume). Abraham Flexner's 1910 report on the status of minority health and minority health professionals reinforced this need. Flexner severely criticized medical education in the United States, noting that many U.S. medical schools had poor facilities, inadequate faculty with little scientific basis for instruction, and functioned principally as "diploma mills." These proprietary schools offered after-hours education and training, and contributed to the tension regarding the social and professional place for inexpensive medical education and primary care (Martensen, 1995). These tensions have not been completely resolved today. In this climate, the medical establishment was agitating for control and educational reform. More than 200 medical schools were founded in the United States between 1800 and 1900 (Stevens, Goodman, and Mick, 1978). At the end of the 20th century, the United States had the highest physician-to-population ratio in the world (Smith, 1999). Flexner believed strongly in the German scientific tradition he had experienced at the new Johns Hopkins University and suggested in the report that only university-based medical schools were appropriate for the responsibility and challenge of training physicians. Regarding the education of Negro physicians, he reports:

"The medical care of the Negro race will never be wholly left to Negro physicians. Nevertheless, if the Negro can be brought to feel a sharp responsibility for the physical integrity of his people the outlook for their mental and moral improvement will be distinctly brightened. The practice of the Negro doctor will be limited to his own race, which in turn will be cared for better by good Negro physicians than poor white ones. But the physical well-being of the Negro is not only of moment to the Negro himself. Ten million of them live in close contact with sixty million whites. Not only does the Negro himself suffer from hookworm and tuberculosis; he communicates them to his white neighbors, precisely as the ignorant and unfortunate white contaminates him. Self-protection not less than humanity offers weighty counsel in this matter; self-interest seconds philanthropy. The Negro must be educated not only for his sake, but for ours. He is, as far as human eye can see, a permanent fact in the nation. He has his rights and due and value as an individual; but he has, besides, the tremendous importance that belongs to a potential source of infection and contagion.

The pioneer work in educating the race to know and practice fundamental hygiene principles must be done largely by the Negro doctor and Negro nurse. It is important they both be sensibly and effectively trained at the level at which their services are now important. The Negro is perhaps more easily 'taken in' than the white; and as his means of extricating himself from a blunder are limited, it is all the more cruel to abuse his ignorance through any sort of pretense. A well-taught Negro sanitarian will be immensely useful; an essentially untrained Negro wearing an M.D. degree is dangerous." (Flexner, 1910, as quoted in Smith, 1999, p. 15).

.

The Flexner report had an enormous impact on medical education and the entire healthcare delivery system. The American Medical Association and major philanthropic organizations closed ranks behind the report. The AMA's Council on Medical Education pushed states to restrict eligibility for state licensure to physicians graduating from approved medical schools (Smith, 1999). Within a few years the number of medical schools was reduced from approximately 155 to 70 (Smith, 1999). The curriculum was lengthened, entrance requirements were raised, and the scientific content of the curricula was increased (Byrd and Clayton 2001). These reforms were costly and many institutions were unable to survive the changes demanded by reformers. These changes, however, forever altered the class background of those trained to become physicians. Many poorer, part-time, and night students found economic barriers to medical education insurmountable, and the proportion of students from working-class and poor families remained steady at approximately 15% for most of the 20th century (Ziem, 1977). Medical education therefore was largely limited to a predominantly upper-class, white, and male population (Ziem, 1977).

This increase in training costs had profound effects on the availability of doctors, particularly in the African-American community. In fact, the physician-to-population ratio among black Americans in 1974, twenty years after the *Brown v. Board of Education* Supreme Court decision that outlawed segregation in schools was worse than in the 1940s (Blackwell, 1977). Further hampering black progress, integration of the nation's medical schools was not seriously addressed until a decade after the 1954 *Brown v. Board of Education* decision. In 1948, for example, one-third of all medical schools were officially closed to blacks and many more failed to accept a single black student until two decades later (Raup and Williams, 1964).

By 1920, only two black medical schools remained, Howard University Medical School and Meharry Medical College (Smith, 1999). The closure of the other black medical schools dramatically reduced the community resource that produced many of their primary care physicians. These closures ensured that the segregation of healthcare in hospitals, in the health professions, and the professional societies would become entrenched in U.S. society. While the black population made up about 10% of the total population in the mid-1950s, for example, black physicians made up only about 2.2% of all physicians (Reitzes, 1958). The nation's overall physician-to-population ratio was 1 to 770. For the nonwhite population, however, the physician-to-population ratio was 1 to 4,567, and the black physician-to-population ratio was 1 to 3,736 (Reitzes, 1958). This disparity was not surprising, given that the burden of training black healthcare professions increasingly fell to only a few institutions. In 1956,

74% of all black medical students attended Howard or Meharry (Ziem, 1977). It was not until 1969 that all of the nation's medical schools enrolled more black students than did Howard or Meharry alone (Ziem, 1977).

During the late 19th and early 20th century, black physicians and community leaders had built their own hospitals in several cities around the country. Many of these hospitals served as major training centers for black health professionals. Medical specialists were in very short supply in the black communities, and access to white hospitals—even for those doctors who graduated from white medical schools—was limited. For African-American physicians, acquiring specialty training or hospital expertise was rare, because these doctors were denied opportunities to access specialty training (Byrd and Clayton, 2001). Failure to acquire the requisite credentials automatically excluded blacks from academic medicine and prestigious hospital staff appointments.

To compound these problems, organized medicine and local specialty societies failed to open doors for minorities to gain equal footing in the profession. The American Medical Association's (AMA) refusal to require its affiliates to desegregate until the mid-1960s made it virtually impossible for most black physicians to gain privileges at white hospitals because local society membership was a prerequisite (Byrd and Clayton, 2001). Smith (1999) described a fear among black medical leaders that the American College of Surgeons standardization efforts could eventually eliminate black hospitals and black medical professionals. In response, the black medical leadership formed its own organization, the National Medical Association (NMA), which was founded in 1895. Blacks were, in effect, excluded from AMA affiliates and the existing medical establishment, unable to fully open the doors to training opportunities until the Civil Rights Era.

THE SETTINGS IN WHICH RACIAL AND
ETHNIC MINORITIES RECEIVE HEALTHCARE

"So you're talking about [the] hospital. I think [large] hospitals, their equipment, [they have] more equipment, I'm talking about [a] large hospital, a hospital versus clinics. I like to go to a place where they have more, a lot of equipment, and complete their services so I don't have to go to different places. I can go to . . . a central place where they'll be able to take care of everything. And then language again, that's important. A Chinese interpreter [is necessary]." (Asian-American patient)

The legacy of racial segregation of healthcare is, in many respects, mirrored in stark racial and ethnic differences in the contexts in which care is received. Rates of health insurance vary greatly among racial and ethnic groups, as do primary sites where care is received, and who delivers this care. Most of these racial and ethnic differences are due to socioeconomic factors. For example, as will be discussed in Chapter 3, patients with Medicaid have difficulty accessing private sector office-based care (Lillie-Blanton et al., 2001) and are more often relegated to public hospitals and clinics. New studies indicate, however, that even when income and education are controlled, minorities are more likely to receive care in the lowest quality facilities with the least likelihood of appropriate follow-up.

Minorities have more difficulty than the majority population in locating a "usual source" of medical care (see Figure 2-9). African-American and Latino patients report greater difficulty than whites obtaining medical care at a consistent location. In 1996, for example, almost a third of Latino patients reported having a regular healthcare provider. Similarly, more minority patients report having little or no choice in where to go for medical care. Twenty-eight percent of African Americans and 30% of Hispanics report this difficulty, compared with 16% of whites and 21% of Asian-American adults (Lillie-Blanton et al., 2001).

In the 1980s, African Americans and Latinos were more likely than their white counterparts to receive care in hospital outpatient departments (particularly teaching and public hospitals), community-based clinics, and emergency rooms as usual sources of care (Lillie-Blanton et al., 2001; Smith, 1999; Gaskin, 1999). Persons with public or no insurance were also more likely to receive care in these settings (Cornelius et al., 1991, as cited

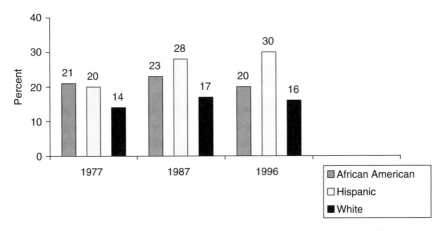

FIGURE 2-9 No usual source of medical care. SOURCE: 1996 Medical Expenditure Panel Survey, as cited in Lillie-Blanton et al., 2001.

in Lillie-Blanton et al., 2001). In a study to assess whether ethnicity is associated with site of care beyond insurance coverage, Lillie-Blanton, Martinez, and Salganicoff (2001) analyzed data from the 1996 Medical Expenditure Panel Survey (MEPS), and found that African Americans and Latinos, regardless of insurance coverage, were almost twice as likely as whites to receive care from a hospital-based provider (Figures 2-10 and 2-11). Those who were uninsured were also more likely to rely on hospitals for care.

Many people from racial and ethnic backgrounds are disproportionately served by safety net urban hospitals, defined as those facilities whose Medicaid utilization rate exceeds one standard deviation above the mean Medicaid utilization rate for urban hospitals in the state. Ethnic minorities comprise 43% of patients seen at these hospitals, but make up only 19% of patients seen at other urban hospitals (Collins et al., 1999). Approximately half of African-American (47%) and Hispanic (53%) adults under age 65 report relying on safety net emergency rooms, outpatient departments, or clinics for their healthcare, compared with 30% of whites.

Children's healthcare service use reveals similar patterns. White children see physicians at twice the rate of minority children (Collins et al., 1999). However, African-American and Latino children are over-represented in emergency rooms and hospital outpatient departments (Table 2-1; Lillie-Blanton et al., 2001). Even across type of insurance, African-

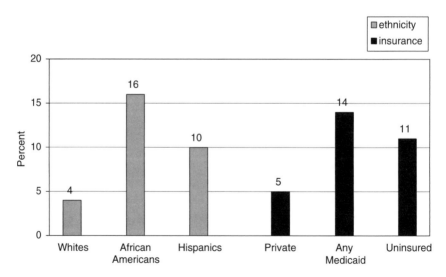

FIGURE 2-10 Site of care: Hospital outpatient departments and emergency rooms. SOURCE: Medical Expenditure Survey, 1997, as cited in Lillie-Blanton et al., 2001.

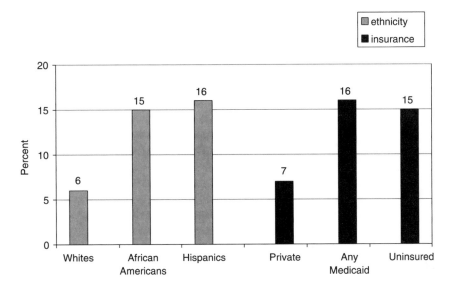

FIGURE 2-11 Site of care: Other non-hospital facilities. SOURCE: Medical Expenditure Survey, 1997, as cited in Lillie-Blanton et al., 2001.

TABLE 2-1 Site of Usual Source of Care by Insurance and Race/ Ethnicity, Children 0–17, 1996

	Office-based		Hospital Clinic or Outpatient Dept.		ER	
	%	(SE)	%	(SE)	%	(SE)
Private Health Insurance						
White	93.6	(0.8)	6.3	(0.8)	0.1	(0.1)
African American	89.5	(2.3)	10.1	(2.2)	0.4	(0.4)
Latino	85.9	(2.4)	13.7	(2.4)	0.4	(0.3)
Medicaid						
White	90.1	(2.3)	9.9	(2.3)	0.0	(0.0)
African American	74.6	(3.8)	22.8	(3.7)	2.7	(1.8)
Latino	80.3	(3.2)	18.8	(3.1)	0.9	(0.6)
Uninsured						
White	90.8	(2.3)	8.3	(2.1)	0.9	(0.6)
African American	73.7	(6.1)	24.1	(6.2)	2.2	(1.9)
Latino	81.6	(3.2)	17.2	(3.1)	1.2	(0.8)

SOURCE: Medical Expenditure Panel Survey, 1996, as cited in Lillie-Blanton et al., 2001.

American and Latino children are more likely to receive care in these settings than their white counterparts.

Racial and ethnic minority patients are also more likely to report experiencing difficulty in accessing specialists. Eight percent of whites, 16% of blacks, 22% of Hispanics, and 26% of Asian Americans report this difficulty (Collins et al., 1999). Within the Asian-American community, Chinese Americans indicated the most difficulty (21%). Among Medicare beneficiaries age 65 and older diagnosed with diabetes, black patients were less likely to have had an office visit with a cardiologist or eye specialist (Collins et al., 1999).

Impact of Community Health Centers on Healthcare in Minority and Medically Underserved Areas

During the 1960s, several new federal efforts were developed to increase healthcare services in poor communities. To this end, services such as the National Health Service Corps and the Community and Migrant Health Centers Program were initiated to help strengthen the workforce in medically underserved communities (Heinrich, 2000). By 1996, 625 community health centers (CHCs) provided services at over 3,900 sites (COGME, 1998). Today, these facilities serve underserved rural areas, migrant and seasonal farm worker communities, and urban communities. These federally funded CHCs include four programs: community health centers, migrant health centers, healthcare for the homeless, and healthcare for residents of public housing (COGME, 1998). CHC services are provided by primary care and other physician specialists, nurse practitioners, physician assistants, certified nurse midwives, dentists, and psychiatrists.

The vast majority (approximately two-thirds) of patients served by CHCs are non-white (COGME, 1998). In some communities, CHCs are the predominant source of care. In others, local governments have created and funded primary care clinics using the federal CHC model, helping to fill the void left by a lack of office-based providers. By the mid-1990s, rates of Hispanic visits to community health centers were 700% higher than for whites. For black, non-Hispanic individuals, visits to CHCs were 550% higher than white, non-Hispanic visits (Table 2-2).

The CHC model has proven effective not only in increasing access to care, but also in improving health outcomes for the often higher-risk populations they serve. The continuity of care has been found to be better in CHCs than in hospital outpatient departments or physician offices, and a study examining preventable hospitalizations among medically underserved communities found that in communities served by federally qualified health centers, rates of preventable hospitalizations

TABLE 2-2 Number of Primary Care Visits Made to Primary Care Delivery Sites in the United States in 1994

	Overall		Community Health Centers		Physician's Offices		Hospital Outpatient Departments	
	In Thousands	Per 100 Persons Per Year	In Thousands	Per 100 Persons Per Year	In Thousands	Per 100 Persons Per Year	In Thousands	Per 100 Persons Per Year
Race/Ethnicity								
Hispanic	28,087 (8.6)	109.1	3608 (31.7)	14.0	21,205 (7.3)	82.4	3275 (15.3)	12.7
Black, non-Hispanic	27,425 (804)	91.0	3356 (29.5)	11.1	19,930 (6.8)	66.1	4140 (19.4)	13.7
Asian/Pacific Islander	11,910 (3.7)	141.0	539 (4.7)	6.4	10,903 (3.7)	129.1	468 (202)	5.5
White, non-Hispanic	257,622 (79.2)	134.9	3891 (34.1)	2.0	240,265 (82.2)	125.8	13,466 (63.1)	7.0
Health Insurance Payer								
Medicare	49,117 (15.1)	N/A	1375 (10.6)	N/A	44,899 (15.4)	N/A	2843 (13.3)	N/A
Medicaid	38,120 (11.7)	N/A	5151 (39.7)	N/A	26,367 (9.1)	N/A	6602 (30.9)	N/A
Private	190,681 (58.7)	N/A	2754 (21.2)	N/A	180,226 (62.0)	N/A	7701 (36.1)	N/A
Uninsured	33,376 (10.3)	N/A	3339 (25.7)	N/A	27,458 (9.4)	N/A	2579 (12.1)	N/A
Other payment	13,758 (4.2)	N/A	350 (2.7)	N/A	11,758 (4.1)	N/A	1623 (7.6)	N/A

SOURCE: Forrest & Whelan, 2000.

Visit counts were multiplied by sampling weights, which account for the multistage sample design and nonresponse of in-scope practitioners, to obtain national estimates. Rates were based on the U.S. Bureau of the Census estimates of the U.S. civilian noninstitutionalized population as of July 1, 1994. N/A indicates that visit rates were not calculated by health insurance payer because denominators were not available.

were lower than in communities not serviced by these centers (Epstein, 2001). Patients in underserved areas served by these centers had 5.8 fewer preventable hospitalizations per 1,000 population over three years than those in underserved areas not served by a federally qualified health center.

While CHCs were developed on the premise that they would service all patients regardless of their ability to pay, limited federal subsidies have forced many clinics to reduce the amount of uncompensated care they provide. Between 1981 and 1991, federal funding increased at half the rate of increase in the urban consumer price index for medical care (Rosenbaum and Dievler, 1992, as cited in COGME, 1998). Changes in the cost of medical technology, shift of services from inpatient to outpatient settings, and Medicare's Prospective Payment System have placed a strain on many hospitals. While most have remained operational, approximately 5% of non-federal community hospitals closed between 1985 and 1988, a rate two to three times higher than in the preceding four years (GAO, 1990). Concerned about loss of their Medicaid patient base, many CHCs have begun participating in managed care arrangements. By 1996, almost half (45%) of CHCs participated in such arrangements (Shi et al., 2000). This shift has generated fears among some that these centers will be less able to serve patients who need care the most, with declines in Medicaid reimbursement and increased difficulty providing non-reimbursable services under managed care (GAO, 1995; Shi et al., 2000). In fact, recent studies suggest that CHCs provide care to a smaller proportion of uninsured patients, while they are serving increasing proportions of Medicaid patients under managed care (Shi et al., 2001).

THE HEALTHCARE PROFESSIONS WORKFORCE IN MINORITY AND MEDICALLY UNDERSERVED COMMUNITIES

Demographics of Healthcare Providers

The historical antecedents of physician and other healthcare provider training, as discussed above, significantly shape the current landscape of health professions education and the healthcare workforce. In this section, data on the demographic profile of healthcare providers that work primarily in racial and ethnic minority communities is reviewed.

Physicians

Minority medical graduates, including African Americans, Asian Americans, Hispanics, and American Indians, represent 9% of the country's physicians. Of these 9%, one-third (33.3%) is African American, 40.1% are

Asian American, one-fourth (24.9%) is Hispanic, and 1.8% is American Indian (AAMC, 2000). These minority graduates are more likely to work in states with large minority populations, such as California, New York, and Texas (AAMC, 2000). Underrepresented racial and ethnic minorities (African Americans, Mexican Americans/Chicanos, mainland Puerto Ricans, and American Indians/Native Americans) represent a smaller subset of this population, as less than 6% of the U.S. physician workforce is composed of individuals from these backgrounds. Significantly, well over 1 in 4 Americans is African American, Hispanic, or American Indian/Alaska Native (U.S. Bureau of the Census, 2000).

Minority physicians are more likely than their non-minority peers to work in hospital-based practices. Whereas only 1 in 5 (21.4%) of all physicians nationally work in hospital-based practices, nearly one-third (32.1%) of African American physicians, over half (50.3%) of Asian American physicians, over 1 in 3 (35%) of Hispanic physicians, and nearly 2 in 5 (39.3%) of American Indian/Alaska Native physicians work in such settings. Non-minority physicians are more likely to work in office-based practices, as 3 in 5 (60.5%) work in such settings, compared with 55.7% of African Americans, 40.8% of Asian Americans, 54.8% of Hispanics, and 53.1% of American Indian/Alaska Natives. Minority physicians are far more likely than non-minorities to be residents or fellows, owing to the generally younger age of minority physicians (AAMC, 2000). In terms of specialty practice, minorities are more likely to be found in family practice (11.5% of African American, 12.7% of Hispanic, and 24.7% of American Indian/Alaska Native physicians are family practitioners, compared with 9.9% of all physicians), obstetrics-gynecology (12.1% of African American, 8.3% of Hispanic, and 7.3% of American Indian/Alaska Native physicians are found in OB/GYN, compared with 6% of all physicians), and pediatrics (10.1% of African American and 11.1% of Hispanic physicians are pediatricians, compared with 8.7% of all physicians), but are poorly represented in other specialties, such as cardiology, surgery, and psychiatry (AAMC, 2000).

Among physicians participating in managed care arrangements, Asian-American physicians are more likely to be in solo practice (56%), while African-American physicians are more likely to practice in staff-model HMOs (19%), white physicians are more likely to be in group practice (45%), and Latino physicians were more likely to be in a hospital- or clinic-based practice (25%). Latino physicians are least likely to have managed care patients compared with physicians of other racial or ethnic groups, even after controlling for their lower rate of board certification. Twenty-six percent of Latino physicians had no managed care patients compared with 10% for African-American physicians, 13% for white physicians, and 14% for Asian physicians (Mackenzie et al., 1999).

Nurses

In 2000, 12.3 percent of registered nurses were racial and ethnic minorities. Nearly 5% of all nurses self-reported as African American, 3.5% as Asian, 2% as Hispanic, 0.5% as American Indian/Alaska Native, 0.2% as Native Hawaiian/Pacific Islander, and 1.2% reported being of two or more racial backgrounds. A larger percentage (86.4%) of minority nurses were employed in nursing, as compared with 81% of white, non-Hispanic nurses. Minority nurses were also more likely to work full-time (U.S. Health Resources and Services Administration, 2001).

Geographically, there are distinct patterns of practice between the minority and non-minority nursing workforce (Table 2-3). Recent estimates revealed that black nurses were more likely to practice in the south and middle Atlantic regions of the country. Hispanic nurses were represented in higher proportions in the west and east south-central areas. Asian/Pacific Islander nurses were more likely to be found practicing in the Pacific and mid-Atlantic states. The west south-central and Mountain areas of the United States were the sites with the highest percentages of American Indian and Alaskan Native nurses. The most common employment setting for minority as well as non-minority nurses was in hospitals (U.S. Health Resources and Services Administration, 2001).

Impact of International Medical Graduates (IMGs)
on the Workforce in Minority Communities

An important phenomenon began to emerge during the 1930s and 1940s that would have a profound effect on the healthcare provided to racial and ethnic minorities, as the numbers of international medical graduates (IMGs) securing residency training positions in U.S. hospitals, especially those serving underserved urban and rural communities, began to increase sharply. Between 1933 and 1940, the composition of the 5,056 immigrant physicians admitted to the United States was predominantly European (Stevens, Goodman, and Mick, 1978). By the 1960s, however, immigration policies had changed such that visas were easily attainable and institutions were beckoning Third World IMGs to the United States for training because of a perceived short supply of physicians (Stevens, Goodman, and Mick, 1978). This movement was occurring as courts ended federally sponsored hospital segregation and as Medicare and Medicaid legislation was passed by Congress. Concurrently, the Civil Rights era laid the groundwork for significant changes in access to healthcare facilities and services for racial and ethnic minorities as well as for the poor and elderly.

TABLE 2-3 Percent Distribution of Registered Nurse Population in Each Geographic Area by Racial/Ethnic Background: March 1996

Race/Ethnicity	U.S.	New England	Middle Atlantic	South Atlantic	East South Central	West South Central	East North Central	West North Central	Mountain	Pacific
Estimated RN population in area	2,558,874	176,951	443,846	460,460	141,705	215,200	452,080	198,952	137,739	331,941
White (non-Hispanic)	89.7	96.5	86.8	87.4	92.1	85.6	93.9	96.6	92.4	83.5
Black (non-Hispanic)	4.4	1.3	5.6	7.3	6.3	5.0	2.8	1.4	1.1	3.1
Asian/Pacific Islander	3.4	0.8	5.4	2.7	0.5	3.8	2.0	0.5	1.7	8.3
American Indian/Alaska Native	0.5	0.1	0.2	0.2	0.3	1.3	0.3	0.6	1.4	0.7
Hispanic	1.6	0.4	1.2	1.4	0.5	3.7	0.7	0.5	2.5	3.5
Other	0.7	0.8	1.0	1.0	0.2	0.5	0.4	0.4	0.8	1.0

SOURCE: National Sample Survey of Registered Nurses, March 2000.

The 1967 report of the National Advisory Commission on Health Manpower (NACHM) sparked renewed efforts to recruit IMGs when it declared a national shortage of physicians (COGME, 1998). The geographic maldistribution of physicians that had been systematically discussed for over 30 years as a problem became a public agenda item. By and large, health professionals had chosen to locate and practice in affluent urban and suburban communities, while large numbers of minorities and the poor had limited access to care. The NACHM report was one of several that led to the rapid expansion of existing undergraduate medical education programs as well as the creation of new medical schools.

Three decades later, the number of students graduating from United States medical schools doubled and the number of IMGs who entered residency training programs each year almost doubled between 1988 and 1994, from 3,600 to 6,700 (COGME, 1996). The number of first-year residency positions filled increased to 140% of the yearly U.S. medical school graduates. The physician-to-population ratio (excluding resident physicians) increased by 65%, from 115 to 190 physicians per 100,000 (COGME, 1996). Most of this increase was in the medical specialties, increasing the specialist physician-to-population ratio 121% from 56 to 123 specialists per 100,000 population (COGME, 1996).

Healthcare expenditures also rose dramatically during this period. Federal spending for all health services just before Medicare and Medicaid was enacted in 1965 was $4 billion, rising to $15.7 billion in 1970, $33.8 billion in 1975, and $65.7 billion in 1980. During the same period of time, state and local spending increased from the pre-Medicare/Medicaid level of $4.8 billion to $31.3 billion. The poor greatly increased their use of healthcare services. By 1976, poor children averaged 65% more physician office visits, poor adults averaged 27% to 33% more visits, and the elderly poor averaged 18% more visits than in 1964. In fact, the poor in each age group increased their use of health facilities more than the non-poor (U.S. Department of Health and Human Services, 1980), contributing to the increased demand for healthcare professionals.

Today, IMGs are a significant part of the U.S. health workforce. The number of residency positions filled by IMGs in 1998-99 was 25,415, or more than one-fourth (26%) of all residents on duty in U.S. hospitals in 1998-99 (COGME, 1999). Many work in minority and medically underserved communities, where few other physicians choose to practice. Verghese (1994) and White (1993) concluded that individual IMGs have established themselves as critical providers of healthcare services in selected rural underserved areas. Most, however, locate in large cities, and practice in urban underserved areas. They are disproportionately distributed in teaching hospitals with high percentages of Medicaid low-pay or no-pay patients. Sixteen percent of all teaching hospitals had an entire resident staff consisting of greater than 40% IMGs (MedPAC, 1999). A detailed survey of the healthcare providers working in nine of the poorest neighborhoods in New York City revealed that greater than 70% of the physicians were graduates of foreign medical schools (Bellochs and Carter, 1990). The data also revealed that only 24% of the practicing physicians were board certified, while the citywide average was 64%. Many other investigators (Fosset et al., 1990; Mitchell, 1991; Mitchell and Cromwell, 1980; Perloff et al., 1986a) have documented that physicians in urban areas who accept Medicaid patients are more likely to be foreign medical graduates and are less likely to be board certified than those who do not accept Medicaid. Ginzberg (1994) summarized his study of healthcare for the poor in four of the nations largest cities:

> A long-term trend of abandonment and avoidance by physicians had drained the low-income neighborhoods in all four metropolitan areas of private practitioners; physician-population ratios were as low as 1: 10,000 to 1: 15,000, in contrast to affluent neighborhoods with ratios of 1: 300 or even higher. Moreover, the majority of practitioners serving the poor consisted of foreign medical graduates, many with indifferent professional competence and language problems that impeded effective communication. Deterred by the low reimbursement rates paid by state Medicaid programs...the majority of U.S. trained physicians refused to accept Medicaid patients or limited the numbers they were willing to treat, leaving the field to group practices with questionable standards (Medicaid mills) that thrived on volume throughput (Ginzberg, 1994, p. 1465).

While from varied geographic locations around the globe, the largest share of IMGs working in the United States today are from South Asian nations. Table 2-4 illustrates the country of origin for the top 10 countries with the highest number of medical graduates in the United States.

TABLE 2-4 Top 10 Countries with Highest Proportion of Medical Graduates in the United States

Country	Percentage of the U.S. IMG Population
India	19.5%
Pakistan	11.9%
Philippines	8.8%
Ex-USSR	3.1%
Egypt	2.6%
Dominican Republic	2.5%
Syria	2.5%
United Kingdom	2.4%
Germany	2.3%
Australia	2.1%

SOURCE: The Educational Commission for Foreign Medical Graduates, 1992.

The cultural, racial, and ethnic diversity of IMG healthcare providers, who constitute more than 25% of the resident physicians in the United States, is broad. Most are new to this country and are learning to live within its vast sociocultural complexities, while also trying to learn to deal with an ambiguous welcome into the U.S healthcare delivery system with its own rigid, complex and demanding subculture (Stevens, Goodman, and Mick, 1978). As these authors note, two-thirds of IMGs are unprepared for the experience, having relied upon friends or family for advice. Many do not have the luxury of selecting a hospital in which to practice; rather, they accept the job that is offered. Often IMGs enter the United States thinking of themselves as "internationally mobile scientists" with knowledge and skills that are transferable anywhere in the world, only to be jolted by the reality of being treated as an alien or outsider inside the hospital (Stevens, Goodman, and Mick, 1978). In one survey (Stevens, Goodman, and Mick, 1978), 13% of IMGs felt that they were inadequately informed about the location of the American hospitals, including the fact that many large hospitals are in high-poverty areas of major cities. For others, complex malpractice claims and standards may pose problems, as well as large caseloads, documentation requirements, long hours, a fast pace, and language difficulties.

The 12th CoGME Report (1999) observed that "when physician and patient differ with respect to race, ethnicity, language, religion and values, ensuring fair, equitable, and culturally sensitive care is more challenging." The opportunity for miscommunication and cultural gaffes between IMGs and minority patients abound and could be manifest in the way healthcare services are provided or received by the communities served. This cultural configuration has existed for nearly 50 years in many of the largest metropolitan teaching hospitals serving millions of racial and ethnic minorities. However, this racial/ethnic interface has been inadequately studied to determine the impact it has on minority patients' perceptions of their healthcare experience, utilization of services, trust, compliance, health status, and quality of care.

THE PARTICIPATION OF RACIAL AND ETHNIC MINORITIES IN HEALTH PROFESSIONS EDUCATION

"I heard an Anglo doctor complaining that his daughter is having trouble getting into medical school. Then another doctor jumps in, another Anglo, "Oh don't worry about it. I know the admissions coordinator. I'll get her in. I'll give him a call and she'll be in." When does a Hispanic or black student have those advantages, the connections? I certainly didn't have any connections, and I still don't have any connections. I couldn't get my son into medical school if I tried." (Hispanic physician)

"When I was in medical school I had a racist comment by one of the white students. He said the only reason why you're here, it wasn't said to me but I overheard it, the only reason why black students are here is because they're black and this that and the other. What was really interesting was that OK, sure I'm black, but I don't take the black test, I don't take the black boards, we take the same exams." (African American physician)

In the late 1960s, many U.S. medical colleges and other health professions organizations began a concerted effort to expand opportunities for careers in the health professions to ethnic minorities who, for a variety of historic, social, political, and economic reasons, had not previously enjoyed such opportunities. The Association of American Medical Colleges (AAMC) and other groups actively encouraged member institutions to improve outreach programs and matriculation efforts targeted to minority students, in the hope that their rates of participation in health professions would achieve parity with the proportion of racial and ethnic minorities in the U.S. population (Nickens and Ready, 1999). This goal was established not only because its attainment would help to rectify inequities in educational opportunities, but also because of a growing appreciation that minority healthcare professionals are more likely to work in minority and medically underserved communities, thereby addressing a growing public health need.

By 1974, 10% of all medical school matriculants were underrepresented minorities (AAMC, 2000). This proportion decreased significantly in the wake of the U.S. Supreme Court's *Bakke* decision in 1976, but other efforts, such as AAMC's "Project 3000 by 2000," initiated in 1990, resulted in significant increases that exceeded 1974 levels. Between 1990 and 1994, the number of underrepresented minority (URM) students increased 36.3% to 2014 students, or 12.4% of the total number of medical school matriculants. Since that time, however, the number and proportion of new URM medical school enrollees has declined significantly. Enrollment of African-American students in medical schools, for example, declined 8.7% between 1994 and 1996 (Carlisle and Gardner, 1998). The greatest declines have occurred in public medical schools, which prior to 1996 enrolled a greater proportion of URM students than private institutions. Over 60% of public institutions experienced declines in URM student enrollment since 1994—a collective decrease of 9.1% in minority student matriculation at these institutions—while only 44% of private medical schools experienced such declines (Carlisle and Gardner, 1998).

While the reasons for these declines are complex, some evidence indicates that the declines have immediately followed significant policy shifts regarding affirmative action and higher education admissions procedures. Several legislative and judicial challenges to affirmative action policies in 1995, 1996, and 1997 (notably, the Fifth District Court of Appeals finding in *Hopwood v. Texas*, the California Regents decision to ban race or gender-based preferences in admissions, and passage of the California Civil Rights Initiative [Proposition 209] and Initiative 200 in Washington state) have forced many higher education institutions to abandon the use of race and gender as factors in admissions decisions. Subsequently, public medical schools in California, Louisiana, Mississippi, and Texas (the latter three states are subject to the *Hopwood* ruling) accounted for 44% of the decrease in URM matriculation in medical schools nationwide (Carlisle and Gardner, 1998a). In 1997, African-American student enrollment in Texas' public medical schools dropped 54% (Carlisle and Gardner, 1998b). And among California's public and private medical schools, URM enrollment declined 32% in 1998 from its peak in the mid-1990s (Grumbach et al., 2001). Because of the large minority populations in these states, much of the nationwide decline in URM enrollment reflects the trends noted above, while more modest minority enrollment declines in states unaffected by legislative or judicial rulings may reflect administrators' greater caution or perceived pressure to scale back affirmative admissions policies.

This decline in the numbers of underrepresented minority students in health professions education programs raises significant concerns regarding the ability of the healthcare workforce to address the nation's future health service needs. Racial and ethnic minorities are four times more likely to receive care from non-white physicians than white physicians (Moy and Bartman, 1995). Further, racial and ethnic minority physicians are more likely to practice in minority and medically underserved communities. A study of physicians' practices in California found that on average, over half (52%) of patients in the practices of African-American physicians were African American, compared with nine percent among non African-American physicians. Among Hispanic physicians, average caseloads approached 55% Hispanic patients, compared with 20% among non-Hispanic physicians (Komaromy, Grumbach, Drake, et al., 1996). Yet African-American and Hispanic physicians constitute less than 6% of the physician workforce.

The racial/ethnic diversity of health professionals also has broader implications for health service costs and improvements in the quality of care. For example:

• Healthcare professionals from racial and ethnic minority groups have generally been more successful in recruiting minority patients to participate in clinical research. Such efforts are critical to link scientific advancements with quality service delivery in underserved communities.

• The quality of healthcare depends as much on physicians' scientific competence as on an understanding of cultural, social, and economic factors that influence the health of patients, the ways in which they seek care, and their response to medical treatment. Racial and ethnic diversity of health professions faculty and students helps to ensure that all students will develop the cultural competencies necessary for treating patients in an increasingly diverse nation (Association of American Medical Colleges, 1998).

• Racial and ethnic minorities disproportionately receive medical care in hospital emergency settings. Such care is more costly than routine medical care and preventive health services. Healthcare professionals from minority and underserved communities may be better poised to tailor preventive health and primary care programs and services to minority populations, thereby reducing associated costs.

SUMMARY

Racial and ethnic disparities in healthcare emerge from an historic context in which healthcare has been differentially allocated on the basis of social class, race, and ethnicity. Unfortunately, despite public laws and sentiment to the contrary, vestiges of this history remain and negatively affect the current context of healthcare delivery. And despite the considerable economic, social, and political progress of racial and ethnic minorities, evidence of racism and discrimination remain in many sectors of American life. This persistent pattern of inequality suggests that interventions to eliminate disparities must be comprehensive and sustained, and that raising public and healthcare provider awareness of the problem is an important first step. Toward this end, a number of public and private organizations have developed educational campaigns targeted toward healthcare consumers, their providers, policymakers, and other "stakeholders." These efforts include, but are not limited to: the public education efforts of U.S. DHHS, which recently launched its "Closing the Health Gap" campaign to heighten awareness of health disparities; Diversity Rx, which provides a clearinghouse of information on language, culture, and improving healthcare services for minorities; and The Henry J. Kaiser Family Foundation, which has developed a number of publications targeted to the general public regarding healthcare disparities.

Finding 2-1: Racial and ethnic disparities in healthcare occur in the context of broader historic and contemporary social and economic inequality, and evidence of persistent racial and ethnic discrimination in many sectors of American life.

Recommendation 2-1: Increase awareness of racial and ethnic disparities in healthcare among the general public and key stakeholders.
Public education to increase awareness of racial and ethnic disparities in healthcare is an important first step toward eliminating these disparities. Media campaigns and other educational efforts to increase awareness of disparities should be targeted to broad audiences, including healthcare consumers, payors, providers, and health systems administrators.

Recommendation 2-2: Increase healthcare providers' awareness of disparities.
Organizations responsible for the education, training, and licensure of health and medical professionals should develop special initiatives to increase levels of awareness of healthcare disparities among current and future healthcare providers.

3

Assessing Potential Sources of Racial and Ethnic Disparities in Care: Patient- and System-Level Factors

The literature reviewed earlier in this report demonstrates that evidence of racial and ethnic disparities in healthcare is persuasive and remarkably consistent across a range of health conditions and procedures, and cannot be fully explained by differences in access to care, such as insurance status. Moreover, the literature suggests several sources for these disparities. This evidence, however, does not suffice for an authoritative, comprehensive, unambiguous account of how disparities arise. A number of uncertainties confound efforts to synthesize what is known empirically about stereotypes and prejudice, doctor-patient relations, clinical judgment and patient preferences, as well as the social, institutional, financial, and legal forces that shape the practice of medicine. Yet an effort at such a synthesis is essential to construct an evidence-based account of how disparities in care emerge, and of what might be done to eliminate these disparities.

To begin, this chapter presents a model of how disparities might occur. This model builds upon the wide foundation of empirical evidence but makes reasoned inferences when they are necessary to explain observed disparities. The committee makes such inferences when, in our judgment, they are more probable than not and when practical consequences, in the form of recommended actions to ameliorate known disparities, follow from these inferences. In doing so, the committee acknowledges that gaps in our understanding about causation remain and that further research has the potential to enhance understanding.

The chapter then presents a review of empirical literature that raises hypotheses regarding potential sources of racial and ethnic disparities in healthcare. This literature is suggestive of a range of sources of dispari- ties, some of which lie just beyond the conscious perception of individual actors (e.g., patients, providers, health systems administrators) in clinical encounters. They include systemic (e.g., those related to health system administration, financing, accessibility and geographic location), patient- level (e.g., the clinical appropriateness of care, patients' attitudes, prefer- ences, and expectations regarding healthcare), and care process-level (e.g., physician biases, stereotyping, and uncertainty) factors. This chapter, however, will focus on the two former sets of variables. As depicted in Figure 1-1, these include "patient-level" variables, and variables related to the operation of healthcare systems and the legal and regulatory con- texts in which health systems function. Chapter 4 will focus the analysis on care process variables, including the roles of clinician bias, prejudice, stereotyping, clinical uncertainty, and patient mistrust. According to the study committee's conceptualization, racial and ethnic *differences* in care may arise from all three sets of variables. *Disparities* in care, however, emerge from the characteristics of and the operation of healthcare sys- tems, as well as the legal and regulatory climate in which care is deliv- ered, and from the process of care (i.e., factors emerging from the pro- vider-patient interaction).

The following section presents a guiding framework that depicts the likely interplay of health systems characteristics, patient-level factors, and care process variables in fostering racial and ethnic disparities in healthcare.

A MODEL: SOURCES OF HEALTHCARE DISPARITIES

The Role of Clinical Discretion

An integrated model of how racial and ethnic disparities in care emerge is presented in Figure 3-1. According to this model, patients present to healthcare providers with varied healthcare needs, expecta- tions, and preferences, some of which are socio-culturally determined. Providers, in turn, possess expectations and beliefs that are shaped both by their professional training and experience, as well as by their social experiences and broader societal norms and structures. These encounters take place within healthcare systems and settings that are broadly influ- enced by institutional design factors (such as the ease of care access), and financial forces (such as incentives to providers and patients to limit ser- vice use and healthcare costs). These systems operate within legal and cultural contexts that influence how healthcare is delivered and the be- havior of both patients and providers.

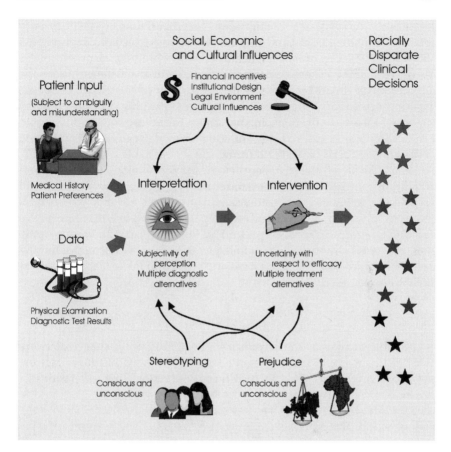

FIGURE 3-1 An integrated model of healthcare disparities.

Central to this model is the role of personal discretion in determining the care that patients receive. Three sets of actors possess and exercise discretion: clinical caretakers, utilization managers remote from the bedside, and patients themselves. Patients' medical histories, physical exam findings, and diagnostic test results often present a level of uncertainty to physicians, and patients vary enormously in their help-seeking behavior, ways of presenting their symptoms and histories, and responses to medical recommendations (Bursztajn, 1990). Clinicians typically have multiple diagnostic and therapeutic options, and choices from among them sometimes do not rest firmly on empirical evidence. In addition, physician perception of clinical signs and symptoms is sometimes incomplete (Eddy, 1996), while decisions concerning diagnostic and therapeutic intervention are no less ambiguous. Significant variations in the incidence of many common medical and surgical procedures have been documented within small geographic areas and between individual practitioners (Wennberg, 1999). These variations reflect, in many instances, both the subjectivity of clinical judgment and the lack of professional consensus about best practice. Further, the lack of firm scientific support for some medical decisions both engenders variations in clinical practice and makes it difficult in many cases to reach evidence-based conclusions concerning the appropriateness of particular practices.

In and of itself, the discretion exercised by patients, providers, and utilization managers does not produce racial and ethnic disparities in healthcare. In most cases, patients and providers are able to work together in an iterative process to match patients' needs with appropriate treatment, regardless of race or ethnicity. Discretion and ambiguity, however, create conditions in which race or ethnicity may become salient in the process of diagnosis and treatment in ways that make disparities more likely to occur, as explained below.

The Patient as Discretionary Actor: Subjectivity and Variability

A substantial research literature in psychiatry and psychology, sociology, and anthropology documents large differences in how people experience, understand, and discuss illness (Goff et al., 1998). Patients' experience and reporting of pain and other symptoms have been found to vary greatly (Bonham, 2001), as has patients' help-seeking behavior relative to health professionals (Milewa et al., 2000). The relationships between such variation and differences in how clinical caretakers go about the diagnosis and treatment of disease have been less well studied. But the subjectivity and incompleteness of clinical perception leave room for differences in patients' experience, understanding, and reporting of symptoms to affect professional judgment and action. These differences, moreover, interact with differences in patients' values and attitudes toward clinical caretakers to shape patients' healthcare choices. To the extent that such variation correlates with patients' race and ethnicity, it is therefore a potential contributor to differences in healthcare use.

Clinical Caretakers as Discretionary Actors: Subjectivity and Uncertainty

Medical care at the dawn of the 21st century has achieved heights thought improbable even a few decades ago. Advances in diagnostic techniques, scientific understanding of the human genome and underlying disease processes, and new, high-tech interventions have led to breakthroughs in treating and preventing disease. Despite these gains, however, many medical decisions must be made in the absence of solid evidence as to the efficacy of diagnostic and therapeutic measures or rigorous scientific understanding of the pathophysiology of disease (Mushlin, 1991). Efforts to better understand pathophysiology are further complicated by variations in clinical expression in individuals with different genetic, environmental, and cultural backgrounds. In addition, even the most technologically sophisticated diagnostic interventions (e.g., magnetic resonance imaging and X-ray and positron tomography) reveal little about the biochemistry and physiology of the diseases they detect. To add to this uncertainty, medicine's diagnostic constructs are themselves limited in their predictive (and thus therapeutic) value by the incompleteness of the pathophysiologic understandings that undergird them (Bloche, 2001).

Moreover, healthcare providers' ability to assess patients' clinical signs and symptoms and gather a relevant medical history is constrained by a number of factors. As noted above, patients' ability to understand and describe their presenting concerns varies not only by cultural, linguistic, and other sociodemographic background factors, but may also vary from day to day. The variability and subjectivity of patients' clinical presentations is compounded by physicians' differences in perception, cultural and psychological sensitivity, and conceptual frameworks for evaluating illness. Similarly, many laboratory tests are open to varying interpretations. Radiologists sometimes give conflicting readings of the same X-ray, tomogram, or other scan, and pathologists sometimes report conflicting interpretations of slides sent for assessment of possible malignancy. Many clinical and laboratory data are likewise open to differing clinical interpretations by physicians with varying conceptual frameworks, perceptions, and biases. As will be discussed in the next chapter, it is reasonable to speculate that the resulting diagnostic subjectivity could permit clinical uncertainty, racial and ethnic biases, and stereotypes to influence the process and outcomes of clinical evaluation, resulting in racial and ethnic disparities in medical diagnosis.

Physicians' decisions regarding appropriate therapeutic interventions introduce still another level of uncertainty, subjectivity, and variability. Despite clinical medicine's gains noted above, accurate, evidence-based prediction of the efficacy of many therapeutic alternatives for most patients is lacking (Bloche, 1999), and geographic variations in clinical practice patterns are common (Wennberg, 1999). In the absence of guidance from prospective and retrospective clinical studies, physicians base their therapeutic judgments on such factors as their training, prior clinical success and failure, and practice norms among professional peers (Bauchner, Simpson, and Chessare, 2001). Inevitably, physicians' subjective under-

standings of their patients' needs play a role; thus psychological sensitivity, cultural and language competency, and conscious and unconscious
stereotypes and biases may also influence therapeutic decision-making.
Further, uncertainty about treatment options in itself, even absent biases
or stereotypes, can lead to disparate treatment of racial and ethnic minority groups, as will be discussed in Chapter 4. In addition, organizational,
financial, and legal influences shape therapeutic judgment. Such institutional and policy forces are often geared toward promoting cost-effective
and efficient care, but may disproportionately and negatively affect minority patients (Bloche, 2001).

Utilization Managers as Discretionary Actors: Uncertainty at a Distance

Variation and subjectivity in healthcare practice may also emerge at
the level of health systems, particularly in managed care arrangements
where utilization managers are charged with authorizing physicians' and
patients' requests for reimbursement for services. Except where contrac-
tually bound by clinical practice protocols, utilization managers evaluate
the necessity of claims from among a range of diagnostic and therapeutic
alternatives acceptable within one or another subset of the medical community. This evaluation often occurs on a case-by-case basis, without the
guidance of recorded precedent or other administrative means for pursuing consistency between utilization management decisions in similar
cases. In some cases, doctors and patients who seek pre-approval for
planned treatments or who pursue internal appeals when pre-approval is
denied know little or nothing about their health plans' past pre-approval
practices in similar cases. Health plans that employ clinical practice protocols as cost management tools sometimes treat these protocols as trade
secrets, not to be disclosed to patients or medical practitioners. The consequence of these administrative arrangements is that there is ample room
(and little visibility) for discretion and inconsistency in the treatment of
clinically similar cases (Bloche, 2001).

The following sections review available empirical evidence and present an analysis of how discretion, subjectivity, and preferences of patients, providers and utilization managers may contribute to healthcare
disparities. Consistent with the committee's model of sources of racial
and ethnic differences in care, these sources are divided into patient-level
variables (such as preferences, needs, and the clinical appropriateness of
care), and factors related to health systems and the legal and regulatory
context of healthcare. Factors arising from the clinical encounter that may
contribute to disparities are addressed in Chapter 4.

PATIENT-LEVEL VARIABLES—PREFERENCES, MISTRUST, TREATMENT REFUSAL, BIOLOGICAL DIFFERENCES, AND OVERUSE OF SERVICES

Patients' Preferences

To a great extent, patients' values, fears and hopes, and other psychological characteristics influence the level and type of care they receive. Patients' trust and doubts about medical advice, as well as their level of comfort with the effectiveness and potential unintended effects of interventions, directly influence their willingness to accept physicians' recommendations. In addition, patients' preferences are influenced by their tolerance for pain and discomfort, attitudes about long-term/short-term tradeoffs, and levels of social and emotional support. These factors also influence physicians' recommendations, in that the physician may directly assess or infer patients' attitudes toward particular interventions and may tailor recommendations accordingly. To the extent that minority patients express greater reluctance to accept physician recommendations, patients' preferences have the potential to contribute to healthcare disparities. Evidence that minority patients are more likely than whites to decline invasive and/or high-tech procedures is reviewed below.

For many racial and ethnic minorities, however, preferences for treatment are often difficult to separate from mistrust of health professions that stems from racial discrimination and the history of segregated and inferior care for minorities (Byrd and Clayton, this volume). Some researchers have not distinguished between these aspects of minority patients' historic experiences and preferences for treatment, and have contrasted "preferences" and racial discrimination as competing explanations for healthcare disparities. This account overlooks the interaction between patients' "preferences" and their experiences of discrimination. As Bloche (2001) notes, "For many African Americans, doubts about the trustworthiness of physicians and healthcare institutions spring from collective memory of the Tuskeegee experiments (Brandt, 2000) and other abuses of black patients by largely white health professionals (Randall, 1996; King, 1998). This legacy of distrust, which, some argue, contributes to disparities in healthcare provision by discouraging African Americans from seeking or consenting to state-of-the-art medical services, is thus itself a byproduct of past racism" (Bloche, 2001, p. 105).

Minority patients' negative experiences with care providers in the clinical encounter can also diminish their preferences for robust treatment, and may thereby contribute to racial disparities. It is reasonable to assume that experiences of real or perceived discrimination in healthcare settings, as evidenced by providers' overt behavior (e.g., as in the examples from focus group data presented in Chapter 2) or more subtle, subjective mistreatment (e.g., healthcare providers' low expectations for compliance or expressions of low empathy for minority patients) can affect patients' feelings about their clinical relationships and thereby dampen their interest in vigorous diagnostic and therapeutic measures. It is therefore necessary to distinguish patient "preferences" from experiences or perceptions of discrimination and not neglect the ways in which patients' preferences can be shaped by provider behavior. In addition, patients' preferences for treatment may be limited by the quality and completeness of information presented by the healthcare provider. Thus, should providers fail to present minority patients with a full range of treatment options, whether out of prejudice, stereotyping, biases, or uncertainty about the diagnosis or appropriate clinical course of action, patients' preferences will be limited by the information they are presented. These dynamics will be addressed in greater detail in Chapter 4.

Minority Patient Preferences Regarding Providers and Racial Concordance

Minority patients' experiences, values, and expectations regarding healthcare may significantly influence their preferences for the race or ethnicity of their providers. A growing body of evidence suggests that racial and ethnic minority patients are generally more satisfied with the care that they receive from minority physicians. Saha, Komaromy, Koepsell, and Bindman (1999), for example, found that African-American patients with African-American healthcare providers were more likely than those with non-minority providers to rate their physicians as excellent in providing healthcare, in treating them with respect, in explaining their medical problems, in listening to their concerns, and in being accessible. Hispanic patients who received care from Hispanic physicians did not rate their physicians as significantly better than Hispanic patients with non-Hispanic healthcare providers, but were more likely to be satisfied with their overall healthcare.

Similarly, Cooper-Patrick and her colleagues (Cooper-Patrick et al., 1999) assessed patients' ratings of the quality of interpersonal care in racially concordant and racially discordant settings. Using a measure of physicians' participatory decision-making (PDM) style, the authors surveyed over 1800 adults (including 43% white, 45% African American, and 12% other race or ethnicity) who were seen in 1 of 32 primary care settings by physicians who were either African American (25% of the physician sample), white (56%), Asian American (15%), or Latino (3%). Overall, African-American patients were found to rate their visits as significantly less participatory than whites, after adjusting for patient age, gender, education, marital status, health status, and length of the patient-physician relationship. Further, patients in race-concordant relationships rated their visits as significantly more participatory than patients in race-discordant relationships.

LaVeist and Nuru-Jeter (in press) examined predictors of racial concordance between patient and provider and the effect of race concordance on satisfaction among a sample of white, African-American, and Hispanic patients. Among all racial and ethnic groups, patients who reported having at least some choice in selecting a physician were more likely to have a race-concordant physician. Having a race-concordant physician was also associated with higher income for African Americans and not speaking English as a primary language among Hispanics. After adjusting for patients' age, sex, marital status, income, health insurance status, and whether the respondent reported having a choice in physician, African-American patients in race-concordant relationships were found to report higher satisfaction than African Americans in race-discordant relationships. Further, Hispanic patients in race-concordant relationships reported greater satisfaction than patients from other racial and ethnic groups in similarly concordant relationships.

While these studies lend important information regarding patients' perceptions of the interpersonal quality of care, few studies have corroborated this data with more objective assessments of the patient-provider interaction in racially concordant and discordant settings. Cooper and Roter (this volume) describe a study that assessed this relationship using post-visit surveys and audiotape analysis among a sample of 143 white and 110 African-American patients seen by 1 of 13 white or 18 African-American primary care doctors. Cooper and colleagues found that the average length of visits was shortest among white physicians with African-American patients (13.2 minutes), and was longest among African-American physicians seeing white patients (18.4 minutes). Visits by African-American patients were characterized by greater physician verbal dominance overall, but physician verbal dominance was highest in visits between white physicians and African-American patients, and lowest among white patients seen by African-American physicians. In addition, visits between white physicians and African-American patients were the least patient-centered, while the African-American physician–white patient interaction was characterized by the highest levels of patient centeredness. However, patients in race-concordant relationships rated their physicians' decision-making styles as more participatory. The finding that African-American physicians were more patient centered and spent more time with white patients, according to Cooper and Roter, suggests two possibilities. One is that African-American physicians, by virtue of their educational success and professional standing, presumably have had greater opportunities to develop skills in communicating with individuals from the dominant culture than white physicians have had to develop communication skills with individuals from minority cultures. This suggests that African-American physicians are likely to be bicultural (i.e., able to function effectively in the dominant culture as well as in minority cultures) or are acculturated (i.e., have assumed traits of the dominant culture). Secondly, African-American physicians may "overcompensate" for perceived deficiencies of their own group by adopting behaviors that indicate less respect for themselves or members of their own group (Cooper and Roter, this volume).

A significant limitation of these studies is the lack of random assignment of patients with physicians, introducing selection factors as a potential confound. In fact, Saha et al. (1999) found that African-American and Hispanic patients who had the ability to choose their provider were more likely to choose a racially or ethnically concordant physician. A significant proportion (42%) of Hispanic patients in this study reported selecting Hispanic physicians because of linguistic barriers with other providers. Nonetheless, these studies demonstrate that racial concordance is associated with greater participatory decision-making, greater patient-centered care, lower levels of physician verbal dominance, and greater patient satisfaction. In turn, evidence from other studies indicates that patient satisfaction is associated with greater patient compliance with treatment regimens, participation in treatment decisions, and use of preventive care services (Cooper and Roter, this volume). For racial and ethnic minorities, according to Cooper-Patrick and colleagues (1999), racial concordance may increase the likelihood that they will "share cultural beliefs, values, and experiences in the society [with their provider], allowing them to communicate more effectively and to feel more comfortable with one another" (p. 588).

Little evidence exists, however, to directly demonstrate that the quality of care provided is better when minority patients and their providers are of the same racial or ethnic group. Evidence of the efficacy of race-concordant patient and provider relationships is only indirect, as patient satisfaction, participation, and patient-centeredness of care are also associated with greater adherence to clinical regimens, greater participation in health screening and preventive medicine, and in some cases, health outcomes (Cooper-Patrick et al., 1999). Chen et al. (2001) suggest the opposite—that racial disparities persist in care even when minority patients are treated by minority physicians. The authors performed a retrospective analysis of data obtained from a sample of Medicare patients hospitalized with acute myocardial infarction (MI) to determine whether racial differences in rates of cardiac catheterization were related to the race of attending physician. Consistent with other studies, the authors found that African-American patients were less likely than white patients to receive catheterization within 60 days after MI. No significant differences were found, however, between African-American and white attending physicians in rates of catheterization among these patients. Among patients treated by African-American physicians, 38 percent of black patients and 50 percent of white patients received catheterization. Among patients treated by white physicians, 38 percent of black patients and 46 percent of whites received the procedure. Chen et al. conclude that "racial discordance between the patient and the physician does not explain differences between black patients and white patients in the use of cardiac catheterization" (2001, p. 1447).

While some newspaper accounts of this study suggested that racial bias is not a likely source of disparities in care (Associated Press, May 9, 2001), this interpretation appears premature. Several methodological problems complicate interpretation of the results obtained by Chen et al. Data on the race of the attending physician were missing for nearly one-third of the initial patient sample. In addition, African-American patients were more likely to be cared for in public or teaching hospitals, where greater barriers exist to receipt of catheterization, such as the availability of the procedure on-site. The most serious methodological problem, however, was the determination of the race of the attending physician ("the clinician who is largely responsible for the care of the patient from the beginning of the hospital episode"). Upon closer examination, it becomes apparent that the African-American physicians of these patients tended to be internists, not cardiologists, when compared with the white attending physicians. While these physicians may all refer patients for the procedure, the determination of who receives the procedure is typically made by the cardiologist. Thus, the authors compare two different physician pools who cared for these African-American patients post-myocardial infarction—African-American internists versus white cardiologists—to assess differences in utilization of a procedure that is specifically performed by and managed by cardiologists. Notably, of the nearly 20,000 cardiologists in the United States during the study period in 1994 and 1995, only 316 (approximately 1.5%) were African American.

Minority Patient Mistrust and Experiences of Discrimination

Some racial and ethnic minorities express greater levels of mistrust of healthcare providers and the medical establishment than white Americans, citing breeches of trust that have previously occurred between minorities and the scientific and medical communities (Swanson and Ward, 1995). In addition, survey research generally indicates that ethnic minority patients perceive higher levels of racial discrimination in healthcare settings than non-minorities. For example, in a survey of 781 African-

American and 1,003 white cardiac patients, LaVeist, Nickerson, and Bowie (2000) found that while the majority of these patients did not tend to endorse the existence of widespread racism in medical settings, African-American patients were four times more likely than whites to believe that racial discrimination is common in doctors' offices, and were significantly more likely to mistrust healthcare systems. Similarly, Lillie-Blanton et al. (2000) found that of a nationwide, random sample of whites and minorities, 30% of Hispanics and 35% of African Americans believe that racism is a "major problem" in healthcare, compared with 16% of whites. Well over half of the minorities in this sample (58% of Hispanics and 65% of African Americans) are "very or somewhat" concerned that they or a family member could be treated unfairly when seeking medical care because of their race or ethnic background, while less than 1 in 4 whites (22%) endorse this view. Finally, nearly three times as many African Americans (64%) as whites (23%) believe that African Americans receive a lower quality of healthcare compared with whites; over twice as many Hispanics (56%) as whites (27%) endorse this view when comparing whites and Hispanics.

In a study of healthcare consumers conducted by the Seattle and King County (WA) Department of Public Health (Hobson, 2001), researchers found that nearly one-third of African Americans report having experienced discrimination at some point in their lifetimes when seeking healthcare, and 16% reported such experiences in the past year. More than one-fifth of Hispanic patients reported similar experiences of discrimination in healthcare settings at any point in their lives, and between 7% and 19% of Asian-American subgroups reported such experiences. Significantly, for almost all ethnic groups, respondents who reported experiences of discrimination were more likely to report a delay in seeking needed healthcare than those who did not report experiences of discrimination; this effect was almost uniform (95%) among African Americans who reported experiences of discrimination.

Patient Refusal of Recommended Treatment

Some researchers have speculated that patient refusal may contribute to disparities in care, noting that African-American and other ethnic minority patients may be more likely to refuse invasive procedures. Schecter et al. (1996), for example, found that African-American patients were more likely than whites to refuse physicians' recommendations that they undergo cardiac catheterization. Similarly, Sedlis et al. (1997) found that 15.4% of African-American patients treated at Veterans' Administration hospitals refused invasive cardiac procedures (surgery or percutaneous transluminal coronary angioplasty) when offered, compared with 8.3% among white patients, a difference that the authors conclude may help to explain observed differences in rates of receipt of procedures. The same study, however, revealed that invasive cardiac procedures were recommended more frequently by physicians for white patients (72.9%) than for African-American patients (64.3%), even following diagnostic cardiac catheterization and initial assessment confirming that all the patients were potential candidates for surgery or angioplasty. Thus, physicians' judgments of suitability for procedures in this study contributed to racial variations in care even before patients were presented with surgical options.

Several other studies find no racial differences in rates of refusal of recommended procedures, or find that patient refusal does not fully account for disparities in receipt of care. Petersen et al. (2002) assessed use of cardiac procedures among a sample of African-American and white VA patients with diagnosed acute MI, and found that black patients were less likely to receive thrombolytic therapy or bypass surgery than whites, even when only patients with high-risk coronary anatomy were examined. Black and white patients did not differ, however, in rates of refusal of angiography, angioplasty, and coronary bypass surgery. Lauori et al. (1997) found that patient refusal of recommended cardiovascular procedures could not explain racial differences in "necessary" revascularization procedure rates. Similarly, Hannan et al. (1999) found that among patients deemed appropriate for a revascularization procedure but who did not receive it, a primary gatekeeper physician did not recommend the procedure in 90% of cases. In a study of African-American and white patients suffering from end-stage renal disease, Ayanian et al. (1999) found that African Americans were less likely than whites to desire a transplant. However, racial differences in rates of renal transplantation remained after adjustment for patients' preferences and expectations about transplantation, sociodemographic characteristics, the type of dialysis facility where they received treatment, perceptions of their care, health status, the cause of renal failure, and the presence or absence of co-morbid illness. Other studies, such as Canto et al. (2000), excluded patients who refused the recommended intervention (in this case, reperfusion therapy), but still found racial differences in receipt of therapy.

In summary, few studies have specifically examined racial differences in rates of refusal of treatment recommendations, or why such differences may occur. Of these studies, the majority find that minority patients are more likely than whites to refuse treatment (particularly invasive treatments). Patient preferences are therefore a likely contributor to racial and ethnic disparities in healthcare. The studies reviewed by the committee, however, find that patient preferences do not fully account for observed disparities, suggesting that other sources of disparities may also be operative, perhaps in interaction with patients' attitudes and preferences. In addition, other studies find that minority patients are more likely than whites to perceive that discrimination is a problem in healthcare settings, and are more likely to believe that minority patients receive poorer care than non-minority patients. Minority patients' greater likelihood of refusal of treatment may therefore be linked to a wide range of factors, including real or perceived negative experiences in healthcare settings, negative experiences in other settings (e.g., housing, employment—see Chapter 2), or the history of inferior treatment that minorities have received by the medical and scientific community (Byrd and Clayton, this volume). Further, as noted in Chapter 1, patients' preferences must be understood in the context of information provided to the patient by his or her healthcare provider. Should providers fail to provide clear, accurate, understandable information about the range of treatment options, then patients' consent for treatment cannot be considered fully informed. It is important to distinguish these sources of patient preferences, because as will be noted in Chapter 4, higher minority patient refusal linked to negative experiences in clinical encounters or incomplete disclosure may constitute discrimination.

Biological Differences That May Justify
Differences in Receipt of Care

Chen et al. (2001) and other researchers speculate that racial differences in clinical characteristics may contraindicate the use of the same therapeutic procedures at similar rates in both African-American and white patients. For example, some African-American patients who have had an MI may be more likely than whites to have negative or unclear electrocardiograms at the time of presentation, complicating diagnosis. In addition, African-American and white patients may respond differently to some therapeutic regimens. Exner et al. (2001), for example, found that African-American patients with left ventricular dysfunction were less likely than whites with the same disorder to benefit from enalapril, an angiotensin-converting-enzyme inhibitor. In this study, similar doses of enalapril therapy or a placebo were provided to matched African-American and white patients. Enalapril was associated with a 44% reduction in the risk for hospitalization for heart failure among white patients, but with no significant reduction in risk for hospitalization among African-American patients.

These racial differences in response to pharamacologic and other therapeutic regimens may reflect genetic differences, differences in the pathogenesis of diseases, and environmental factors, such as differences in diet and health-related behaviors. Genetic differences may reflect differences in the distribution of polymorphic traits—including drug receptors or drug-metabolizing enzymes—across all racial and ethnic groups, rather than traits unique to any one group (Wood, 2001). Further research is needed to determine racial differences in response to pharmacologic intervention to assist physicians in weighing individual patients' likely treatment response. It is important to note, however, that many therapeutic regimens have proven efficacious for minority as well as non-minority populations. As noted in Chapter 1, several studies document that these procedures are provided at lower rates to African-American and minority patients where racial differences in response to treatment cannot justify differences in application (Canto et al., 2000; Todd et al., 2000; Bach et al., 1999; Gregory et al., 1999; Hannan et al., 1999; Peterson et al., 1997; Allison et al., 1996; Ball and Elixhauser, 1996; Gornick et al., 1996; Herholz et al., 1996; Imperato et al., 1996; Harlan et al., 1995; Ayanian et al., 1993).

Overuse of Clinical Services by White Patients

Several researchers have suggested that racial and ethnic disparities in care may arise in part from the overuse of services among white patients, rather than differences in service utilization arising from clinical necessity. White patients enjoy generally higher levels of education and may have greater access to and means of gathering information about their presenting concerns and possible diagnostic and treatment options. They may also feel more comfortable advocating for themselves and urging their physician to provide desired services. Racial differences would therefore be expected to be pronounced for optional or non-essential services and procedures. As noted in Chapter 1, however, several studies have tested the "overuse" hypothesis by examining use of clinical procedures relative to established criteria for necessity. These studies demonstrate that in the case of essential services, African-American and minority patients tend to receive a lower quality of care than whites when assessed relative to established quality criteria. Hannan et al. (1999), for example, assessed rates of coronary artery bypass grafting (CABG) among 1,261 post-angiography patients who would benefit from CABG according to RAND appropriateness and necessity criteria. Controlling for age, gender, severity of disease, patient risk status, type of insurance, and other clinical characteristics, the authors found that African-American and Hispanic patients were 36% less likely than whites to undergo CABG. Similarly, Laouri et al. (1997) used RAND/UCLA criteria for necessity of revascularization procedures and found that African Americans were half as likely as whites to undergo necessary CABG and one-fifth as likely to undergo percutaneous transluminal coronary angioplasty (PTCA). In a larger study, Canto et al. (2000) studied the use of reperfusion therapy among more than 26,000 patients meeting eligibility criteria as a result of acute MI. After controlling for clinical and demographic characteristics, the authors found that African Americans were slightly less likely than whites to undergo reperfusion therapy. Further, Schneider et al. (2001b) found that while overuse of PTCA was greater among white men than among minorities, this difference did not fully account for racial differences in revascularization.

To further address the question of whether racial disparities in receipt of revascularization procedures reflect clinical necessity or merely overuse among whites, Peterson et al. (1997) assessed racial differences in receipt of coronary angioplasty and CABG among patients with documented coronary disease, and assessed whether differences were associated with survival. The investigators followed 12,402 patients seen at Duke University Medical Center, and found that African Americans were 13% less likely than whites to undergo angioplasty and 32% less likely to undergo CABG. Racial differences in procedure rates were more marked among patients with severe disease. Analysis of survival benefit of surgery also revealed racial differences; among patients expected to survive more than one year, 42% of African Americans underwent surgery, compared with 61% of whites. Finally, analysis of the adjusted five-year mortality rate among patients revealed that African-American patients were 18% more likely than whites to die.

HEALTH SYSTEMS-LEVEL VARIABLES

Aspects of health systems—such as the ways in which systems are organized and financed, and the "ease" of accessing services—may exert different effects on patient care, particularly for racial and ethnic minorities. Complicated reimbursement procedures and structures, for example, may deter patients with low literacy or limited English proficiency from seeking care. Similarly, time pressures on physicians may hamper the ability of providers to accurately assess presenting symptoms of minority patients, especially where cultural or linguistic barriers are present. Further, the geographic availability of healthcare institutions—while largely influenced by economic factors that are outside the charge of this study—may have a differential impact on racial and ethnic minorities, independently of insurance status. This means that even among minorities and non-minorities insured at the same level, the ease of accessing services and racial differences in where care is typically received may contribute to disparities. Perhaps most significantly, rapid changes in the financing and delivery of healthcare services—such as the dramatic shifts brought by cost-control efforts and the movement to managed care—may pose greater barriers to care for racial and ethnic minorities than for non-minorities (Rice, this volume). Increasing efforts by states to enroll Medicaid patients in managed care systems, for example, may disrupt traditional community-based care and displace providers who are familiar with the language, culture, and values of ethnic minority communities (Leigh, Lillie-Blanton, Martinez, and Collins, 1999). Finally, legal and regulatory policy with regard to healthcare can create a context in which healthcare disparities are not tolerated or implicitly accepted. These potential influences on the quality of care for racial and ethnic minority patients are discussed below, along with supporting evidence.

Language Barriers

As noted in Chapter 2, nearly 14 million Americans are not proficient in English. Linguistic concordance between patient and provider is important, however, as language allows the provider to construct an accurate medical and social history, and assess the patient's belief about health and illness. Language is also an important tool for clinicians to establish an empathic connection with patients (Woloshin et al., 1995), and to reach agreement with patients on treatment decisions and prescribe a course of action. The failure of patients and providers to communicate effectively with each other may result in misunderstandings of patients' concerns, misdiagnosis, or unnecessary testing. In addition, miscommunication can result in poor patient compliance, inappropriate follow-up, and poor patient satisfaction. To the extent that healthcare systems and institutions fail to address language barriers and assist communication between patients and providers, language mismatches are a fertile source of racial and ethnic disparities in care.

Several studies suggest that care processes and outcomes are affected by linguistic barriers. Perez-Stable, Napoles-Springer, and Miramontes (1997), for example, assessed the effects of ethnicity and language concordance between patients and their physicians on health outcomes, use of health services, and clinical outcomes among a sample of Spanish-speaking and non-Spanish-speaking Hispanic and non-Hispanic patients at a university-affiliated general medicine practice. Of the 74 Spanish-speaking Latinos, 60% were treated by clinicians who spoke Spanish, while 40% were treated by non-Spanish-speaking clinicians. After controlling for patient age, gender, education, number of medical problems, and number of prescribed medications, the authors found that having a language-concordant physician was associated with better patient self-reported physical functioning, psychological well-being, health perceptions, and lower pain.

Baker et al. (1996) surveyed 467 native Spanish-speaking and 63 English-speaking patients presenting with non-urgent medical problems in a hospital emergency department to assess patients' reports of the use and need for interpretation. Interpretation, which is usually provided at the discretion of healthcare workers, was provided for only 26% of the Spanish-speaking patients. Just over half (52%) of the Spanish-speaking patients who were seen without a translator felt that interpretation was not necessary, but an additional 22% of the patients who did not receive interpretation felt that it was necessary. Of the patients who received interpretation services, almost half (49%) received interpretation services by a physician or a nurse. But when both the providers' Spanish and the patients' English were poor, interpretation was not called in over one-third (34%) of encounters. In these instances, 87% of patients felt an interpreter should have been called.

Baker et al. (1996) went further to assess patients' understanding of their medical condition and treatments. They found that only 38% of patients who did not have an interpreter when they thought one was necessary reported that their understanding of their condition was good or excellent. Nearly 3 in 5 (58%) reported that their understanding of their treatment was good or excellent, and 90% wished that their examiner had explained their diagnosis or treatment better. However, when patients' knowledge of their diagnosis and treatment were assessed objectively using a standardized measure, no significant differences were found between those who received interpretation and those did not have an interpreter and thought one was necessary (Baker et al., 1996).

David and Rhee (1998) examined the impact of language barriers on patient compliance with medication, satisfaction with care, and preventive testing. Spanish-speaking patients who possessed good English skills and did not need an interpreter were more likely than Spanish-speaking patients who had low English skills and used an interpreter to report that the side effects of medications were explained, and reported greater satisfaction with medical care. Surprisingly, while large majorities of both "cases" (Spanish-speaking patients with low English proficiency who used interpretation) and "controls" (Spanish-speaking patients who reported not needing interpretation) reported that their doctors discussed mammography and clinical cancer screening tests, significantly more cases than controls received these screening tests, leading the authors to speculate that testing served as a substitute for verbal communication.

Interpretation in healthcare settings has commonly been provided in one of several ways. Professional interpretation, using formally trained interpreters who demonstrate proficiency in mediating communication between languages and an understanding of medical terminology, remains rare. Without such services, one of three "sub-optimal" (Woloshin et al., 1995) strategies may be used: 1) the language skills of patients and providers; 2) the skills of family or friends; or 3) ad hoc interpretation from non-clinical employees (e.g., a clerk, aide, or custodian) or bilingual bystanders (e.g., other patients). These strategies are less desirable than professional interpretation because they can interfere with the patient-provider relationship and introduce error into interpretation. Ebden et al. (1988), for example, recorded and analyzed ad hoc interpretation encounters and found that 23% to 52% of words and phrases were incorrectly interpreted. Perhaps more importantly, ad hoc interpretation raises significant concerns regarding patient privacy. The use of bystanders, friends, or family, particularly children, as interpreters undermines patient privacy and may suppress the patient's willingness to discuss sensitive concerns (U.S. DHHS Office for Civil Rights, 2000).

Availability and Access to Services

Literature reviewed in Chapter 1 suggests that the quality of care for minority and non-minority patients may differ in part as a function of where these patients receive care. Even among equally insured patient populations, studies note differences in the quality of care provided, with private, teaching, and high-volume settings generally providing better quality care than public, non-teaching institutions. Significantly, minorities' access to better quality facilities is often limited by the geographic distribution of care facilities and patterns of residential segregation (see Chapter 2), which results in higher-quality facilities being less accessible to minorities.

Leape et al. (1999) tested this hypothesis by assessing racial differences in revascularization procedures as a function of hospital characteristics among 631 patients admitted to 13 New York City hospitals. Revascularization procedures were deemed clinically necessary for all 631 patients, according to RAND criteria. The authors found no significant racial differences in rates of revascularization procedures among African-American patients, (72%), Hispanic patients (67%) and white patients (75%). Rates of revascularization were significantly lower, however, among patients initially seen in hospitals that did not provide revascularization services (and therefore had to refer patients to other hospitals) than those treated in settings that did provide revascularization.

Similarly, Kahn et al. (1994) assessed the quality of care received by nearly 10,000 poor and/or African-American Medicare patients aged 65 years or older admitted to one of 297 acute care facilities for treatment of congestive heart failure, acute myocardial infarction, pneumonia, or stroke. For all patients, processes of care (as assessed by measures of physician and nurse clinical decision-making, technical diagnostic and therapeutic processes, and monitoring processes) were of lower quality in rural hospitals and best in urban teaching hospitals. No overall differences in the quality of care or mortality rates were found by race and poverty status. The authors note, however, that African-American patients and those who were from poor neighborhoods were 1.8 times as likely as whites and those not from poor neighborhoods to receive care in urban teaching hospitals, which generally provide better quality care. After adjusting for sickness at admission, patient and hospital characteristics (i.e., removing the effect of blacks and people from poor neighborhoods receiving better care in urban teaching hospitals), and other clinical factors, African-American patients and those who were from poor neighborhoods received a lower overall process-of-care and were 1.4 times more likely to be discharged in an unstable condition. The authors conclude that "the greater frequency of use of urban teaching hospitals by patients who are black or poor almost completely offsets the worse process of care they receive within each hospital. This phenomenon . . . should be considered in studying the care received for groups of patients whose care may be influenced by the setting in which it is provided" (Kahn et al., 1994, p. 1172).

Geographic factors have also been found to contribute to minorities' lower rates of access to pharmaceutical products. Morrison et al. (2000) examined the relationship between the racial and ethnic composition of New York City neighborhoods and the availability of opioid supplies of pharmacies to assess patients' ease of filling palliative care prescriptions. After controlling for the proportion of elderly persons at the census-block level and for crime rates at the precinct level, the authors found that only 25% of pharmacies in predominantly non-white neighborhoods (those in which less than 40% of residents are white) had sufficient opioid supplies to treat patients in severe pain. In contrast, 72% of pharmacies in predominantly white neighborhoods (those characterized by over 80% white residents) carried sufficient opioid supplies to treat patients in severe pain.

Maneuvering Through Clinical Bureaucracies

Racial and ethnic differences in rates of referral for specialty medical care can emerge in any of several steps in the process of care. Maneuvering through the bureaucratic and administrative "maze" commonly found in modern hospitals and clinics is essential in accessing clinical resources, yet some racial and ethnic groups, for a variety of reasons, may experience less success in navigating through such bureaucracies. Clinical caretakers, for example, are critical actors in helping patients access clinical resources. If these caretakers' advocacy efforts are adversely influenced by clinical uncertainty, stereotypic thinking, and/or lesser personal engagement with patients (to be discussed in the next chapter), it is reasonable to surmise that racial and ethnic minorities will be at a disadvantage in negotiating the medical bureaucracy. Thus, despite formal "equality" in access, minorities may experience differences in the rates with which they receive clinical services. To compound these difficulties, to the extent that minority patients are more likely to experience a subjective sense of disempowerment—whether because of a lack of cultural or linguistic familiarity with the "culture" of medicine (Good et al., this volume), or because of perceived discrimination—these patients may be expected to less vigorously assert their needs or "to feel bitter, even resentful, and to act in a manner that conveys this bitterness, rendering clinical administrators less empathic" (Bloche, 2001, p.106). As yet, however, little empirical data are available to support these hypotheses. An important aspect of navigation through healthcare systems—the clinical referral—is discussed next.

Referral Patterns and Access to Specialty Care

As noted in Chapter 2, racial and ethnic minorities report greater difficulty in obtaining referral and accessing specialty care. Einbinder and Schulman (2000), drawing on empirical literature and theory, illustrate how patient race or ethnicity may influence the referral process for invasive cardiac procedures. The initial step in the process involves the patient's recognition of symptoms that may suggest coronary artery disease. Some evidence, the authors note, indicates that racial and ethnic minorities are less likely than whites to recognize the symptoms of coronary artery disease, and therefore may delay seeking medical treatment. Such delays may limit treatment options. A second step involves obtaining access to healthcare providers, and varies by patient race or ethnicity because of differences in insurance status, as well as the local availability of providers (minority patients are more likely than whites to live in physician shortage areas). In addition, minority patients are less likely than whites to have a regular care provider. The lack of an on-going relationship with a healthcare provider may affect referral because the evaluation and referral process requires regular medical follow-up. In the third step, patient race or ethnicity may influence the presentation of symptoms, and the ability of care providers to recognize them (this topic will be discussed in greater detail in Chapter 4). Physicians' subsequent assessments and recommendations may therefore be based on incomplete information, or can be influenced by assumptions or unconscious stereotypes and biases, according to the authors. Patients' acceptance of physician recommendations also plays a minor role in racial differences in referral rates, as minority patients may refuse referral for invasive testing at higher rates than whites, and physicians may not have the time or interest in discussing patients' concerns or questions about unfamiliar procedures (see earlier discussion of patient refusal). A sixth step identified by Einbinder and Schulman—referral for noninvasive diagnostic evaluation—may be influenced by whether the patient is being followed by a primary care provider or a cardiac specialist, and the relationship that this provider has with other specialists in order to obtain referral. Referral for cardiac catheterization is affected by many factors, according to the authors, including the availability of catheterization services and access to high-technology hospitals, the presence of co-morbid conditions, patient preferences, advanced age, or social factors that may limit patients' ability to comply with therapeutic interventions. All of these factors may disproportionately limit minority patients' ability to undergo catheterization (Einbinder and Schulman, 2000).

Few studies have empirically assessed racial disparities in medical referral. A recent study by Hargraves and colleagues (Hargraves, Stoddard, and Trude, 2001), however, assessed minority physicians' experiences in both obtaining referrals for their patients to specialists and gaining hospital admissions. As noted earlier, racial and ethnic minority physicians are disproportionately more likely to serve minority patients, and therefore play a key role in enhancing access to care for minority populations. Hargraves et al. (2001) surveyed a nationally representative sample of African-American, Hispanic, and white physicians, and asked them how often they were able to arrange referrals to specialists and obtain admissions for their patients. Controlling for physician characteristics (e.g., years in practice, gender, specialty, group or private practice, revenue from managed care, Medicaid, and Medicare) and market characteristics (e.g., local physician participation in managed care, supply of hospital beds, and specialists per capita), minority physicians were found to have greater difficulty in gaining access to care for their patients. Hispanic physicians were more likely to report problems with obtaining referrals for specialty care than their white colleagues, and African-American physicians reported experiencing greater difficulty than white physicians in arranging hospital admissions for their patients. Hargraves et al. (2001) conclude that because physicians' training, type of practice, and other local characteristics were taken into account, only a few variables, such as physicians' prestige or clout, the proximity of hospitals and specialists to their patients, or discrimination directed at the physicians or their patients could account for these differences. The study's findings are limited, however, by a lack of direct measures of characteristics of the physicians' panel of patients. Given the fact that minority physicians are more likely to work in lower-income and minority communities, their patients might differ in disease status, preferences for treatment, and health insurance status.

Fragmentation of Healthcare Systems

"Fragmentation" of healthcare can occur when patients, even those privately insured, encounter different levels of plan coverage that influence the kinds and quality of services they receive. Multiple coverage options offered by health plans are often characterized by different types of benefits packages and different degrees of provider choice. In addition, coverage options vary in levels of pre-authorization review and financial incentives to physicians to practice frugally. At the lowest level of coverage, beneficiaries may face greater constraints in their choice of providers, settings in which care is received, and types of covered services. These differences imply that even within health plans, the medical marketplace is segmented by personal wealth and health status as well as consumer and employer preference (Bloche, 2001). This effect is seen most profoundly in the case of managed care plans comprised largely or entirely of Medicaid recipients and other poor Americans. Such plans have expanded coverage for the neediest (Rosenbaum, this volume), but further segmented the market.

There is little empirical data bearing on the question as to whether less costly, more restrictive health plans provide a poorer (or better) quality of care than more costly, less restrictive plans. However, lower per capita plan budgets mean fewer resources per capita for clinical services, given that care must be provided within a budget. On average, population groups disproportionately represented in less costly, more restrictive plans receive a lower intensity of care. Significantly, much of the research on racial and ethnic disparities in healthcare cited in Chapter 1 controls for insurance status at only a crude level (e.g., insured versus uninsured, privately insured versus publicly insured, etc.), and has not adequately controlled for variations in levels of insurance coverage. They therefore leave open the possibility that racial disparities in care result to some degree from the disproportionate presence of socioeconomically disadvantaged groups in less costly plans.

Furthermore, fragmentation of healthcare financing and provision may foster the development of disparate clinical practice norms, arising from distinct institutional cultures and provider and patient characteristics as well as from different levels of fiscal constraint. The fragmentation ensuing from the Medicaid program's statutory design merits mention as a special case. Because of Medicaid's low reimbursement rates for doctors and hospitals, its poor, disproportionately minority beneficiaries are subject to largely separate, often segregated systems of hospital and neighborhood clinics (Rosenbaum, this volume; Watson, 1995). These systems often adopt their own norms of medical practice, shaped by tight resource constraints. In addition, Medicaid's low reimbursement rates drastically restrict Medicaid beneficiaries' ability to access private physicians, and prevents many Medicaid patients from being admitted to hospitals in the absence of a private doctor with hospital admitting privileges (Rosenbaum, this volume), unless admitted as "community service" inpatients. Even in these instances, such patients are more likely to be cared for primarily by house staff as opposed to private attending physicians. Congress further reinforced Medicaid's low payment scales and largely separate systems of care with repeal of the Boren Amendment, which required Medicaid payments to doctors and hospitals to be "reasonable and adequate" and gave healthcare providers a federal cause of action against state Medicaid programs[1] (Bloche, 2001).

U.S. Department of Defense and Veterans Administration Healthcare Systems

Additional evidence of the impact of health systems on the ability of racial and ethnic minority patients to receive quality healthcare emerges from studies of large healthcare systems run by the U.S. Department of Defense (DoD) and Department of Veterans Affairs (VA). While findings are mixed, some studies suggest that racial and ethnic healthcare disparities are reduced or eliminated in these systems. These findings appear more consistently in studies of DoD systems, which ensure universal access to care, than in VA systems, which significantly reduce financial barriers to care among veterans. Taylor et al. (1997), for example, found no racial differences in rates of catheterization or revascularization among more than 1,400 military patients seeking care for acute myocardial infarction. And as noted above, Optenberg et al. (1995) studied more than 1,600 African-American and white active duty military personnel, their dependents, or military retires with prostate cancer served in DoD healthcare facilities. They found no significant racial differences in waiting time to receive treatment after initial diagnoses, type of treatment, and survival rates once stage of presentation and other clinical and demographic

---

[1]42 U.S.C.A. §1396a(a)(13)(C) (1982 & Supp. V 1987), repealed by Balanced Budget Act of 1997, Pub. L. No. 105-33, §4712(c), 111 Stat. 509 (1997). A state plan for medical assistance must "provide . . . for payment . . . of hospital services, nursing facility services, and services in an intermediate care facility for the mentally retarded provided under the plan through the use of rates (determined in accordance with methods and standards developed by the State . . .) which the State funds, and makes assurances satisfactory to the [Health and Human Services] Secretary, are reasonable and adequate to meet the costs which must be incurred by efficiently and economically operated facilities in order to provide care and services in conformity with applicable State and Federal laws, regulations, and quality and safety standards and to assure that individuals eligible for medical assistance have reasonable access . . . to inpatient hospital services of adequate quality."

factors were considered. In a study of prenatal birth outcomes among civilian and military women, Barfield et al. (1996) found that rates of prenatal care utilization were lower, and rates of low birth weight and fetal and neonatal mortality higher among African-American women than white women, but that these racial disparities were lower (but still significant) among the military population. In addition, a recent study of VA systems found modest racial differences in mortality rates among African-American and white patients admitted for pneumonia, angina, congestive heart failure, chronic obstructive pulmonary disease, diabetes, or chronic renal failure, but these differences suggested *better* survival rates for minority patients (Jha et al., 2001).

Other studies, however, note significant racial differences in VA systems in rates of procedures such as cardiac catheterization. Peterson et al. (1994), Mirvis et al. (1994), Whittle et al. (1993), and Mirvis and Graney (1998) all found African-American VA patients less likely to receive cardiovascular procedures than white VA patients. Sedlis et al. (1997) found that therapeutic cardiac procedures (surgery or PTCA) were offered more frequently for white VA patients (72.9%) than African-American VA patients (64.3%). This difference could not be explained by simple clinical differences between the two groups. Conigliaro et al. (2000) found that although African-American VA patients were less likely then white VA patients to undergo CABG and PTCA, when RAND appropriateness criteria were considered, African Americans were still less likely to receive CABG when deemed "necessary." Oddone et al. (1999) studied racial differences in rates of carotid artery imaging among patients diagnosed with transient ischemic attack, ischemic stroke, or amaurosis fugax seen at one of four VA Medical Centers. After controlling for patients' age, co-morbid factors, clinical presentation, anticipated operative risk, and hospital, African-American patients were found to be half as likely as whites to receive carotid imaging.

Evidence for racial and ethnic disparities in care in VA systems is therefore mixed, but suggests that financial, structural and institutional factors of these systems, as well as the universally available care for military personnel in DoD systems may serve to attenuate some disparities in care. For example, physicians in both DoD and VA systems are salaried, eliminating the role of financial incentives to physicians to recommend or withhold specialized procedures (Okelo et al., 2001). In addition, other practices of these health systems related to larger quality improvement goals may also serve to attenuate disparities. The VA, for example, has instituted clinical decision support programs for physicians, which provide automated, time-sensitive and context-sensitive clinical reminders at the point of care, such as prescription checks and preventive care information. These clinical supports rely on a computerized patient record system that provides patients' medical and social histories, discharge summaries and progress notes, allergies, prior laboratory results, and other information. Clinical reminder notifications provided through these computerized data systems are largely based on the VA's national clinical practice guidelines. In addition, clinical care is evaluated relative to performance measures in six domains (quality, functional status, patient satisfaction, access, cost, and healthy communities). Most of the measures used to assess progress in these domains are based on "best practices" formally supported by evidence-based medicine (Swift, 2001). Such practice guidelines, as will be discussed in Chapter 5, may help to reduce variations in care due to clinical discretion and/or uncertainty.

Significantly, some evidence also suggests that when patients' race or ethnicity is unknown (e.g., when treatment decisions are made by a group of conferring physicians based solely on clinical data), racial and ethnic disparities in care may be attenuated. Okelo et al. (2001) assessed whether racial differences in recommendations for cardiac revascularization persisted when patients' race or ethnicity is unknown. The authors described the treatment decision-making procedures of cardiologists at the Cleveland VA Medical Center, who review clinical data of each patient considered for revascularization absent information about patients' race or ethnicity. Following this procedure, Okelo et al. found no overall racial differences in recommendation for revascularization. After adjusting for patients' age, co-morbidities, location and number of coronary stenoses, left ventricular function, and previous CABG, the authors found that white patients were more likely to undergo CABG and African-American patients were slightly (but not significantly) more likely to undergo PTCA. These findings lead Okelo et al. to conclude that "when only clinical factors are considered, the rates of recommendations for revascularization will be similar for white and African-American patients; but the type of revascularization procedure may differ by ethnicity and may depend, in part, on clinical factors" (Okelo et al., 2001, p. 698).

The Managed Care Revolution

Managed healthcare remains the predominant model of cost containment in an era of continuing escalation of healthcare costs and overall health expenditures. Most managed care organizations employ various forms of either supply-side (i.e., incentives to healthcare providers to practice frugally) or demand-side (i.e., incentives to patients to constrain the use of services) cost containment strategies, or combinations of both as part of managed competition strategies (Rice, this volume). As part of broader efforts to contain costs, improve the quality of care, and increase market share, some managed care organizations employ standardized practice protocols and collect data on patient satisfaction and outcomes of care. As such, managed care offers the potential to help eliminate disparities in healthcare. In many other areas, however, managed care has introduced new institutional dynamics that may enhance the conditions in which racial and ethnic disparities in healthcare can occur.

Utilization review and practice guidelines, for example, may be used by some managed care organizations (MCOs) to ensure that physicians provide services deemed medically appropriate. In this vein, it may be assumed that prospective utilization management, when applied in a standardized fashion, offers the prospect of ensuring that clinical care is consistent across patient groups. As noted earlier in this chapter, however, the subjectivity and ambiguity of clinical situations make standardized practice difficult, and guidelines cannot be developed for all clinical contingencies (Bloche, 2001). As a result, utilization managers must, in many instances, authorize reimbursement under conditions where considerable ambiguity and uncertainty exist. Under these conditions, advocacy by committed clinical caretakers may influence utilization managers' decisions. Typically, such advocacy is more likely to occur where patients and their providers have an established relationship and where providers have the time and resources to pursue claims. Minority patients, as noted below, are less likely than whites to receive care from private physicians and are less likely to have a regular primary care provider—even when compared to whites at the same insurance level (Lillie-Blanton et al., 2001). It is therefore possible that minorities may be less likely to benefit from the advocacy of their provider. The outcomes of competition for resources within a plan also hinge on utilization managers' discretion. With the exception of the studies cited below (see, for example, Lowe et al., 2001), there has been little research into subjective influences on utilization reviewers' decisions in ambiguous cases. Possible influences may include different degrees of sponsorship and advocacy on behalf of patients from their provider, which may be associated with patients' socioeconomic status, and utilization managers' assumptions about which patients are most likely to appeal utilization decisions (Bloche, 2001).

Another supply-side constraint employed by many MCOs is the practice of cost control via devolution of financial risk, thereby shifting responsibility for cost control to practicing physicians. Economic rewards for frugality and penalties for costly tests, treatments, and referrals have become common in contemporary clinical practice (Rice, 1997; Rice, this volume). The result has been increased reliance on the discretion of gatekeeping clinical caretakers to set limits and manage scarce resources. As noted in the model depicted in Figure 3-1, such discretion may allow cognitive, affective, social and cultural factors to influence clinical discretion in racially disparate ways. It may also affect medical resource allocation decisions, in that physicians' suspicions and fears about which patients will protest or sue if denied a test or treatment may influence (even at a subconscious level) the distribution of resources (Bloche, 2001).

While more research must be conducted to fully test these hypotheses, evidence indicates that low-income and ethnic minority patients are less likely to have a regular provider, are more likely to be denied claims, and are less satisfied with many aspects of the care they receive in managed care settings. In a study of low-income African-American, Hispanic, and white patients enrolled in managed care and fee-for-service plans in four states, Leigh and colleagues found that for all three groups, those enrolled in managed care plans were less likely to have a regular provider than those enrolled in fee-for-service plans (Leigh, Lillie-Blanton, Martinez, and Collins, 1999). African-American and Hispanic patients enrolled in managed care plans, however, were more likely than whites enrolled in MCOs to lack a regular provider, as approximately two of every five (38% among African Americans and 42% among Hispanics) lacked a regular provider, compared with 27% of whites enrolled in such plans. In addition, African-American patients enrolled in managed care plans were more than twice as likely as African Americans enrolled in fee-for-service plans to report that they did not obtain needed care. Further, when asked about "the extent to which your physician cares about you," Hispanic patients enrolled in managed care plans were nearly twice as likely as Hispanics enrolled in fee-for-service plans to rate their physicians' level of concern as "fair" or "poor" (Leigh, Lillie-Blanton, Martinez, and Collins, 1999).

Similarly, Phillips et al. (2000) used 1996 Medical Expenditure Panel Survey (MEPS) data to compare the experiences of 22,087 African-American, Hispanic, Asian-American, and non-Hispanic white patients enrolled in either managed care plans or other types of health systems (e.g., fee-for-service plans). Overall, survey respondents reported generally high levels of satisfaction with care, but minorities reported experiencing greater barriers to care than white patients. In particular, Hispanics experienced the greatest difficulty of the surveyed groups in obtaining care (24%), followed by Asian Americans (16%). Three in ten Hispanics reported lacking a usual source of care, as did two in ten African Americans and 21% of Asian Americans. Whites were least likely to report these barriers to care. In addition, and in contrast to Leigh et al. (1999) above, Phillips et al. found that among all racial and ethnic groups, those enrolled in managed care plans were more likely to report having a usual source of care than those enrolled in non-managed care plans. Minorities enrolled in managed care plans, however, tended to experience greater dissatisfaction with their usual source of care than those not enrolled in managed care plans. Asian Americans enrolled in managed care plans were 10 times more likely than Asian Americans enrolled in other types of plans to express dissatisfaction with their usual source of care; Hispanics enrolled in managed care plans were 4 times more likely to express this belief; while whites enrolled in managed care plans were only 1.5 times more likely than whites enrolled in non-managed care plans to endorse this view.

Research also suggests that managed care organizations' gatekeeper policies may pose greater barriers to care for minority patients. Lowe et al. (2001), for example, assessed racial differences in rates of gatekeeper approval for emergency department (ED) services sought by more than 15,000 African-American and white patients at an urban hospital. Nearly three-fourths (73%) of the ED visits analyzed were by African-American patients, and over two-thirds (67%) of visits were by Medicaid beneficiaries. Following a triage assessment by ED staff, 4.4% of visits were denied authorization for services, most commonly because they were deemed "minor" or non-urgent. African-American patients were more likely to receive low triage scores upon presentation; however, after adjusting for patients' age, gender, day and time of ED visit, type of MCO and triage score, African Americans were nearly 1.5 times more likely to be denied authorization for care. Patients who were covered by a Medicaid MCO or those covered by MCOs with mixed Medicaid and commercial patient populations were also more likely than those covered by purely commercial MCOs to be denied authorization for care. The authors note it unlikely that the gatekeepers who approved or denied authorization knew the race or ethnicity of patients presenting in the ED, as they generally did not know the patients and were not informed by ED staff of the patients' race. Therefore, these disparities could have emerged from other sources, such as ED staff's initial triage assessments, advocacy efforts by primary gatekeepers on behalf of patients (as discussed above), or other unmeasured factors (Lowe et al., 2001).

Finally, some of the most significant support for the hypothesis that managed care may pose greater barriers to care for racial and ethnic minorities than whites is provided by Tai-Seale and colleagues (Tai-Seale, Freund, and LoSasso, 2001). Using a "natural experiment," the authors assessed the differential effects of mandatory enrollment in managed care plans on use of clinical services by African-American and white Medicaid beneficiaries. A "difference-in-differences" econometric approach controlled for both time trends in demand for services and for fixed characteristics of beneficiaries that may have affected their use of services. African-American beneficiaries, including both children and adults, experienced significant declines in the use of physician services relative to whites. This relationship was found even when trends in service use unrelated to managed care were controlled by comparing service use to beneficiaries not subject to mandatory enrollment in managed care plans (Tai-Seale et al., 2001).

Supply-Side Cost Containment and Demand for Clinical Services

When patients are well insured, demand for clinical services is not constrained by demand-side prices. Because of low co-payment and/or generous insurance coverage of healthcare expenses, these patients will tend to display a higher demand for clinical services. Such is the case when previously uninsured or underinsured patients are provided with better health insurance, as their use of services (and subsequently, their healthcare costs) increases. In these circumstances, health plans will often use supply-side constraints to encourage doctors to engage in more frugal practice. These cost-containment efforts may involve capitation (providing a set fee for all patients seen in a health system or practice), devolution of financial risk to providers, or other practices (Rice, this volume). Similarly, limitations on the availability of physicians or resources within hospitals or clinics may also induce supply-side constraints. These supply-side constraints can engender demand-supply mismatches within hospitals (Joskow, 1981) and other clinical institutions, as patients will be less able to access all desired providers or services.

These demand-supply mismatches have the potential to contribute to racial and ethnic disparities in care. Excess demand for a hospital's services creates multiple internal queues for these services (Harris, 1979). Competition for these services within institutions may turn on the ability of providers to use their influence in advocating for their patients. As Bloche (2001) observed, "Absent bright-line, easy-to-apply criteria for prioritizing among patients in a queue, the politics of personal influence and professional hierarchy shape resource allocation. Attending physicians with the professional stature and/or political skills to push to the head of the queue in clinically ambiguous situations will do so on behalf of the patients to whom they feel most committed. Conversely, house staff and less influential attending physicians will have more difficulty making their way up the queue" (Bloche, 2001, p. 107).

As noted above, racial and ethnic minority patients are less likely to be seen by a private physician, or to have a regular primary care provider, even when insured at the same level as whites (Lillie-Blanton et al., 2001). Moreover, they are more likely to receive care in hospital clinics and other settings characterized by rapid staff turnover and lack of continuity of care providers. Under these circumstances, it is reasonable to assume that physician advocacy on behalf of patients will be less likely, either because the physician is less familiar with patients that he or she does not regularly treat, or because resource constraints such as capitation prevent physicians from meeting all patients' demands for services (Rice, this volume). Therefore, patients cared for by physicians in settings that support continuity of clinical relationships may have preferred access to services when demand-supply mismatch conditions exist.

Legal and Regulatory Policy and Healthcare Disparities

A number of legal and regulatory mechanisms exist that, in theory, may serve to remedy discriminatory healthcare practice. In some cases, however, these mechanisms are insufficient by themselves to address discriminatory practices, or cannot be implemented without addressing significant obstacles. A few of these mechanisms are briefly described below, as a means of providing examples of how legal and regulatory tools, while well-intended, often fail to address the complexity of racial and ethnic discrimination in healthcare.

Medical Tort Law and Clinical Discretion

Medical malpractice law, in some cases, has served as an effective response to departures from standards of competent practice. Its application to the problem of healthcare discrimination, however, has been limited.

In theory, medical malpractice law prescribes a unitary level of care, regardless of health insurance status or ability to pay. Tort doctrine assumes that a "correct" standard of care can be discerned from physician-experts through the adversary process. Yet, as noted above, clinical practice patterns and styles vary widely. Without high-quality data about the efficacy of alternative approaches, physician-experts cannot provide testimony that distinguishes scientifically between "correct" and "incorrect" clinical practice variations. So long as the care at issue in a medical malpractice case adhered to one or another widely accepted practice variation, it can be defended by resorting to like-minded physician-experts. Without empirical evidence that the practice variation at issue is "wrong," the requirement that plaintiffs shoulder the burden of proof on the issue of negligence in tort cases poses a high barrier to legal success. The lack of such evidence poses another obstacle to malpractice plaintiffs. Plaintiffs must shoulder the burden of proof as to whether the negligence they allege was in fact the cause of the harm that occurred. In the absence of high-quality evidence concerning the comparative efficacy of alternative courses of treatment, proof that a defendant physician's choice of one treatment over another resulted in harm (or a diminished probability of a favorable outcome) is more difficult. Racial disparities in care that fall within the range of widely accepted clinical practice variations are thus not easily amenable to correction through the operation of medical malpractice law (Bloche, 2001).

Moreover, only a small proportion of arguable errors of clinical judgment—arguable based on empirical grounds for preferring one approach over another—result in medical malpractice suits (Weiler, 1993). Even smaller proportions yield monetary settlements or judgments, and poor people and members of disadvantaged minority groups are less likely than other Americans to sue their doctors (Burstin et al., 1993). Medical malpractice law is therefore of weak utility as a mechanism to address racial and ethnic discrimination in healthcare.

Emergency Medical Treatment and Active Labor Act

The federal Emergency Medical Treatment and Active Labor Act (EMTALA)[2] requires federally funded hospitals (e.g., those that participate in Medicare or Medicaid) that operate emergency rooms to screen all emergency room patrons for "emergency medical conditions" regardless of patients' ability to pay, and to provide stabilizing treatment for emergency conditions. Further, these hospitals are required to refrain from discharging patients or transferring them to other facilities (also known as "patient dumping") on economic grounds. Judicial interpretation of EMTALA, however, has been criticized as having weakened the law's force as a deterrent to disparate treatment in the emergency room (Bloche, 2001). Federal appellate court panels in several circuits have ruled that the mandatory emergency screening examination required by EMTALA need not meet national standards of care, but rather, should conform only to the screening hospital's regular practice. Plaintiffs, as a result, commonly experience difficulty pursuing suits alleging violations of EMTALA, as they must challenge local hospital policy, often without the assistance of physicians familiar with emergency room screening practice at the hospital they intend to sue or other evidence of violations of hospital emergency room procedures. As Bloche (2001) notes, "the resulting 'code of silence' problem is obvious: avoidance of the 'code of silence' barrier was a principal reason for the shift from community to national standards of care in medical malpractice law" (Bloche, 2001, p. 110). The difficulties encountered by plaintiffs in suing to enforce EMTALA may lead to cursory evaluation and transfer or discharge of members of disproportionate numbers of minority patients, whether because of no or insufficient insurance, racial discrimination, or unconscious bias. To add to this difficulty, state laws mandating

---

[2]EMTALA, 42 U.S.C. §1395dd (1995).

emergency room screening have generally been construed and applied with similar permissiveness (Rosenblatt et al., 1997).

The Unfulfilled Potential of Title VI

Title VI of the Civil Rights Act of 1964 bars discrimination in health-care and other services by all entities that receive federal funds. Title VI therefore applies to the vast majority of U.S. hospitals and clinics, given the large percentage of these care settings that rely significantly or in part on Medicaid or Medicare reimbursement. Significantly, the law extends beyond intentional discrimination to prohibit many facially neutral practices that may result in disparate negative effects on racial and ethnic minorities and other disadvantaged groups. The impact of Title VI in desegregating healthcare and ensuring the equitable treatment of all patients has been enormous. Despite resistance to desegregation in the early years following the law's passage, for example, the enforcement of Title VI by federal investigators, aided by activists and health professionals, resulted in many previously segregated hospitals opening their doors and wards to all patients who could pay (Smith, 1999). Evidence of discrimination in some sectors of the healthcare industry, however, remained. Discriminatory practices such as denial of admitting privileges to African-American physicians,[3] refusal of admission to patients lacking attending physicians with staff privileges, high prepayment requirements for black patients, and discriminatory routing of ambulances continued in some instances (Smith, 1999). In these cases, the DHHS Office for Civil Rights (OCR) has enacted such measures as revising requirements for staff privileges, eliminating prepayment requirements, and requiring changes in ambulance routes (Rosenbaum et al., 2000).

Despite these gains, some argue that Title VI has yet to fulfill its potential as a tool to eliminate discrimination in healthcare (Perez, this volume; Bloche, 2001). For example, the federal regulations promulgated pursuant to Title VI did not offer detailed compliance instruction to healthcare institutions (Rosenbaum, 2000; U.S. Commission on Civil Rights, 1999), making it difficult for even the well-intended institutions to assess what practices may run afoul of the law. More significantly, federal Title VI regulations held that Medicare's payments to physicians do not constitute "federal financial assistance" under Title VI. This rule

---

[3]Some hospitals pursued the facially neutral strategy of refusing to grant privileges to physicians who were not members of their local medical societies. The difficulty for African-American doctors (and their patients) in some localities, was that these medical societies (which received no "federal financial assistance" and were thus beyond Title VI's reach) refused admission to blacks (Smith, 1999).

meant that private physicians were not subject to Title VI, despite the fact that virtually all other federal payments to private actors are treated by the regulations as "federal financial assistance," triggering Title VI protections (Rosenbaum, 2000). If physicians who accept Medicare were subject to Title VI, the law would have given DHHS (and private plaintiffs) a powerful civil rights enforcement tool, applicable not only to racial disparities in the care provided to Medicare patients but also to disparate treatment of non-Medicare patients by physicians who accept Medicare. Given that most physicians accept Medicare, and given their important role as key decisionmakers with respect to use of hospital resources and services, extending the reach of Title VI to Medicare coverage of physician services would subject most of the private healthcare sector to Title VI enforcement.

The reach and effectiveness of Title VI can be improved by addressing these gaps. More specific regulatory guidance, based on empirical research regarding potential disparate impact and means to improve access to and quality of care for minority patients, will enable healthcare institutions to develop more finely crafted policies and will help enforcement efforts by drawing distinctions between allowable and potentially illegal practices (Bloche, 2001). More robust DHHS monitoring and enforcement, similar in scope to the early efforts of the Department following passage of Title VI, can help to re-establish federal leadership work toward the elimination of care disparities (Smith, 1999). In addition, application of Title VI to private physicians who accept Medicare would extend the law's reach to a significant segment of the healthcare industry.

Furthermore, the application of Title VI beyond intentional discrimination to include policies that may create disparate racial impacts could be an important tool for civil rights enforcement. Disparate impact could be assessed using institution-specific statistical evidence of disparities in healthcare provision. Such evidence may suffice to state a *prima facie* case of discrimination, requiring a healthcare provider to justify policies and practices that result in racially disparate clinical decisions (Barnes and Weiner, 1999). Establishing proof of institution-specific disparities—and of causal links between such disparities and particular policies and practices—will pose significant challenges. The possibility of institution-specific databases sufficiently powerful to serve this probative purpose is speculative, but the ongoing effort to establish electronic clinical record-keeping (see Chapter 7) may make such evidence increasingly accessible to civil rights enforcement authorities.

Despite the promise of this type of data, however, new challenges have emerged within the last year that will limit private parties' ability to seek legal relief under Title VI from policies with disparate racial impact (Perez, this volume). In *Alexander v. Sandoval*, the U.S. Supreme Court

held that Title VI did not create a private right of action concerning policies with disparate impact, absent discriminatory intent. This action therefore places the greatest burden of civil rights enforcement with U.S.
DHHS, which will shape Title VI's future as a health policy tool through
its civil rights enforcement policies.

SUMMARY

This chapter presents a review of evidence regarding potential sources
of racial and ethnic differences in healthcare, once access-related factors
such as patient education, income, and insurance status are held constant.
Consistent with the committee's definitions of *differences*, *disparities*, and
discrimination in care, several sources are identified. Those related to patients' preferences, needs, and racial or ethnic differences in the clinical
appropriateness of care may contribute to differences in the quality or
intensity of care provided, but these are not sources of healthcare disparities, as they do not imply undue differential treatment on the basis of race
or ethnicity. Disparities in care, on the other hand, likely emerge from a
range of sources, such as characteristics of healthcare systems and the
legal and regulatory context of healthcare delivery. In the next chapter,
sources of disparities arising from the clinical encounter will be examined
in greater detail.

Finding 3-1: Many sources—including health systems, healthcare
providers, patients, and utilization managers—may contribute to
racial and ethnic disparities in healthcare.
Evidence suggests that several sources may contribute to healthcare
disparities, including healthcare providers, patients, utilization managers and healthcare systems. In the current era of healthcare delivery, clinical decision-making increasingly involves this large number of individuals, who are subject to an array of systems influences
that may contribute to healthcare disparities.

4

Assessing Potential Sources of Racial and Ethnic Disparities in Care: The Clinical Encounter

Previous chapters have assessed the extent of racial and ethnic disparities in healthcare, and have identified potential sources of these disparities. Disparities are found to arise from an historic and social context in which racial and ethnic minorities received inferior healthcare, reflecting broader socioeconomic disadvantage among minorities and societal discrimination. When seen by a healthcare provider, minorities typically have been treated in segregated healthcare systems that today remain largely segmented by socioeconomic class. When differences in treatment attributable to insurance, access to care, health status, and other factors are eliminated, however, racial and ethnic healthcare disparities still remain.

As discussed in Chapter 3, factors related to patients' needs and preferences, as well as the characteristics of health systems and the legal and regulatory contexts in which care is delivered, may explain some of the racial and ethnic differences in care that remain once access-related factors are controlled. In this chapter, aspects of the clinical encounter that may contribute to disparities—including patients' and providers' attitudes, expectations, and behavior—are assessed. When these encounters systematically produce racial and ethnic disparities, they may constitute discrimination. As noted in Chapter 1, the study committee defines *discrimination* as differences in care that emerge from biases and prejudice, stereotyping, and uncertainty in communication and clinical decision-making. It should be emphasized that this definition is not intended in a legal sense. Different sources of federal, state and international law define discrimination in varying ways, with some focusing on intent and others emphasizing disparate impact.

Three mechanisms might be operative in producing discriminatory patterns of healthcare from the provider's side of the exchange: 1) bias (or prejudice) against minorities; 2) greater clinical uncertainty when interacting with minority patients; and 3) beliefs (or stereotypes) held by the provider about the behavior or health of minorities (Balsa and McGuire, 2001a). Patients might also react to providers' behavior associated with these practices in a way that contributes to disparities. If minority patients mistrust doctors' advice, they may be less likely to follow it, potentially accounting for some part of healthcare disparities.

To many observers, the mechanism behind disparities that comes most immediately to mind is provider prejudice: doctors and other providers might have a lower regard for minority patients and treat them less well. Prejudice is the least subtle of the mechanisms likely involved in clinical disparities, and does not require a sophisticated understanding of doctor-patient interaction to see how it might work. The same is not true, however, for other mechanisms. Clinical uncertainty and stereotypes lead to disparities through processes requiring some understanding of medical decision-making. To appreciate how these second and third mechanisms might work, and how patient response affects clinical interactions, it is necessary to keep in mind some salient features of the medical encounter.

MEDICAL DECISIONS UNDER TIME PRESSURE
WITH LIMITED INFORMATION

In the process of healthcare, doctors and other healthcare providers often must reach judgments about patients' conditions and make decisions about treatment without complete and accurate information. Moreover, they frequently must do so under severe time pressure and resource constraints. These conditions contribute to clinical uncertainty, as providers must weigh a vast array of information, presented both by the patient and from diagnostic test data. This uncertainty opens the possibility that medical decisions and the course of treatment will reflect subjective variability and preferences of the physician (Eisenberg, 1986; Wennberg, 1999). Under conditions of time pressure, problem complexity, and high cognitive demand, physicians' attitudes may therefore shape their interpretation of this information and their expectations for treatment, such as the likelihood of patient compliance.

To add to this uncertainty, as clinicians and their patients work together, both parties are involved in highly complex processes of decision-making, requiring the acquisition of a wide array of diverse information and the weighting of these data on various dimensions of salience. The assembly and use of these data are affected by many influences, including various heuristics that introduce significant problems for recall and weighting. In conditions such as these, it may be assumed that cognitive shortcuts have significant value to any decision-maker. Physicians, in fact, are commonly trained to rely on gestalts that functionally resemble the application of "prototypic" or stereotypic constellations. That is, physicians use clusters of information in making diagnostic and other complex judgments that must be arrived at without the luxury of the time and other resources to collect all the information that might be relevant. These conditions of time pressure and resource constraints are common to many clinical encounters, and map closely onto those identified as producing negative outcomes due to lack of information, to stereotypes, and to prejudice (van Ryn and Burke, 2000; van Ryn, 2002).

Patients may also hold stereotypes of clinicians that would come into play under these conditions of stress and demand for rapid and complex cognition. These stereotypes may paint the physician as an arrogant clinician, or as "the white man who experiments on minority patients," or as a person who cannot be trusted to provide the whole truth. Even if the parties would, upon direct inquiry, deny the reality of such stereotypes in the particular circumstance, they may still unconsciously act from these perspectives in a pressured situation. The following sections present a more detailed discussion of the mechanisms by which disparities can arise in the clinical encounter. We explain how the mechanisms work, and consider the evidence in support of the empirical importance of each mechanism.

HEALTHCARE PROVIDER PREJUDICE OR BIAS

Prejudice is defined in psychology as an unjustified negative attitude based on a person's group membership (Dovidio et al., 1996). Prejudice, when held explicitly, may become part of a "reasoned" and normative pattern of behavior that becomes discriminatory. While it is reasonable to assume that the vast majority of healthcare providers find prejudice morally abhorrent and at odds with their professional values, healthcare providers, like other members of society, may not recognize manifestations of prejudice in their own behavior. Socially conditioned implicit prejudice may be manifested in healthcare providers' nonverbal behaviors reflecting anxiety (e.g., increased rate of blinking), aversion (e.g., reduced eye contact) or avoidance (e.g., more closed postures) when interacting with minority rather than white patients.

Empirical support for the presence of biased or prejudicial attitudes among healthcare providers is limited but growing. Some research suggests that differences in care may result from conscious or unconscious biases on the part of physicians and other healthcare providers. Schulman et al. (1999), for example, assessed physicians' recommendations for management of chest pain after they viewed vignettes of "patients" (actually actors) who complained of symptoms of coronary artery disease. "Patients" varied only in race (black or white), sex, age (55 or 70 years), level of coronary risk, and the results of an exercise stress test. As originally reported in the published findings, Schulman et al. found that physicians were less likely to recommend cardiac catheterization procedures for women (odds ratio = 0.6, suggesting that they were 40% less likely to be recommended for catheterization) and African Americans (odds ratio = 0.6, again suggesting that this group was 40% less likely to referred for catheterization) than for whites and men.

These results as reported, however, overstated the likelihood of referral for African Americans and women relative to whites and men. In a rebuttal to Schulman et al., Schwartz, Woloshin, and Welch (1999) demonstrated that had the study authors calculated the relative chance of referral using risk ratios, rather than odds ratios, the probability of African Americans being referred for cardiac catheterization was only 7% lower than for whites. In addition, Schwartz et al. demonstrated that significantly lower rates of referral were found only in the case of African-American women, whose rate of referral was approximately 12% less than that for white men, white women, and African-American men. There were no significant differences in rates of referral among the latter three groups, suggesting that a more accurate interpretation of the data would be that the effect of race on physician's referral patterns is modified by gender. Furthermore, Schwartz et al. contend that referral rates for catheterization alone do not constitute a "gold standard" of care; to the contrary, these authors assert, the assumption that "more testing"—i.e., catheterization for all patients who present with cardiac symptoms—represents better care is unfounded. Less testing, in some instances, may result in more appropriate care (Schwartz et al., 1999).

In a reply to Schwartz et al. (1999), Schulman, Berlin, and Escarce (1999) agree that calculation of risk ratios would have been more appropriate as a means of assessing differences in referral rates. They note, nonetheless, that the findings of the study are consistent with the hypothesis that clinical decision-making may be influenced by physicians' conscious or subconscious perceptions on the basis of patients' race and gender, rather than on objective data. And while catheterization may not be appropriate for all patients even given similar objective preliminary test results, Schulman and colleagues, referring to the robust findings of studies that indicate lower rates of referral among blacks for catheterization, write, "we doubt that the lower utilization rates observed consistently among black patients reflect an effort to provide more appropriate care to these patients" (Schulman, Berlin, and Escarce, 1999, p. 286).

In another experimental design, Abreu (1999) assessed whether conscious or non-conscious stereotypes would influence the clinical impressions of mental health professionals. Abreu "primed" these clinicians with either African-American stereotypes (e.g., "Negroes," "blacks," "blues," "rhythm") or neutral words (e.g., "water," "then," "about," "things") flashed on a computer screen for 80 milliseconds. Clinicians were then asked to evaluate the same hypothetical patient on a number of dimensions, including general impressions as well as clinical features. Abreu found that therapists primed with stereotype-laden words rated the patient significantly less favorably on hostility-related attributes than therapists exposed to neutral words, demonstrating that "therapists can be affected by African-American stereotypes in ways that produce negative or positive first impressions, depending on the nature of the attribute that is rated" (Abreu, 1999, p. 387).

Another experimental study using patient vignettes also found variations in physician recommendations when patient demographic variables were manipulated, although results were mediated by physician gender. In a study of primary care physicians' recommendations for pain management, Weisse et al. (2001) presented vignettes of patients suffering from identical symptoms of kidney stone pain, lower back pain, and as a control condition, sinusitis. Nearly 80% of the physician sample was white, while 15% were Asian American or Pacific Islander. In each case, only the race (African American or white) and gender of the "patient" was manipulated. The authors found that male physicians prescribed higher doses of hydrocodone for white "patients" than black "patients" suffering from back pain and renal colic, while female physicians prescribed higher doses of analgesic for black "patients" than white "patients." In both cases, findings were robust: male physicians prescribed twice as much hydrocodone to white patients than black patients, while female physicians prescribed the reverse. No other patient-physician race and gender interactions were observed. These findings, the authors suggest, imply that male and female physicians may react differently to gender and/or racial cues. While few other studies have replicated this finding, the study also implies that healthcare providers' perceptions of and attitudes towards patients are potentially influenced by a range of factors, and illustrates the complexity of disentangling the effects of race, ethnicity, and gender as they influence patient-provider interaction. More research is needed to better understand these processes, and to specifically assess how physicians' race, ethnicity, or gender may influence their attitudes toward and perceptions of patients.

Another experimental study, using first- and second-year medical students as subjects, assessed whether the race and gender of hypothetical patients influenced students' perceptions of presenting symptoms. Rathore et al. (2000) randomly assigned 164 medical students to view a video of either a black female or white male actor who presented with the same symptoms of angina. Students were then asked to rate the patients' health status, based on their assessment of how the patients' presenting symptoms would affect their quality of life. They were also asked to provide a diagnosis of "definite" or "probable" angina. The authors found that students were more likely to provide a diagnosis of "definite" angina for the white male patient than the black female patient, but rated the health status of the black female patient as lower than that of the white male. Thus, these subjects assessed the while male patient's cardiac symptoms to be more severe, yet perceived the black female patient's quality of life to be lower, despite objectively similar presentations from the two "patients." Minority students, however, did not rate the health status of the black female patient as significantly different than that of the white patient. When examined by students' gender, Rathore et al. found that the male students tended to rate the black female's health status as lower than the white male, while female students did not rate the two patients' heath status differently (Rathore et al., 2000).

In a study conducted in a clinical setting, Finucane and Carrese (1990) assessed when and how patients' race was referenced during house staff case presentations. In this study, the chief medical resident surreptitiously recorded oral case presentations during a 2-month period, and assessed, using *a priori* criteria, whether and how often the patient's race was mentioned, and whether potentially "unflattering characteristics" (e.g., low intelligence, uncooperativeness, unkemptness) were also noted. Race was noted in the vast majority (16 of 18) of cases involving black patients, but only in about half (19 of 36) of cases involving white patients. Among patients to whom house staff ascribed unfavorable characteristics, race was mentioned in 10 of 10 cases involving black patients, but in only 4 of 9 cases involving white patients. Findings of this study must be interpreted with caution, however, as the study suffers from a very small sample size and is limited by the single study setting. In addition, the authors employed no objective means of assessing whether the unfavorable characteristics ascribed to patients resulted from a true difference in the prevalence of these characteristics, rather than from racial bias.

In another study based on actual clinical encounters, van Ryn and Burke (2000) surveyed 193 physicians to assess their perceptions of 842 patients (57% white and 43% African American) following post-angiogram hospital visits. The authors asked physicians to rate their patients on a variety of personal characteristics such as intelligence, self-control, education level, pleasantness, rationality, independence, and responsibility. In addition, the authors asked physicians to rate their feelings of affiliation toward the patient and their perceptions of their patients' degree of social support, tendencies to exaggerate discomfort, likelihood of complying with medical advice, likelihood of drug or alcohol abuse, as well as other characteristics. van Ryn and Burke also surveyed patients and assessed their frailty/sickness, depressive symptoms, social assertiveness, feelings of self-efficacy, and perceived social support. These variables, along with information about physicians' age, sex, race, and medical specialty were entered into logistic regression analyses to control for the impact of these variables on physicians' assessments of patients. The results supported the authors' hypotheses that patient race and socioeconomic background do influence physicians' perceptions, even when controlling for differences in patients' socioeconomic status, personality attributes and degree of illness. African-American patients were rated as less intelligent, less educated, more likely to abuse drugs and alcohol, more likely to fail to comply with medical advice, more likely to lack social support, and less likely to participate in cardiac rehabilitation than white patients. Furthermore, African-American patients were two-thirds as likely as whites to be perceived as the kind of person with whom the physician could see him/herself being friends. Finally, a significant interaction of race and socioeconomic status was found, in that at low socioeconomic (SES) levels, black patients were rated as less pleasant and less rational than whites.

These studies lend support to the hypothesis that physicians' diagnostic and treatment decisions are influenced by patient race. In addition, they suggest that these influences are complex, and that both patient and provider gender may significantly influence physicians' perceptions. They do not, however, elucidate the mechanisms by which these attitudes, biases, and stereotypes may result in differences in clinical treatment, or the degree to which these attitudes might affect the outcome of patient care. It therefore remains unclear what degree of racial and ethnic disparities may be explained by this mechanism.

As noted above, there is no evidence that any significant proportion of healthcare professionals in the United States harbors overtly prejudicial attitudes. Health professionals in general are well educated and subscribe to a professional ethic that should mitigate against discrimination on the basis of race or ethnicity. How then, could a well-meaning group of healthcare professionals, working in their usual circumstances with diverse populations of patients, create a pattern of care that appears (on the now substantial weight of available scientific evidence) to be discriminatory? In other words, is it possible for physicians and other healthcare professionals to act in a racially biased manner without knowing it?

To begin to address this question, the following section offers a hypothesis about clinical uncertainty, and how it may affect healthcare providers' decision-making, and ultimately influence the care provided to minority patients.

Clinical Uncertainty

Theory and research on clinical decision-making suggest that ambiguities in physicians' understanding and interpretation of information from patients may contribute to disparities in care (Balsa and McGuire, 2001a). Any degree of uncertainty a physician has about the condition of a patient may, by itself, result in disparities in treatment. A doctor's decision-making process is nested in uncertainty. Doctors must depend on inferences about severity based on what they can see about the illness and on what else they observe about the patient (e.g., race). The exact same symptom information can lead the physician to make different clinical decisions depending on the other characteristics of the patient. Physicians can therefore be viewed as operating with prior beliefs about the likelihood of their patient's conditions, "priors" that will be different according to age, gender, SES, and possibly race/ethnicity. These priors—which are taught as a cognitive heuristic to medical students—as well as the information gained in a clinical encounter both influence medical decisions.

A doctor starting with a prior and supplementing this with new clinical information must weigh both in coming to an initial hypothesis about the source of the patient's problem. Formal models of medical decision-making view this as an application of the rules of probability (Weinstein et al., 1980).[1] In particular, "Bayes' rule" describes how a decision-maker combines prior beliefs with new information to make the best guess about the likelihood of some phenomenon. Among other things, Bayes' rule says that the relative weights placed on the prior and the new information depend on the strength of the evidence behind the prior and on the quality of the new information.

As an example, consider the case of a Latino male patient and a white male patient, both 50 years old and otherwise healthy. Suppose their doc-

---

[1] A number of other explicit decision-theoretic approaches explore clinical decision-making. For other examples, see Mushlin et al. (1997) or Fendrick et al. (1995).

tor believes that the prior probability of either patient having heart problems is low and regards it to be the same for both patients. Now, suppose the Latino and the white patient both experience exactly the same symptom(s) and describe their pain to the doctor. Will the doctor come to the same clinical decision for the Latino and the white? Expression of pain symptoms differs among cultural and racial groups (Bonham, 2001). White doctors may simply understand pain reports better from members of their own racial group. When the white male talks to the doctor, the doctor relates easily to the patient's report; when the Latino tells his story, the doctor follows less well, and picks up fewer implicit clues. If we apply the terms of the Bayesian model of medical decision-making to the Latino patient, the reliability is lower because the potential error in the symptom report is higher than in the case of the white patient. With more uncertainty in the symptom report from the Latino, the Bayesian doctor puts more weight on his or her prior. The consequence could be that the white patient is referred for testing, and the Latino patient is not. Differences in medical decisions from the uncertainty mechanism can arise when the doctor has the same regard for each patient (no prejudice) and when there is no difference in the prior beliefs (stereotypes or clinical heuristics) the doctor holds for patients from the two groups. Differential treatment can therefore result from greater uncertainty associated with clinical information alone.

The effect of elevated uncertainty intervening between the patient's symptoms and the doctor's understanding of those symptoms depends on several factors (Balsa and McGuire, 2001a) and can lead to minorities getting either more or less care than whites. Suppose a psychiatrist in an emergency situation must decide whether to commit a patient after a failed suicide attempt. Unless the psychiatrist can get sufficient information to be assured that the patient is no longer a threat to harm himself, hospitalization is indicated. A black or Latino patient who is less well understood by the doctor is, in this case, more likely to be hospitalized because without sufficient information, the doctor must go with the prior that the patient might be a danger to himself.

Although the uncertainty hypothesis does not always imply that minorities receive less care, it can explain why they might sometimes receive less (and sometimes not). It also leads to the prediction that although the quantity of care for minorities may be more or less, the *match of care to need* will in general be worse for minorities because doctors have less good information with which to modify their priors about the patient's problem. Thus, the uncertainty hypothesis implies that outcomes will be worse for minorities (because of the poor match), and it also implies that minorities will rationally demand less healthcare, seek care at lower rates, and comply less frequently, since they anticipate that the care will be less well-matched to their needs.

Provider Beliefs and Stereotypes

The mechanism of stereotypes is the most complicated of the three discussed in this chapter. We begin by briefly examining the functions of stereotypes and attitudes in general, exploring their origins, and then considering the interpersonal consequences of stereotypes in a health context. The mechanisms are illustrated by examples from the extensive body of psychological research on these processes.

Functions of Stereotypes and Attitudes

Stereotyping can be defined as the process by which people use social categories (e.g., race, sex) in acquiring, processing, and recalling information about others. The beliefs (stereotypes) and general orientations (attitudes) that people bring to their interactions serve important functions. Primarily, they help organize and simplify complex or uncertain situations and give perceivers greater confidence in their ability to understand a situation and respond in efficient and effective ways. People tend to categorize others into social groups because of the complexity of the social environment and our limited cognitive resources to organize and manage this complexity. These categories are often based on readily apparent, salient similarities, such as physical characteristics associated with sex or race (Dovidio, 1999).

The development of social stereotypes results from an individual's need to understand, to predict, and potentially to control one's environment (Mackie, Hamilton, Susskind, and Rosselli, 1996). Studies indicate that once categorization occurs, members of a group tend to be viewed as more similar to one another (the out-group homogeneity effect) and as having common characteristics. Personal traits (dispositional attributions), rather than situational or environmental attributions, are often overemphasized in stereotypes because they offer more stable explanations for the group's behavior and enhance feelings of predictability (Dovidio, 1999).

Biases in Social Stereotypes and Attitudes

Although functional, social stereotypes and attitudes also tend to be systematically biased. Humans are social animals, and people tend automatically to classify others into important, essential social categories, typically relating to dimensions such as age, gender, and skin color. These biases may exist in overt forms, as represented by traditional forms of bigotry. However, because of their origins in virtually universal social categorization processes, they may also exist, often unconsciously, among people who strongly endorse egalitarian principles and truly believe that they are not prejudiced (Dovidio and Gaertner, 1998). For example, Devine (1989) assessed the reactions of both high- and low-prejudiced (as assessed by a pre-test) white college students to ambiguous behavior described in a vignette (e.g., an individual demanding money back from a sales clerk) after subliminally priming the students with words reflecting both African American stereotypes (e.g., "Negroes," "lazy," "blues," "ghetto") and neutral words. Both the high- and low-prejudiced participants interpreted the described behavior as more hostile after being primed with stereotype-laden words than when primed with neutral words. Other studies reveal that among people who endorse egalitarian principles, racial bias may be expressed in subtle and indirect ways that can be rationalized on the basis of factors apparently other than race, or in the form of discomfort and uncertainty in interactions involving racial and ethnic minorities (Dovidio, 1999).

Other studies of social categorization reveal that when people or objects are categorized into groups, actual differences between members of the same category tend to be perceptually minimized and often ignored in making decisions or forming impressions (Fiske, 1998). Members of the same category seem to be more similar than they actually are, and more similar than they were before they were categorized together. This forms the basis for the development of stereotypes. In addition, although members of a social category may be different in some ways from members of other categories, studies show that these differences tend to become exaggerated and overgeneralized (Fiske, 1998). Thus, categorization enhances perceptions of similarities within groups and differences between groups (particularly with respect to one's own group), which emphasizes social difference and group distinctiveness. This process is not benign because these within- and between-group distortions have a tendency to generalize to additional dimensions (e.g., character traits) beyond those that differentiated the categories originally. Furthermore, as the salience of the categorization increases, the magnitude of these distortions also increases (Turner et al., 1987).

Moreover, in the process of categorizing people into two different groups, people typically classify themselves *into* one of the social categories and *out of* the other (Operario and Fiske, 2001; Fiske, 1998). Upon social categorization of individuals into in-groups and out-groups, people spontaneously experience more positive feelings toward the in-group. They also favor in-group members directly in terms of evaluations and resource allocations. In addition, in-group membership increases the psychological bond and feelings of "oneness" that facilitate the arousal of empathy in response to others' needs or problems. As a consequence, assistance is offered more readily to in-group than to out-group members. Furthermore, studies indicate that people are more likely to be cooperative and exercise more personal restraint when using endangered common resources when these are shared with in-group members than with others, and they work harder for groups they identify as their in-group (Tajfel and Turner, 1979). Self-categorization in terms of collective identity, in turn, increases the likelihood of the development of intergroup biases and conflict.

A number of studies demonstrate just how powerfully mere social categorization can influence differential thinking, feeling and behaving toward in-group versus out-group members. Mackie, Devos, and Smith (2000), for example, assessed whether college students who were assigned membership to a social group would develop feelings of anger, fear, and contempt toward students in other, similarly assigned groups. The investigators manipulated interactions between the groups, and found that collective support for the in-group was associated with increased feelings of anger toward the out-group and a willingness to argue, confront, oppose, and attack the out-group (Mackie, Devos, and Smith, 2000).

Consequences of Stereotypes

Stereotypes and attitudes toward members of social groups, such as those based on race and ethnicity, significantly shape the outcomes of interpersonal interactions with members of these groups. In general, individual differences in both racial stereotypes and prejudice systematically predict whites' discriminatory actions toward blacks (Dovidio, Brigham, Johnson, and Gaertner, 1996). They do so in a variety of convergent ways and different mechanisms. For instance, studies show that people not only tend to interpret the behaviors of others in ways that are consistent with their stereotypes and attitudes about the group, but these biases also influence the way that information is subsequently recalled. When people do not have a strong memory for particular information about a group member, they "recall" information in stereotype-consistent ways (Dovidio, 1999).

People also develop expectations about others substantially on the basis of their group membership and the associated stereotypes and attitudes. Stereotypes are particularly likely to influence expectations, inferences, and impressions when people are not motivated to attend to individuating information or are limited in their capacity to process information due to other demands on their attention and thoughts (for review of this research, see Biernat and Dovidio, 2000). Because stereotypes shape interpretations, influence how information is recalled, and guide expectations and inferences in systematic ways, they tend to be self-perpetuating. They also can produce self-fulfilling prophecies in social interaction, in which the stereotypes of the perceiver influence the interaction in ways that conform to stereotypical expectations (Jussim, 1991).

Recent evidence indicates that people do not have to be aware of their attitudes or consciously endorse stereotypes for these factors to influence their thoughts, feelings, and behaviors. Whereas "explicit" stereotypes and attitudes operate in a conscious mode, "implicit" stereotypes commonly function in an unconscious fashion (Fiske, 1998). Implicit stereotypes and attitudes develop with repeated pairings, either through direct experience or social learning of the association, between the category or object and evaluative and descriptive characteristics. In the United States, because of shared socialization influences, there is considerable research evidence that even well-meaning whites who are not overtly biased and who may not believe that they are prejudiced typically demonstrate, on average, unconscious implicit negative racial attitudes and stereotypes (Dovidio, 1999). For example, an experiment by Dovidio, Kawakami, and Gaertner (2002) found that white college students' egalitarian explicit racial attitudes were reflected in a bias of their verbal behavior toward black compared with white confederates and their perception of their own friendliness toward white as compared with black partners. In contrast, white subjects' implicit attitudes (as measured following subliminal presentation of black or white faces) reflected a systematic bias against blacks, particularly when spontaneous, non-verbal behaviors were assessed.

Stereotypes and Healthcare Disparities

Negative stereotypes about minorities, held explicitly or implicitly by physicians, can contribute to healthcare disparities in a number of ways. In some cases, healthcare providers may be consciously aware of their negative stereotypes of minorities, but may nonetheless view these stereotypes as accurate, functional, and appropriate for their clinical work. In these cases, the research cited above suggests that these providers will selectively attend to and recall information that confirms their stereotypes, and will tend to allow such stereotypes to enter into clinical decisions regarding the diagnosis and appropriate course of treatment.

Such cases, however, likely represent only a small minority of healthcare professionals. While the study committee could find no survey data to elucidate racial attitudes of providers, it is likely that the vast majority endorse egalitarian and non-racist attitudes. But even among these individuals, research suggests that stereotyping and social categorization are prevalent, universal processes. Subtle and unintentional types of biases exist even among highly educated whites who support egalitarian ideals and are not consciously racially prejudiced (Biernat and Dovidio, 2000). These biases have their origins in normal and pervasive processes associated with social categorization and thus can operate without conscious awareness or control. Stereotypes, whether consciously endorsed or not, are heuristics that typically efficiently guide the perception, interpretation, storage, and retrieval of information, particularly under conditions of high cognitive demand (Mackie et al., 1996). Similarly, when individuals do not have the time, capacity, opportunity, or motivation to assess situations fully and deliberately, implicit attitudes automatically shape people's responses to objects, individuals, and groups. These conditions of time pressure, high cognitive demand, and stress are common to many healthcare settings, making these settings "ripe" for the activation of stereotypes.

van Ryn and Burke's (2000) work shows that physicians believe blacks are less likely to comply with treatment and more likely to engage in destructive health behaviors (e.g., drug abuse) that may interfere with the value of treatment. When doctors hold these beliefs, they may be less likely to recommend treatment to blacks (e.g., "it is wasteful if the patient fails to follow the treatment regimen"), or less likely to put as much effort into discerning the nature of the black patient's problem if the patient will not take care of himself (e.g., "why should I work hard for a self-destructive patient?"). These stereotypes do not have to be consciously endorsed to influence such decisions (Devine, 1989), and they typically may influence decisions without physicians being aware of their presence. These stereotypical expectations, in turn, can shape the nature of interactions in ways that lead patients to respond in stereotype-confirming ways (Sibicky and Dovidio, 1986).

Questions remain, however, about the nature of these stereotypes and how they affect clinical decisions. For example, do healthcare professionals sometimes make more benevolent, but nonetheless stereotyped assessments of minority patients, such as assuming that co-morbid factors such as alcohol or drug use are present and may complicate treatment, or that minority patients will not comply with treatment regimens? Stereotypes may also reflect well-meaning, but nonetheless harmful judgments on the part of healthcare providers. For example, physicians may be less aggressive in seeking minority patients' consent for certain medical procedures, out of a heightened (but nonetheless stereotyped) concern that minority patients' wishes to avoid aggressive or new healthcare technologies should be respected, or because of a desire to foster a sense of empowerment among minority patients relative to treatment decisions.

A general issue in the stereotyping literature is the question of whether the stereotypes are "accurate." What if the doctors studied by van Ryn and Burke (2000) are correct in their belief that African Americans are less likely to comply with treatment? If this is true, how can a "stereotype" held by providers be regarded as a "cause" of the disparities? Is it not more correct to say that the provider's belief is the result of racial differences in underlying patterns of health behavior? This important question can be answered at two levels. First, based on the general literature on stereotyping, we would expect that any "true" differences among racial/ethnic groups would tend to be exaggerated, particularly if the belief is negative. This "exaggeration of negative attributes" would tend to be reinforced through selective attention and recall of stereotype-confirming evidence.

Second, stereotypes can lead to unfavorable treatment of minorities, even when there are no underlying differences in healthcare attitudes of minorities and whites (Balsa and McGuire, 2001a). Providers' expressions of implicit or explicit stereotypes can evoke responses in minority patients that can "cause" the stereotypes to be confirmed. Thus, doctors might believe that "blacks comply less frequently," and this belief might be confirmed in their own experience. Nonetheless, the *cause* of the problem could be the belief itself, in the sense that acting with this belief, doctors may treat African-American patients differently, and this differential (less favorable) treatment may lead African Americans to comply with treatment less frequently. Thus, even without the "exaggeration/bias" feature of stereotyping behavior by the perceiver, stereotyping can persist and be harmful. This can be demonstrated with the tools of game theory (Balsa and McGuire, 2001b) to illustrate that even when two groups (blacks and whites) are objectively identical, a differential belief held by doctors may lead to differential patterns of treatment recommendations and compliance that is rational for all parties, but leads to disparities in treatment. Stereotypes—beliefs held by the doctor—can therefore turn a situation of *a priori* equality into one of *ex post* disparity.

PATIENT RESPONSE: MISTRUST AND REFUSAL

As noted above, racial and ethnic minority patients' responses to healthcare providers are also a potential source of disparities. Little research has been conducted on how patients may influence the clinical encounter. It is reasonable to speculate, however, that if patients convey mistrust, refuse treatment, don't adhere or comply poorly with treatment, providers may become less engaged in the treatment process, and patients are less likely to be provided alternative treatments and services. As noted in Chapter 3, some evidence suggests that patient refusal may contribute to disparities in care. For example, African American and other minority patients may be more likely to refuse invasive procedures. This higher rate of refusal of recommended treatments may reflect patients' experiences of discrimination in other sectors or mistrust of authority. Some mistrust and refusal, however, might be a "rational" reaction to explicit discrimination, aversion, or disregard displayed by the provider. If minority patients perceive that their provider has a lower regard for them, they will be less likely to comply with treatment recommendations.

It should be noted, however, that despite ethnic minority patients' generally higher levels of mistrust of the medical and research establishment, most minority patients appear to be satisfied with and have confidence in their healthcare providers (Shi, 1999). Further, as Geiger (this volume) and others have noted, mistrust or perceived discrimination alone is unlikely to cause ethnic minority patients to reject potentially life-saving or highly recommended procedures that promise to improve health and decrease symptoms of illness. Therefore, future analyses of patient attributes that may be related to healthcare disparities must carefully consider the roots of these attitudes in historic and contemporary social and cultural forces, in and outside medical practice, that play a role in minority patients' perceptions of healthcare institutions.

In the absence of careful study as to how patients may influence the clinical encounter and contribute to disparities in healthcare, the committee is reluctant to speculate on how and to what extent such processes occur. It may be reasonable to assume, however, that patients' and providers' behavior and attitudes influence each other reciprocally and reflect the attitudes, expectations, and perceptions that each has developed in a context where race and ethnicity are often more salient than these participants recognize. In addition, it is clear that the healthcare provider, rather than the patient, is the more powerful actor in clinical encounters. Providers' expectations, beliefs, attitudes, and behaviors are therefore likely to be a more important target for intervention efforts.

CONCLUSION

In the previous sections, we have considered factors arising out of doctor-patient interactions that may account, at least in part, for racial and ethnic disparities in healthcare. The committee's focus has been on understanding the *processes* that may underlie these biases. We propose that these processes have their origins in pervasive and normal distinctions based in social categorization (stereotypes, prejudice, and uncertainties in intergroup communication) and do not necessarily involve either awareness or conscious motivations to discriminate. Thus, even highly educated and socially conscious individuals, such as doctors, are susceptible to these biases. Moreover, the types of situations that promote these biases—time pressure, incomplete information, high demand on attention and cognitive resources—are those that frequently occur in the context of doctor-patient interactions. We supported these propositions with research and illustrated their likely effects.

Beyond identifying the pervasiveness and importance of these factors in healthcare outcomes, this perspective emphasizes two other fundamental issues. First, this approach highlights the fact that disparities in healthcare services may not necessarily be a matter of "less." Within the models of bias, with the exception of the simple prejudice mechanism, the implications of the other mechanisms may be more or less in terms of quality of services. The importance of disparities in services is that minorities may have healthcare services poorly matched to their needs. A focus on the issue of matching needs to services is a more general and pertinent framework than simply focusing on equal amounts of services.

A second implication of this perspective is that it suggests different types of policies and interventions to address disparities based on different processes. The research on healthcare disparities to date does not consistently differentiate among the various mechanisms that may operate in doctor-patient interactions and underlie the disparities. At a general level, making good choices about alleviating disparities should be based on a good idea as to what causes disparities.

In summary, the committee found no direct evidence that racism, bias, or prejudice among healthcare professionals affects the quality of care for minority patients, such as that which might be available from audit studies where "testers" from different racial or ethnic groups present in clinical settings with similar clinical complaints, histories, and symptoms to assess possible differences in the quality of their treatment. In addition, no survey data suggest that even a small minority of physicians, nurses, or other healthcare professionals harbors biases or prejudices against minorities. Both of these forms of evidence present methodologic (and in the case of paired testers, ethical and legal) challenges to investigators, making it unlikely that such evidence will be available in the near future.

In the meantime, the committee is confronted with several "streams" of evidence that, while not definitive, collectively provide a sufficient base from which to draw inferences. To summarize the evidence presented in this chapter and the previous two chapters that provider prejudice, stereotyping, and biases may influence clinical care:

1. With increasing sophistication, several recent studies of racial and ethnic disparities in receipt of health services have controlled for possible confounding variables or other possible explanations for racial and ethnic differences in care, including patient preferences, overuse of services by whites, health insurance status, type of health system, patient income and education, severity or stage of disease, co-morbidity, hospital type, and

resources. These studies generally find that disparities remain and cannot be fully explained by these variables. While this literature does not provide any measure of evidence that provider biases and stereotyping explain disparities, they do illustrate that disparities cannot be "reduced" to patients' preferences or other explanations.

2. Racial and ethnic disparities in healthcare emerge from an historic context in which healthcare has been differentially allocated on the basis of social class, race, and ethnicity. Unfortunately, despite public laws and sentiment to the contrary, vestiges of this history remain and negatively affect the current context of healthcare delivery. And despite the considerable economic, social, and political progress of racial and ethnic minorities, evidence of racism and discrimination remain in many sectors of American life.

3. Evidence from patient surveys indicates that racial and ethnic minority patients are far more likely than white patients to believe that discrimination is a problem in healthcare, and that they have personally experienced discriminatory treatment. Data from the focus groups conducted by the study committee suggest that minority patients may perceive both overt, as well as subtle forms of discrimination when seeking care.

4. There is considerable evidence that even well-meaning whites who are not overtly biased and who do not believe that they are prejudiced typically demonstrate, on average, unconscious implicit negative racial attitudes and stereotypes (e.g., Dovidio, Brigham, Johnson, and Gaertner, 1996). Both implicit and explicit stereotypes significantly shape interpersonal interactions, influencing how information is recalled and guiding expectations and inferences in systematic ways. They also can produce self-fulfilling prophecies in social interactions, in which the stereotypes of the perceiver influence the interaction with others in ways that conform to stereotypical expectations (e.g., Jussim, 1991).

5. Experimental evidence indicates that healthcare providers are influenced by patients' race or ethnicity, and possibly gender (Schulman et al., 1999; Weisse et al., 2001), or when providers are "primed" with racial stereotypes (Abreu, 1999). Preliminary evidence also suggests that female physicians may respond to racial cues differently than male physicians (Weisse et al., 2001; Rathore et al., 2000). Minority race or ethnicity is found to be associated with generally more negative evaluations or lower rates of referral for clinical services, even when "patients" present with the same clinical condition. In addition, a survey of physicians following actual clinical encounters demonstrates that physicians endorse stereotypes about their African-American patients (who were characterized as "less intelligent, less educated, more likely to abuse drugs and alcohol, more likely to fail to comply with medical advice," and less likely "to be . . . the kind of person the physician could see him/herself being

friends with"), even after controlling for patients' socioeconomic status, personality variables, and perceived social support (van Ryn and Burke, 2000).

6. The conditions in which many medical encounters take place—characterized by time pressure, resource constraints, and high cognitive demand—have been identified in the social psychological literature as conditions that may promote stereotyping due to the need for cognitive "shortcuts" and lack of full information to adequately assess patients.

These streams of evidence lead the committee to conclude that bias, stereotyping, prejudice, and uncertainty on the part of healthcare professionals cannot be ruled out—and indeed, appear among the many patient-level, system-level, and clinical encounter-level factors to contribute to racial and ethnic disparities in healthcare.

> **Finding 4-1: Bias, stereotyping, prejudice, and clinical uncertainty on the part of healthcare providers may contribute to racial and ethnic disparities in healthcare.** While indirect evidence from several lines of research supports this statement, a greater understanding of the prevalence and influence of these processes is needed and should be sought through research.
>
> Indirect evidence indicates that bias, stereotyping, prejudice, and clinical uncertainty on the part of healthcare providers may be contributory factors to racial and ethnic disparities in healthcare. Prejudice may stem from conscious bias, while stereotyping and biases may be conscious or unconscious, even among the well intentioned. Ambiguities in the interpretation of clinical data, barriers to patient-provider communication, and gaps in evidence of the efficacy of clinical interventions contribute to uncertainty, and therefore may promote the activation of prejudice and stereotypes. However, few studies have attempted to assess these mechanisms, and therefore direct evidence bearing on the possible role of these factors, especially prejudice, is not yet available. The committee finds strong, but circumstantial evidence for the role of bias, stereotyping, prejudice, and clinical uncertainty from a range of sources, including studies of social cognition and "implicit" stereotyping, but urges more research to identify how and when these processes occur.

Patients' refusal or acceptance of recommendations for treatment, like other patient decisions, is the result of many influences, including information about their condition, information about treatment effectiveness and risks, trust of the clinician, preferences for treatment type and outcome, and advice of significant others. Overall, such preferences for care should be developed by patients and their families on the basis of full and accurate information presented by a healthcare provider, but the acquisition and use of such information may be influenced by the quality of patient-provider communication and interaction, patients' expectations, values and beliefs, as well as the values and beliefs of patients' communities. To the extent that minority patients are more likely than whites to refuse treatment, such behaviorally expressed preferences may be considered a source of healthcare disparities. A small number of studies suggest that racial and ethnic minorities are slightly more likely than whites to refuse treatment, but this research has yet to distinguish the sources of minority patients' higher rates of refusal (i.e., general mistrust of healthcare providers, real or perceived experiences of discrimination in healthcare settings, or patient treatment decisions based on incomplete information from providers). These sources must be better understood to fully understand the role of patient preferences in healthcare disparities.

Finding 4-2: A small number of studies suggest that racial and ethnic minority patients are more likely than white patients to refuse treatment. These studies find that differences in refusal rates are generally small and that minority patient refusal does not fully explain healthcare disparities.
A small number of studies suggest that racial and ethnic minorities are more likely to refuse treatment. These studies find that differences in refusal rates are generally small and that minority patient refusal does not fully explain healthcare disparities. However, research has yet to distinguish the sources of minority patients' higher rates of refusal (i.e., general mistrust of healthcare providers, real or perceived experiences of discrimination in healthcare settings, or patient treatment decisions based on incomplete information from providers). These sources must be better understood to fully comprehend the role of patient preferences in healthcare disparities.

5

Interventions: Systemic Strategies

The preceding analysis of sources of racial and ethnic disparities in healthcare reveals that many participants—including patients, their providers, utilization managers, and health system administrators—make decisions on a daily basis that contribute to gaps in care. These individuals operate within many contexts, including clinical care settings and health system settings that set policies for access to and utilization of services, and at a larger level, are affected by laws and policies regulating the healthcare industry. Given the role of patient, provider, and contextual factors in shaping the quality of patient care, systemic interventions directed at multiple levels offer promise to modify conditions in which healthcare disparities occur.

Systemic interventions to improve healthcare delivery for diverse populations include organizational accommodations that may promote equity in healthcare, policies that reduce administrative and linguistic barriers to care, and practices that enhance patients' knowledge of and roles as active participants in the care process. These efforts are likely to be most effective when applied in a systematic, simultaneous, multi-level, coordinated fashion, and follow a well-developed strategic plan that has support and "buy-in" from all actors involved in healthcare, including patients, their families, and the communities in which they live; clinicians; administrative staff; and health systems leadership. Systemic interventions also include changes to healthcare law and policy that promote equality of healthcare delivery.

There are many reasons why health systems may choose to adopt comprehensive strategies to eliminate racial and ethnic disparities in healthcare. First, they may react to comply with growing state and federal guidelines that encourage, and in some cases, mandate greater responsiveness on the part of health systems to the growing diversity of the U.S. population (Brach and Fraser, 2000). Second, they may view such strategies as integral to help achieve the U.S. Department of Health and Human Services' goal of eliminating racial and ethnic disparities in health (U.S. DHHS, 2000). Third, health systems may find that developing and implementing culturally competent systems of care are consistent with the "business case" of increasing market share among racial and ethnic minority populations (Brach and Fraser, 2000). Increasingly, health plan purchasers are also finding that health system responsiveness to the needs of racial and ethnic minority patients makes good business sense. Given that over 2 of every 5 new workers is a racial or ethnic minority, many employers find that health plan efforts to improve services for these populations and narrow the healthcare gap can attract better workers and increase employee productivity (Washington Business Group on Health, 2001).

Many of these system-wide intervention objectives are reflected in the culturally and linguistically appropriate services standards (CLAS) for healthcare issued by the U.S. DHHS Office of Minority Health (OMH) in December 2000 (U.S. DHHS, 2000). These standards, which are listed in Box 5-1, are primarily directed at healthcare organizations, but OMH encourages individual providers to familiarize themselves with the standards and incorporate them into their practices.

Further, while the standards are intended to help improve care for racial and ethnic minority populations, by implication they suggest that greater attention to the importance of culture and language in healthcare settings will improve the quality of care for all populations. Noting that culture and language define how healthcare information is given and received and shape the expression and understanding of health and illness, the agency states that "healthcare is a cultural construct, arising from beliefs about the nature of disease and the human body," and that "cultural issues are . . . central in the delivery of health services treatment and preventive interventions" (U.S. DHHS, 2000, p. 80863).

A significant evidence base has accumulated for many aspects of health systems-level interventions that may improve the quality of care for minority patients. The remainder of this chapter explores several such strategies.

LEGAL, REGULATORY, AND POLICY INTERVENTIONS

As noted in Chapter 3, institutional design and legal and regulatory governance will not eliminate racial and ethnic disparities in healthcare,

BOX 5-1
U.S. Department of Health and Human Services Standards for
Culturally and Linguistically Appropriate Services

1. Healthcare Organizations should ensure that patients/consumers receive from all staff members effective, understandable, and respectful care that is provided in a manner compatible with their cultural health beliefs and practices and preferred language.
2. Healthcare Organizations should implement strategies to recruit, retain, and promote at all levels of the organization a diverse staff and leadership that are representative of the demographic characteristics of the service area.
3. Healthcare Organizations should ensure that staff at all levels and across all disciplines receive ongoing education and training in culturally and linguistically appropriate service delivery.
4. Healthcare Organizations must offer and provide language assistance services, including bilingual staff and interpreter services, at no cost to each patient/consumer with limited English proficiency at all points of contact, in a timely manner during all hours of operation.
5. Healthcare Organizations must provide to patients/consumers in their preferred language both verbal offers and written notices informing them of their right to receive language assistance services.
6. Healthcare Organizations must assure the competence of language assistance provided to limited English proficient patients/consumers by interpreters and bilingual staff. Family and friends should not be used to provide interpretation services (except on request by the patient/consumer).
7. Healthcare Organizations must make available easily understood patient-related materials and post signage in the languages of the commonly encountered groups and/or groups represented in the service area.

but institutions and law make a large difference, in that they exert a broad influence over the kinds of conditions that may foster healthcare disparities. In this section, the committee suggests how healthcare institutions, legislators, and regulators might respond pragmatically to the problem of racial and ethnic disparity even as they pursue other important policy goals.

"De-Fragmentation" of Healthcare Financing and Delivery

Many of the studies cited earlier in this report have not taken detailed account of variations among health plans, and therefore the dispropor-

8. Healthcare Organizations should develop, implement, and promote a written strategic plan that outlines clear goals, policies, operational plans, and management accountability/oversight mechanisms to provide culturally and linguistically appropriate services.
9. Healthcare Organizations should conduct initial and ongoing organizational self-assessments of CLAS-related activities and are encouraged to integrate cultural and linguistic competence-related measures into their internal audits, performance improvement programs, patient satisfaction assessments, and outcomes-based evaluations.
10. Healthcare Organizations should ensure that data on the individual patient's/consumer's race, ethnicity, and spoken and written language are collected in health records, integrated into the organization's management information systems, and periodically updated.
11. Healthcare Organizations should maintain a current demographic, cultural, and epidemiologic profile of the community as well as a needs assessment to accurately plan for and implement services that respond to the cultural and linguistic characteristics of the service area.
12. Healthcare Organizations should develop participatory, collaborative partnerships with communities and utilize a variety of formal and informal mechanisms to facilitate community and patient/consumer involvement in designing and implementing CLAS-related activities.
13. Healthcare Organizations should ensure that conflict and grievance resolution processes are culturally and linguistically sensitive and capable of identifying, preventing, and resolving cross-cultural conflicts or complaints by patients/consumers.
14. Healthcare Organizations are encouraged to regularly make available to the public information about their progress and successful innovations in implementing the CLAS standards and to provide public notice in their communities about the availability of this information.

tionate presence of members of disadvantaged minority groups in lower-end health plans may be a major source of disparities in healthcare provision. As noted in Chapter 2, some racial and ethnic minorities are disproportionately represented in publicly financed health insurance programs (Phillips et al., 2000). And even within a broad federal program such as Medicare, for example, tiers of health systems exist (e.g., more than 60% of Medicare beneficiaries possess supplemental coverage), with minorities typically congregated at lower levels. Further, as noted in Chapter 3, low per capita resources associated with lower-end plans may result in differences in the intensity of care between lower and higher end health plans. Studies consistently demonstrate an association between insurance status and use of healthcare resources. For example, patients seen in emergency departments following head injury are more likely to be admitted to the hospital and have a longer length of stay if they are privately insured, rather than publicly insured or uninsured (Svenson and Spurlock, 2001), and Medicare patients without supplemental coverage are approximately 10% less likely to have influenza vaccination, cholesterol testing, mammography, or Pap smears than those with supplemental coverage (Carrasquillo, Lantigua, and Shea, 2001). Fragmentation also engenders different clinical cultures, with different practice norms, tied to varying per capita resource constraints. The relationship between racial and ethnic maldistribution in tiered health plans, differences in the intensity and the quality of care provided by these plans, and clinical outcomes should be a national research priority (see Chapter 8). Until such research is conducted, it is reasonable to surmise that efforts to reduce the socioeconomic segmentation of the medical marketplace would help to diminish racial and ethnic disparities in healthcare provision (Bloche, 2001).

Equalizing access to high-quality plans can limit fragmentation. Public healthcare payors such as Medicaid should strive to help beneficiaries access the same health products as privately insured patients. This recommendation is reflected in the IOM *Crossing the Quality Chasm* report's strategies for focusing health systems on quality, in its call to "eliminate or modify payment practices that fragment the care system" (IOM, 2001a, p. 13). Expanding access for publicly funded beneficiaries to high-quality health plans will be expensive. Rising healthcare costs, however, threaten to increase the likelihood of fragmentation, and subsequently threaten to increase the racial and ethnic gap in healthcare.

Recommendation 5-1: Avoid fragmentation of health plans along socioeconomic lines.
Medical care financing arrangements should discourage fragmentation of healthcare provision into separate tiers of providers who adhere to different standards of care and disproportionately serve separate racial and ethnic minority segments of American society. Medicaid and other government programs that mandate enrollment of beneficiaries in managed care should be prepared to pay plans at rates that give Medicaid enrollees access to the same health plan products serving substantial proportions of privately insured patients.

Strengthening Doctor-Patient Relationships

Several lines of research suggest that the consistency and stability of the doctor-patient relationship is an important determinant of patient satisfaction and access to care. Having a usual source of care is associated, for example, with use of preventive care services. In addition, having a consistent relationship with a primary care provider may help to address minority patient mistrust of healthcare systems and providers, particularly if the relationship is with a provider who is able to bridge cultural and linguistic gaps (LaViest, Nickerson, and Bowie, 2000). Further, as noted in Chapter 3, several lines of evidence suggest that a patient's access to clinical resources within a hospital or health plan may partly reflect his or her doctor's stature, skill, and commitment as an advocate. This suggests that minority patients may benefit from stronger bonds with physicians who understand the cultural and linguistic barriers to care faced by many minority patients navigating through health systems, and who are positioned and willing to play the advocate's role vigorously. Health systems should attempt to ensure that every patient, whether insured privately or publicly, through Medicare or Medicaid, has a sustained relationship with an attending physician able to help patients navigate the healthcare bureaucracy effectively (e.g., to help patients obtain referral and secure appropriate specialty care). This is not meant to imply that physicians should navigate health systems for their patients; rather, it is an acknowledgement that primary care providers sometimes wield great influence and leverage in helping their patients to access specialty care, clinical trials, and other healthcare resources.

Several strategies can help to promote the stability of patient and provider relationships in publicly funded health plans. Federal and state performance standards for Medicaid-managed care plans, for example, should include guidelines for the stability of patients' assignments to primary care providers and these providers' accessibility. These guidelines should also encourage reasonable patient loads per primary physician and time allotments for patient visits. Regulations governing health plans' participation in Medicare should include similar guidelines, as should private accrediting bodies' prerequisites for all health plans (Bloche, 2001).

Recommendation 5-2: Strengthen the stability of patient-provider relationships in publicly funded health plans.
Policies that strengthen provider-patient relationships in publicly funded health plans and that promote the consistency of these relationships should be adopted. These include guidelines for:
• **the stability of patients' assignments to primary care providers and these providers' accessibility;**
• **reasonable patient loads per primary physician; and**
• **reasonable time allowances for initial and follow-up patient visits (and health providers' flexibility to take additional time when needed to communicate adequately).**

Strengthening patient and provider relationships will also benefit from greater racial and ethnic diversity in the health professions. Racial concordance of patient and provider is associated with greater patient participation in care processes, higher patient satisfaction, and greater adherence to treatment (Cooper-Patrick et al., 1999). In addition, racial and ethnic minority providers are more likely than their non-minority colleagues to serve in minority and medically underserved communities (Komaromy et al., 1998b). Evidence of these benefits of diversity in health professions fields weighs in favor of robust commitment to affirmative action in medical school admissions, residency recruitment, and professional specialty training. This is not intended to suggest, however, that racial concordance of patients and providers should be encouraged as a matter of policy. Rather, it is expected that the benefits of diversity in the health professions will accrue broadly, as this diversity helps to expand the disciplines' ability to conceptualize and respond to the health needs of increasingly culturally and linguistically diverse populations.

Recommendation 5-3: Increase the proportion of underrepresented U.S. racial and ethnic minorities among health professionals.
To the extent legally permissible, affirmative action and other efforts are needed to increase the proportion of underrepresented U.S. racial and ethnic minorities among health professionals.

Patient Protections

Much of the political focus on Capitol Hill in the summer of 2001 was devoted to managed care regulation. To one extent or another, the various bills debated all would extend protections to enrollees in private managed care organizations, providing avenues for appeal of care denial decisions, improving access to specialty and emergency department care, and providing other legal remedies to resolve disputes. These bills were crafted on the assumption that due process protections of patient choices were necessary, despite a lack of empirical evidence that overall quality of care is inferior in managed care plans relative to fee-for-service systems. Extensive reviews of the literature do not establish whether the quality of care provided within managed care plans is worse (or better) than other health systems. However, there is some evidence that managed care may provide better care for some patient populations. For example, results of a review by Miller and Luft (1997) suggest a significantly better quality of care for some subsets of managed care enrollees, such as patients in the intensive care unit, elderly Medicare patients, and patients with acute appendicitis or cancer.

As discussed in Chapter 3, however, there are reasons and empirical evidence to be concerned about how financial incentives and decision-making within managed health plans may differentially affect racial and ethnic minority groups. Some evidence indicates that low-income and ethnic minority patients enrolled in managed care plans are less likely to have a regular provider than similar patients in fee-for-service plans (Leigh, Lillie-Blanton, Martinez, and Collins, 1999), are more likely than whites to be denied claims for emergency department visits (Lowe et al., 2001), and are less satisfied with many aspects of the care they receive in managed care settings (Phillips et al., 2000). Other studies find that the intensity of care is lower for some populations within managed care settings relative to other care systems. Tai-Seale, LoSasso, Freund, and Gerber (2001), for example, found that prenatal care use was lower among women enrolled in Medicaid managed care systems relative to women in fee-for-service systems.

Given that many minorities are disproportionately represented among the publicly insured who receive care within managed care organizations, extending the same due process protections proposed in current legislation may help to address these disparities. Other factors, however, may also justify extending the same protections, regardless of payor source. Extending legal protections only to those enrolled in private managed care plans raises concerns about the unequal application of law. As Hashimoto (2001) writes, "The [current proposals'] emphasis on individual choice, due process protections, and limiting its jurisdiction to private health plans will result in an important regulation that largely benefits the employed middle class . . . it is unfair to guarantee special legal protections to members of private managed care plans while failing to provide these same guarantees to members of publicly financed managed care programs" (Hashimoto, 2001, pp. 83-84).

Recommendation 5-4: Apply the same managed care protections to publicly funded HMO enrollees that apply to private HMO enrollees.

Civil Rights Enforcement

The committee believes that education and training of healthcare providers, administrators, and consumers is an important first step as part of a comprehensive, multi-level intervention strategy to address racial and ethnic disparities in healthcare. Enforcement of regulation and statute is also an important component of such a strategy, but unfortunately has been too often relegated to low-priority status. The U.S. DHHS Office for Civil Rights (OCR) is charged with enforcing several relevant federal statutes and regulations that prohibit discrimination in healthcare (principally

Title VI of the 1964 Civil Rights Act). The agency, however, has suffered from insufficient resources to investigate complaints of possible violations, and has long abandoned proactive, investigative strategies (Smith, 1999). Complaints to the agency have increased in recent years, while funding has remained constant in actual dollars but has decreased in fiscal year 2000 to less than 60% of fiscal year 1981 funding, after adjusting for inflation (U.S. Commission on Civil Rights, 2001). This decrease in spending power has severely and negatively affected OCR's ability to conduct civil rights enforcement strategies, such as on-site complaint investigations, compliance reviews, and local community outreach and education. The agency should be equipped with sufficient resources to better address these complaints. In addition, OCR should resume the practice of periodic, proactive investigation, both to collect data on the extent of civil rights violations and to provide a deterrent to would-be lawbreakers. As will be discussed in Chapter 7, LaVeist and Gibbons (2001) suggest a two-tiered strategy in which routine data collection and monitoring can be used to identify health systems that display persistent disparities, followed by field investigations—possibly by trained, paired testers.[1] While audits of healthcare facilities are largely untested and methodologies must be developed for fair and appropriate assessment of discrimination in healthcare settings, such a strategy offers a promising "last line" of defense against civil rights violations.

Recommendation 5-5: Provide greater resources to the U.S. DHHS Office for Civil Rights to enforce civil rights laws.
Congress and the U.S. Department of Health and Human Services should provide adequate funding to the U.S. DHHS Office for Civil Rights to expand the agency's capabilities to address civil rights complaints and carry out its oversight responsibilities.

HEALTH SYSTEMS INTERVENTIONS

Research suggests that a variety of interventions applied at the level of health systems may be effective as a part of a comprehensive, multi-level strategy to address racial and ethnic disparities in healthcare.

---

[1] Paired testing strategies, in which auditors of differing race, ethnicity, or gender are matched for a variety of socioeconomic and personality characteristics, have been used successfully to identify discrimination in housing, employment, and mortgage lending practices. This strategy is discussed in Chapter 2.

Evidence-Based Cost Control

As discussed in Chapter 3, medical science has made tremendous advances that have transformed clinical practice. Many innovations are available to healthcare providers, and the use of evidence-based practice guidelines to improve and standardize care has increased. Despite these developments, variations in practice patterns are still observed across geographic areas and types of healthcare institutions, and utilization managers still exert considerable discretion in making decisions regarding healthcare resource allocation. To the extent possible, given the gaps in knowledge about medical care's efficacy and the difficulty of anticipating all clinical contingencies, clinical practice and utilization decisions should be based on evidence-based guidelines. Such application of evidence to healthcare delivery can help to address the problem of potential underuse of services resulting from capitation or per case payment methods, as noted in the IOM *Quality Chasm* report (IOM, 2001a). Practice guidelines may be a useful tool in the effort to eliminate racial and ethnic disparities in healthcare, given the advantages of guidelines over general, discretionary standards—including consistency, predictability, and at least the appearance of objectivity.

A pragmatic balance must be sought, however, between the advantages and limitations of guidelines. The goal of standardized care must be weighed against the need for clinical flexibility. One means to address this balance—disclosing health plans' clinical protocols—would aid both private sector and public efforts in balancing the virtues of rules and discretion. Private accrediting entities and state regulatory bodies could require that health plans' clinical practice protocols be published—with supporting evidence—and thus open them to professional and consumer review.

Clinical guidelines that are not backed by evidence and argument should not be entitled to deference in administrative or legal proceedings that involve challenges to health plans' application of such guidelines. But where guidelines do have empirical support, even if the evidence is at best debatable, administrative and legal decision makers should give substantial weight to the social importance, in a racially and culturally diverse nation, of making allocative choices in a manner that achieves some consistency in appearance and practice (Bloche, 2001).

Recommendation 5-6: Promote the consistency and equity of care through evidence-based guidelines.
To the extent possible, medical care allocative decisions should be driven by evidence-based clinical guidelines to insure consistency of care. These guidelines should be published, along with their supporting evidence base, to allow public and professional scru-

tiny, and used to examine the quality of care for racial and ethnic minorities.

Financial Incentives in Healthcare

As discussed in Chapter 3, financial factors, such as capitation and plan incentives to providers to practice frugally, can pose greater barriers to racial and ethnic minority patients than for whites, even among patients insured at the same level. Low payment rates inhibit the supply of physician (and other healthcare provider) services to low-income groups, disproportionately affecting ethnic minorities. Inadequate supply takes the form of too few providers participating in plans serving the poor, and provider unwillingness to spend adequate time with patients. In Chapter 4, the committee linked this time pressure to the underlying problem of poor information exchange between physicians and members of minority groups. Where employers have an interest in providing an attractive benefit package, market forces protect middle and upper income groups against health plans "going too far" in rationing care. These protections are not available to all low-income groups, who must rely on balanced public policy to induce adequate supply of care.

More finely crafted provider incentives can have a positive role in efforts to reduce disparities in care. Greater economic rewards for time spent engaging patients and their families can contribute to overcoming barriers of culture, communication, and empathy. Payment schemes that reward providers for high scores on measures of patient satisfaction would further encourage the bridging of barriers related to racial and ethnic difference. Incentives to adhere to evidence-based protocols for frugal practice and to engage in age- and gender-appropriate disease screening would generally encourage efficient, quality care and penalize deviations regardless of race or ethnicity. Further, payment linked to favorable clinical outcomes, where reasonably measurable (e.g. control of diabetes, asthma, and high blood pressure), would provide additional such encouragement. Industry movement toward more nuanced incentive schemes along these lines could be catalyzed by private accrediting bodies, encouraged by business and professional leaders, and even initiated by public payors. Again, this recommendation is consistent with the IOM *Quality Chasm* report, which called for healthcare organizations, clinicians, purchasers, and other stakeholders to "align the incentives inherent in payment and accountability processes with the goal of quality improvement" (IOM, 2001a, p. 10).

Recommendation 5-7: Structure payment systems to enhance available services to minority patients, and limit provider incentives that may promote disparities.

Payment systems to providers should ensure an adequate supply of services to racial and ethnic minority patients. Financial incentives to restrict care and pass liability to providers should be limited, to reduce conditions in which racial and ethnic stereotypes and biases may be exacerbated or reinforced.

Recommendation 5-8: Enhance patient-provider communication and trust by providing financial incentives for practices that reduce barriers and encourage evidence-based practice.
Economic incentives should be considered for practices that enhance provider-patient communication and trust, and that reward appropriate screening, preventive, and evidence-based clinical care.

Interpretation Services

As noted in Chapter 2, nearly 14 million Americans are not proficient in English. In 1995, the Commonwealth Fund estimated that language differences are problematic for 21% of racial and ethnic minority group members who receive healthcare (Commonwealth, 1995). This percentage is almost certainly higher today given recent increases in immigration to the U.S. from many parts of the world. Language barriers may affect the delivery of adequate care through poor exchange of information, loss of important cultural information, misunderstanding of physician instruction, poor shared decision-making, and ethical compromises, such as difficulty obtaining informed consent (Woloshin et al., 1995). In addition, low English reading proficiency may disproportionately and negatively affect many racial and ethnic minority patients' ability to read and understand written material from health plans and healthcare providers if appropriate translation is not provided. As discussed in Chapter 3, there is significant evidence that language affects variables such as follow-up compliance and satisfaction with services (Carrasquillo et al., 1999). Linguistic difficulties may present a barrier to the use of healthcare services (Derose and Baker, 2000), decrease adherence with medication regimes and appointment attendance (Manson, 1988), and decrease satisfaction with services (Carrasquillo et al., 1999; David and Rhee, 1998). For example, a recent survey of Spanish-speaking Latinos and English speakers of varying ethnicities who used emergency department services found that among patients who reported at least one physician visit in the previous three months, Latinos with fair or poor English proficiency reported 22% fewer visits than English-speaking non-Latinos, after controlling for reason for the visit (Derose and Baker, 2000). These associations were similar for patients in poor health, those with no usual source of care, and those without insurance. Other investigators have found independent effects of language concordance on health outcomes, such that having a physician who spoke Spanish resulted in higher ratings of physical and psychological well being, higher health perceptions, and lower perceptions of pain (Perez-Stable, Napoles-Springer, and Miramontes, 1997).

A few studies examining the effectiveness of interpretation services have been conducted, with mixed results. Although mostly uncontrolled, some studies suggest that the use of interpreters for patients with limited English skills results in greater satisfaction (as compared to patients who said an interpreter should have been used; Baker, Hayes, and Fortier, 1998) and better medical outcomes (Tocher and Larson, 1998). However, in the investigation by Baker and colleagues (1998), while patients who used interpretation services rated their care as better than patients who would have liked services and did not receive them, they still rated their provider as less friendly, less respectful, less concerned, and felt less comfortable than patients who did not need an interpreter. These results suggest that interpretation services are necessary, but that both interpreters and providers should be aware that the mere availability of the service may not be adequate to improve satisfaction and outcomes. It has also been suggested that the use of remote language services, in which the interpreter is not physically in the room, may be preferable (for both patients and providers) to in-person interpretation services (Hornberger et al., 1996). While outcomes are somewhat variable, it is generally agreed that professional interpreters are necessary for many patients and that the use of family members, minors, or friends should be avoided as it may represent a breach of confidentiality, inhibit the patient from fully expressing symptoms or difficulties, or lead to errors in transmitting medical information.

The importance of interpretation services is underscored in guidelines offered by the Office for Civil Rights of the Department of Health and Human Services (U.S. DHHS) to prevent discrimination against limited-English proficient persons (U.S. DHHS, 2000). These guidelines pertain to any entity that receives direct or indirect financial assistance from HHS. Four key elements for compliance with the guidelines include: an assessment of the needs of the population; comprehensive written policies on language access (including hiring of bilingual staff and interpreters, arranging for telephone interpreters); training of staff; and monitoring of programs to ensure people with limited English proficiency are adequately served. Further, if the covered entity/agency suggests, requires, or encourages the use family members, minors, or friends as interpreters, it may expose them to liability under Title VI. Similarly, as noted above, the Office of Minority Health's national standards on culturally and linguistically appropriate services (CLAS) in healthcare also emphasize the importance of language access services.

An important issue for future consideration is the establishment of minimum standards for training of translators and interpreters. Significantly, the U.S. DHHS and some accreditation bodies are beginning to assess the feasibility of establishing minimum standards for interpreters and interpretation services. Selected federal laws and regulations, such as the Disadvantaged Minority Health Improvement Act, require the development of interpreter programs to increase the access of limited English proficient individuals to healthcare services. In addition, associations such as the Massachusetts Medical Interpreter Association (MMIA) in conjunction with Education Development Center, Inc., have published standards of practice focused on areas of interpretation, cultural interface, and ethical behavior. The recently established National Council on Interpretation in Healthcare has charged its Standards, Training and Certification (STC) Committee to draft standards, recommendations and informational materials concerning the interpreter role and performance as well as interpreter services and programs of interpreter education and assessment. Similarly, the California Healthcare Interpreters Association (CHIA) has recently released draft standards of ethical principles, protocols, and guidance for healthcare interpreters within the state.

Finding 5-1: As a result of the increasing linguistic diversity in the United States, professional interpretation services are increasingly needed to assist low-English proficient racial and ethnic minority patients in healthcare settings.

Recommendation 5-9: Support the use of interpretation services where community need exists.
Professional interpretation services should be the standard where language discordance poses a barrier to care. Greater resources should be made available by payors to provide coverage for interpretation services for limited-English proficient patients and their families. Future research should identify best practices where the availability of interpretation services is limited.

Community Health Workers

Community health workers have been acknowledged participants in healthcare systems since the 1960s (Witmer et al., 1995). These individuals, often termed lay health advisors, neighborhood workers, indigenous health workers, health aids, consejera, or promotora, fulfill multiple functions in helping to improve health outcomes. They have been defined as being "community members who work almost exclusively in community settings and who serve as connectors between healthcare consumers and providers to promote health among groups that have traditionally lacked access to adequate care" (Witmer et al., 1995). The training of lay health workers varies and typically depends on the nature of services they will provide. Generally, the length of training varies from a few weeks to six months and includes lectures and supervised practical/field experiences (for review see Jackson and Parks, 1997; Witmer et al., 1995). One of the greatest assets of lay health programs is that they build on the strengths of community ties to help improve outcomes for its citizens.

In addition to increasing access to services, some evidence suggests that lay health workers can help improve the quality of care and reduce costs (Witmer et al., 1995). Lay workers can facilitate community participation in the health system, serve as liaisons between patients and providers, educate providers about community needs and the culture of the community, provide patient education, promote consumer advocacy and protection, contribute to continuity and coordination of care, assist in appointment attendance and adherence to medication regimens, and help to increase the use of preventive and primary care services (Brownstein et al., 1992; Earp and Flax, 1999; Jackson and Parks, 1997). Programs that utilize lay health workers have sought to improve healthcare delivery for a variety of conditions including stroke and hypertension (Richter et al., 1974), breast and cervical cancer screening (Brownstein et al., 1992; Dignan et al., 1998; Earp and Flax, 1999), and the use of prenatal services (Meister et al., 1992). Lay health workers have also been used to address broader issues such as improving healthcare organizations' ability to identify needs of the community (Baker et al., 1997) and improve general wellness through informing community members about resources and facilitating their access to and negotiation through services (Rodney et al., 1998).

During its inception, the concept of using lay health workers included collaborations between lay health workers and public health departments, homeless programs, and community health centers (Richter et al., 1974). More recently, partnerships have been formed with academic medical centers (see for example, Levine et al., 1994). This movement has been accompanied by increased efforts to evaluate the effectiveness of lay workers in improving patient satisfaction and increased use of services. Results indicate that use of lay health workers can increase awareness of and screening for breast cancer (Bird et al., 1998; Navarro et al., 1998; Slater et al., 1998) and cervical cancer (Bird et al., 1998; Dignan et al., 1998; Navarro et al., 1998). For example, among a population of Vietnamese-American women in California, the use of lay health workers significantly increased women's awareness of and utilization of Pap smear and mammography (Bird et al., 1998). The use of lay health workers in a diabetes education program improved completion, regardless of financial status or language spoken, over conducting the education program without lay health workers (Corkery et al., 1997). However, the health workers did not have a significant effect on diabetes knowledge, self-care behavior, or glycemic control, although the small sample size ($n = 64$) may have limited the investigators' ability to find statistically significant relationships with these outcomes.

In order for community health worker programs to be successful, they must be designed properly and workers must be adequately trained and supervised. Barriers to their effective use have included a lack of consistent, widely accepted definition of who they are and what services they can provide (e.g., scope of practice, qualifications), lack of consideration by degreed health professionals for their services, and lack of consistent funding for lay health programs (Witmer et al., 1995). Some literature provides guidance regarding the design of community health worker programs (Brownstein et al., 1992; Giblin, 1989; Jackson and Parks, 1997; Richter et al., 1974; Witmer et al., 1995), but rigorous evaluations of specific program components and their impact on service utilization are needed.

Finding 5-2: Community health workers offer promise as a community-based resource to increase racial and ethnic minorities' access to heathcare and to serve as a liaison between healthcare providers and the communities they serve.

Recommendation 5-10: Support the use of community health workers. Programs to support the use of community health workers (e.g., as healthcare navigators), especially among medically underserved and racial and ethnic minority populations, should be expanded, evaluated, and replicated.

Multidisciplinary Teams

Research demonstrates that multidisciplinary team approaches—utilizing physicians, nurses, dietitians, and others—have proven effective in optimizing risk reduction strategies. This effect is found in randomized controlled studies for patients with coronary heart disease (Multiple Risk Factor Intervention Trial Research Group, 1982), hypertension (Hypertension Detection and Follow-up Program Cooperative Group, 1979), and other diseases (SHEP Cooperative Research Group, 1991; Pedersen et al., 1994; Treatment of Mild Hypertension Study Research Group, 1993), and has extended to strategies for reducing risk behaviors such as smoking and sedentary lifestyle and managing obesity (Hill and Miller, 1996). Multidisciplinary teams coordinate and streamline care, enhance patient adherence through follow-up techniques, and address the multiple behavioral and social risks that patients face, particularly racial and ethnic minority patients. They may save costs and improve the efficiency of care by reducing the need for face-to-face physician visits and improve patients' day-to-day care between visits. Further, such strategies have proven effective in improving health outcomes of minorities previously viewed as "difficult to serve" (Hill and Miller, 1996). Multidisciplinary team approaches should be more widely instituted as strategy for improving care delivery, implementing secondary prevention strategies, and enhancing risk reduction.

Recommendation 5-11: Implement multidisciplinary treatment and preventive care teams.
Multidisciplinary teams offer promise as a means to improve and streamline care for racial and ethnic minority patients, and therefore should be more widely implemented.

PATIENT EDUCATION AND EMPOWERMENT

Skill-building and training for providers of healthcare has been a traditional avenue for helping to improve outcomes (see for example Roter and Hall, 1994; Roter et al., 1995; Williams and Deci, 2001), increase patient satisfaction with care (Roter et al., 1996), and decrease the incidence of lawsuits (Levinson et al., 1997; Mock, 2001). However, as issues of improved patient-provider communication/relationship have moved to the forefront, patient education, participation, activation, and empowerment have received more attention. Information that flows in both directions is deemed important for increasing patient cooperation, engagement, and adherence to medical regimes (Korsch, 1994).

Patient education has taken many forms including provision of books, pamphlets, in-person instruction, CD-ROM, and Internet-based information. Books such as that by Korsch and Harding (1998) help guide patients through typical office visits and provide information about asking the right questions, communicating with the provider when instructions are not understood or cannot be followed, and being an active participant in decision making. The guide also helps patients understand the nature of medical training and its impact on provider behavior. Other mediums such as entertainment television (Cooper, Roter, and Langlieb, 2000) and computer-based education programs (McRoy, Liu-Perez, and Ali, 1998) have been initiated. In addition, private and academic institutions offer information systems to assist patients in navigating healthcare systems. For example the Bayer Institute has developed a program called PRE-PARE, a six-step program using a self-administered audiotape and guidebook to help patients prepare for office visits. Complementary materials were also developed for use by providers of healthcare to support and encourage use of the program. In addition, some medical institutions, such as the Ohio State University Medical Center and Cincinnati Children's Hospital Center, have established Internet-based programs to help answer patient questions about topics such as pain management, medications, medical procedures, nutrition, and health promotion.

As patient education approaches become more widely used, efforts to evaluate their effectiveness have increased, and have demonstrated positive results. In one of the earliest papers examining the beneficial effects of patient education, Roter (1977) assessed the effects of a health education intervention to increase patient question-asking during office visits. In this study, which was conducted with an urban and predominantly black population, patients were randomly assigned to intervention and non-intervention groups. There were also two non-randomized control groups. Results indicated that patients in the intervention group asked more direct questions and fewer indirect questions than did non-intervention group patients. However, within the intervention group, there was more negative affect, anxiety, and anger in the patient-provider interaction, while in the placebo group, patient-provider interaction was characterized as mutually sympathetic. In addition, the intervention group patients were less satisfied with care received in the clinic on the day of their visit than were placebo patients, but they demonstrated higher appointment-keeping (accounting for average number of appointments made) during a 4-month prospective monitoring period. These results suggest that efforts directed at increasing patient activation must also target physician behavior and how providers receive and respond to patients' increased participation.

A recently developed CD-ROM reproductive health education program for adolescents with diabetes has been evaluated for its effectiveness in altering knowledge, attitudes, skills, and behaviors. Initial results indicate that the use of the CD-ROM was associated with changes in knowledge, attitudes, and beliefs over the use of a self-instruction packet or standard care. Similarly, an individual education and coaching program in pain self-management for cancer patients was demonstrated to improve ratings of pain severity over patients who did not receive the intervention. However, no changes were observed in functional impairment resulting from pain, frequency of pain, or pain-related knowledge.

In a review article, Roter and colleagues (1998) summarized results of 153 studies evaluating the effectiveness of interventions to improve patient compliance. Many of these studies were patient education-based and included strategies such as individual and group teaching, use of written and audiovisual materials, mailed materials, and telephone instructions. Overall, the most striking results were seen for behavior strategies (e.g., skill building, practice activities, modeling and contracting, rewards, mail and telephone reminders) and those that combined education and behavior strategies. In general, interventions that combined strategies were more successful than single-focus interventions. Significant results, though varied in magnitude, were found for refill records, pill counts, utilization, and improved health outcomes. While most studies cited were not specifically targeted toward communities of color, positive results from patient education programs offer promise for their use with racial and ethnic minority patients. However, it is crucial that interventions be adapted with cultural and linguistic considerations in mind and also address physician responses to their patients' increased activation, to ensure collaborative interactions.

Finding 5-3: Culturally appropriate patient education programs offer promise as an effective means of improving patient participation in clinical decision making and care-seeking skills, knowledge, and self advocacy.

Recommendation 5-12: Implement patient education programs to increase patients' knowledge of how to best access care and participate in treatment decisions.
Culturally appropriate patient education programs tailored to specific racial and ethnic minority populations should be developed, implemented, and evaluated.

6

Interventions: Cross-Cultural Education in the Health Professions

BACKGROUND

The 2000 U.S. Census confirmed what demographers had been predicting all along—our country has become more diverse than ever before (U.S. Census, 2000). Our expansion has been fueled by growth of our minority populations, in addition to significant immigrant influx (Immigration Statistics, 2001). How will the United States respond to this increasing diversity? Ultimately, our success as a nation hinges on how we meet the challenges diversity poses, while capitalizing on the strengths it provides. Many sectors have responded proactively to our demographic evolution, understanding that there are financial and market imperatives to better understanding, communicating, servicing, and partnering with those from diverse backgrounds. This has resulted in major educational efforts, through training and corporate development, as to how better to "manage" diversity at the workplace and in business/service relations (Chin, 2000).

How will one of our largest industries—healthcare—respond? There is a growing literature that delineates the impact of sociocultural factors, race, and ethnicity on clinical care (Berger, 1998; Hill et al., 1990). Clinicians aren't shielded from diversity, as patients present varied perspectives, values, beliefs, and behaviors regarding health and well-being. These include variations in patient recognition of symptoms, thresholds for seeking care, ability to communicate symptoms to a provider who understands their meaning, ability to understand the management strategy, expectations of care (including preferences for or against diagnostic and therapeutic procedures), and adherence to preventive measures and medications (Einbinder and Schulman, 2000; Flores, 2000; Betancourt et al., 1999; Denoba et al., 1998; Gornick, 2000; Coleman-Miller, 2000; Williams and Rucker, 2000).

CROSS-CULTURAL COMMUNICATION: LINKS TO RACIAL/ETHNIC DISPARITIES IN HEALTHCARE

Sociocultural differences between patient and provider influence communication and clinical decision-making (Eisenberg, 1979). Evidence suggests that provider-patient communication is directly linked to patient satisfaction, adherence, and subsequently, health outcomes (Figure 6-1) (Stewart et al., 1999). Thus, when sociocultural differences between patient and provider aren't appreciated, explored, understood, or communicated in the medical encounter, the result is patient dissatisfaction, poor adherence, poorer health outcomes, and racial/ethnic disparities in care (Flores, 2000; Betancourt et al., 1999; Stewart et al., 1999; Morales et al., 1999; Cooper-Patrick et al., 1999; Langer, 1999). And it is not only the patient's culture that matters; the provider "culture" is equally important (Nunez, 2000; Robins et al., 1998b). Historical factors for patient mistrust, provider bias, and its impact on physician decision-making have also been documented (Gamble, 1997; Schulman et al., 1999; van Ryn and Burke, 2000). Failure to take sociocultural factors into account may lead to stereotyping, and in the worst cases, biased or discriminatory treatment of pa-

Evidence Linking Communication to Outcomes

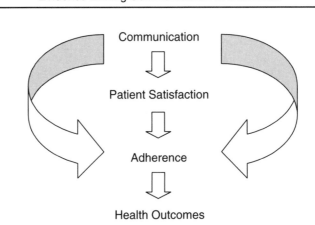

FIGURE 6-1 Evidence linking communication to outcomes.

tients based on race, culture, language proficiency, or social status (Schulman et al., 1999; van Ryn and Burke, 2000; Donini-Lenhoff and Hedrick, 2000). Two studies for physicians highlight these points.

First, Schulman et al. (1999) showed that differential referral to cardiac catheterization was based on race and gender. Second, van Ryn and Burke (2000) illustrated that physicians have different attitudes about patients based on race, as well. Similarly, one study involving 116 nursing students found that negative attitudes about racial/ethnic minorities was related to the absence of prior exposure, suggesting that these issues are not limited to physicians (Eliason, 1998).

THE FOUNDATION AND EMERGENCE OF CROSS-CULTURAL EDUCATION

The meaning of "culture" has been widely debated and broadly defined, with certain common themes emerging. To summarize, culture can be seen as an integrated pattern of learned beliefs and behaviors that can be shared among groups and include thoughts, styles of communicating, ways of interacting, views on roles and relationships, values, practices, and customs (Robins et al., 1998b; Donini-Lenhoff and Hedrick, 2000). Culture shapes how we explain and value our world, and provides us with the lens through which we find meaning (Nunez, 2000). It should not be considered "exotic" or about "others" (Shapiro and Lenahan, 1996; Like et al., 1996), but as part of all of us and our individual influences (including socioeconomic status, religion, gender, sexual orientation, occupation, disability, etc.). We all are influenced by and belong, to multiple cultures that include, but go beyond, race and ethnicity.

Sociocultural factors are critical to the medical encounter, yet cross-cultural curricula have been incorporated into undergraduate, graduate and continued health professions education only to a limited degree (Carrillo et al., 1999). Their goal is to enhance learners' awareness of sociocultural influences on health beliefs and behaviors, and to equip them with skills to understand and manage these factors in the medical encounter (Carrillo et al., 1999; Culhane-Pera et al., 2000; Zweifler and Gonzalez, 1998). This includes understanding population-specific disease prevalence and health outcomes and ethnopharmacology (Lavizzo-Mourey, 1996; Zweifler and Gonzalez, 1998).

Although cross-cultural medicine has gained recent attention, it has been discussed in the literature since the 1960's during the advent of the community health and civil rights movement. There was a clear call then for responsiveness to cultural differences in health attitudes, beliefs, behavior, and language (Chin, 2000). In the 1970's, the seminal work of Kleinman et al. solidified the important link between culture, illness and healthcare (Kleinman et al., 1978). In the 1980's and 1990's, the focus shifted from "cultural sensitivity" to a demand for "cultural competence," a more skill-focused paradigm (Rios and Simpson, 1998; Welch, 1998; Lavizzo-Mourey 1996). Early work in the field is found in the literature of nursing, mental health, and family medicine (Shapiro and Lenahan, 1996; Kai et al., 1999; Kristal et al., 1983). An international interest in the intersection between culture and health has arisen, with work done in Australia, Great Britain, and Canada, among others (Louden et al., 1999).

Looking at undergraduate medical education over this time, we see interesting parallels. Since 1978, four surveys/literature searches have been conducted to determine whether medical schools were teaching cross-cultural issues in their curriculum (Louden et al., 1999; Wyatt et al., 1978; Lum and Korenman, 1994; Flores et al., 2000) (Table 6-1). Although each study was limited by not determining curriculum specifics (whether a course was required, contact hours, approaches, etc.), the trend shows a decrease in specific cross-cultural courses, and an increase in incorporation of these issues into the overall curriculum. This last finding is deceiving, as it's unknown to what extent cross-cultural issues are dealt with in other courses. This could simply mean that there are optional noon lectures or electives that cover cross-cultural issues during some part of the standard health professional academic year. Experts in the field remain skeptical about the results, which show a "mainstreaming" of cross-cultural education, and are concerned about how effectively these issues are addressed during medical education (Kai et al., 1999; Flores et al., 2000). There is no literature to document the extent to which these issues are covered in graduate or continuing medical education for either residents or practicing providers. The literature in nursing education is similarly sparse. Although material related to cultural diversity is considered an

TABLE 6-1 Cross-Cultural Curricula in Undergraduate Medical Education

1978 (Wyatt):
    20% med schools offered specific "sociocultural courses"
    40% covered issues within other courses, 40% offered none
1992(Lum):
    13% offered separate "sociocultural course" (only 1 required)
    60% integrated sociocultural factors into broader curriculum
1998(Flores):
    8% offered separate course
    87% integrated sociocultural factors into curriculum
1999(Loudon)
    17 programs teaching "cultural diversity" identified (US, UK, Canada, Australia).

NOTE: Cultural competence or cross-cultural medicine not used as search terms.

important part of baccalaureate curricula, there is virtually no information published on the extent to which cultural competence is included in undergraduate courses or the specifics of the material that is included (Clinton, 1996; Janes and Hobson, 1998).

Cross-cultural education for health professionals has emerged because of three major factors. First, cross-cultural education has been deemed critical in preparing our providers to meet the health needs of our growing, diverse population (Welch, 1998). Second, it's been hypothesized that cross-cultural education could improve provider-patient communication and help eliminate the pervasive racial/ethnic disparities in medical care seen today (Einbinder and Schulman, 2000; Williams and Rucker, 2000; Brach and Fraser, 2000). Third, in response to the Institute of Medicine Report on Primary Care which states that "there should be an understanding of cultural belief systems of patients that assist or hinder effective healthcare delivery," and in response to the Pew Health Professions Commission, which states that "cultural sensitivity must be a part of the educational experiences of every student," accreditation bodies for medical training (i.e., Liaison Council on Medical Education, Accreditation Council on Graduate Medical Education) now have standards that require cross-cultural curricula as part of undergraduate and graduate medical education (Liaison Committee on Medical Education, 2001; Accreditation Council for Graduate Medical Education, 2001; Committee on the Future of Primary Care, 1994; Pew Health Professions Commission, 1995). Although these standards are general in their language, they are being expanded in detail and remain enforceable. Similarly, leaders in nursing education recognize the importance of culture in the health of populations and patients. As early as 1977, the National League for Nursing required cultural content in nursing curricula and in 1991, the American Nursing Association published standards specifically indicating that culturally and ethnically relevant care should be available to all patients.

APPROACHES TO CROSS-CULTURAL EDUCATION

Training in cross-cultural medicine can be divided into three conceptual approaches focusing on *attitudes, knowledge,* and *skills.* Like the proverbial three-legged stool, each approach plays a crucial role, but is unable to support any weight when not fully supported by the other two.

A Focus on Attitudes: The Cultural Sensitivity/Awareness Approach

The foundation of cross-cultural care is based in the *attitudes* central to professionalism—humility, empathy, curiosity, respect, sensitivity, and awareness of all outside influences on the patient (Bobo et al., 1991;

TABLE 6-2 Conceptual Approaches to Cross-Cultural Education

Sensitivity/Awareness Approach

- Primary focus on provider **attitudes**
  - o Goal is to increase provider awareness of impact of sociocultural factors on individual patients' health values, beliefs, behaviors, and ultimately quality of care and outcomes
- Exploration and reflection on culture, racism, classism, sexism, etc.
  - o Discussion of these factors as they relate to the provider and the patient culture, and what impact they may have on clinical decision-making
  - o Importance of curiosity, empathy and respect in the medical encounter highlighted
- Approach primarily taught in early in medical school and in certain residencies

Gonzalez-Lee and Simon, 1987). The added importance of these attitudes in cross-cultural medical encounters, where the desire to explore and negotiate divergent health beliefs and behaviors is paramount, has given rise to curricula designed to build or shape them within providers. The cultural sensitivity/awareness approach (see Table 6-2) incorporates educational exercises and techniques that promote self-reflection, including understanding one's own culture, biases, tendency to stereotype, and appreciation for diverse health values, beliefs, and behaviors (Culhane-Pera et al., 1997). Examples include open conversations exploring the impact of racism, classism, sexism, homophobia, and other types of discrimination in healthcare; determining how providers have themselves dealt with feeling "different" in some way; attempting to identify, using patient descriptors or vignettes, hidden biases we may have based on subconscious stereotypes; determining our reaction to different visuals of patients of different races/ethnicities; and discussing ways in which our family members have interacted with the healthcare system (Berlin, 1998; Donnini-Lenhoff, 2000; Tervalon and Murray-Garcia, 1998).

From a practical perspective, efforts to change attitudes are labor intensive, difficult, charged, complex to evaluate, and can seem abstract to those who are more clinically oriented (Kai et al., 1999). Nevertheless, attitudes such as curiosity, empathy, respect, and humility are critical to engaging in effective communication during the clinical encounter, whether the patient is from a similar or a distinct cultural background.

A Focus on Knowledge: The Multicultural/Categorical Approach

Traditionally, cross-cultural education has focused on a "multicultural" or "categorical approach," providing *knowledge* on the attitudes, values, beliefs, and behaviors of certain cultural groups (Paniagua, 1994). For example, methods to care for the "Asian" patient or the "Hispanic" patient would present a list of common health beliefs, behaviors, and key practice "do's and don'ts." With the huge array of cultural, ethnic, national, and religious groups in the United States, and the multiple influences such as acculturation and socioeconomic status that lead to intragroup variability, it is difficult to teach a set of unifying facts or cultural norms (such as "fatalism" among Hispanics, or "passivity" among Asians) about any particular group (Chin, 2000; Hill et al., 1990). These efforts can lead to stereotyping and oversimplification of culture, without a respect for its fluidity (Donini-Lenhoff and Hedrick, 2000; Carrillo et al., 1999). Research has shown that teaching "cultural knowledge" can be more detrimental than helpful if it is not done carefully (Shapiro and Lenahan, 1996).

There are two instances where focusing on a knowledge-based approach can be effective. First, following the basic tenets of community-oriented primary care and community assessment, students and practitioners can learn about the surrounding community in which they train or practice. Some important factors include the social and historic context of the population (new immigrants or longstanding residents), the predominant socioeconomic status, the immigration experience (was the immigration chosen or forced), nutritional habits (diet high in protein, fiber, or fat), common occupations (i.e., blue collar or service industry), patterns of housing (i.e., housing development), folk illnesses and healing practices (i.e., *empacho*, "coining"), and disease incidence and prevalence. Several such models are described in the literature focusing on communities in U.S.-Mexican border towns, communities with a new influx of a specific immigrant group, and Native-American reservations (Kristal et al., 1983; Nora et al., 1994).

The second instance of an effective knowledge-based approach is knowledge that has a specific, evidence-based impact on healthcare delivery. Examples include ethnopharmacology; disease incidence, prevalence, and outcomes among distinct populations; the impact of the Tuskegee Syphilis Study and segregation as the cause of mistrust in African Americans; the effect of war and torture on certain refugee populations and how this shapes their interaction with the healthcare system; and the common cultural and spiritual practices that might interfere with prescribed therapies (such as Ramadhan—the sunup-to-sundown fast observed by Muslims—and how this might affect people with diabetes), to name a few.

When learning facts about "cultural groups," it's important for providers to ask themselves several questions to avoid falling prey to ecologic fallacy. How accurate and generalizable are these group assumptions? How current are they, given the fluidity of culture and diversity among groups? What are the limitations? How can I use this knowledge

TABLE 6-3 Conceptual Approaches to Cross-Cultural Education

Multicultural/Categorical Approach

- Primary focus on increasing provider **knowledge** of cross-cultural issues
  o Previous focus on teaching unifying cultural characteristics of cultural groups
     (patients of culture x believe. . . and behave . . .)
- New focus on teaching methods of community assessment and evidence-based factors
  o These include disease incidence/prevalence among groups, ethnopharmacology,
     and historical factors that might shape health behaviors
- Taught in undergraduate, graduate, and continuing medical education

to deliver better care? (Shapiro and Lenahan, 1996). In summary, if a knowledge-based approach (see Table 6-3) is taught, it should focus on community oriented or specific, evidence-based factors. Absent this, learning as much as possible about the patient's own sociocultural context and perspectives while minimizing the reliance on generalizations is ideal.

A Focus on Skills: The Cross-Cultural Approach

The cross-cultural approach teaches providers *skills* that meld those of medical interviewing with the ethnographic tools of medical anthropology (Shapiro and Lenahan, 1996; Carrillo et al., 1999). These framework-based approaches focus on communication skills, and train providers to be aware of certain cross-cutting cultural issues, social issues, and health beliefs, while providing methods to deal with information clinically once it is obtained (Nunez, 2000; Berlin and Fowkes, 1998; Clinton, 1996). Curricula have focused on providing methods for eliciting patients' explanatory models (what patients believe is causing their illness) and agendas, identifying and negotiating different styles of communication, assessing decision-making preferences, the role of family, determining the patient's perception of biomedicine and complementary and alternative medicine, recognizing sexual and gender issues, and being aware of issues of mistrust, prejudice, and racism, among others (see Table 6-4) (Carrillo et al., 1999; Hill et al., 1990; Zweifler and Gonzalez, 1998; Culhane-Pera et al., 1997). For example, providers are taught that while it is important to understand all patients' health beliefs, it may be particularly crucial to understand the health beliefs of those who come from a different culture or have a different healthcare experience. As such, frameworks including questions to obtain this and other information are taught. Instead of applying a deductive approach that applies broad rules and generalizations about cultures to the individual, this inductive approach

TABLE 6-4 Conceptual Approaches to Cross-Cultural Education

Cross-Cultural Approach

- Primary focus on developing **tools and skills** for providers
- Process-oriented instruction that melds medical interviewing and communication skills with sociocultural and ethnographic tools of medical anthropology
  - Approaches to elicit patient's explanatory model (patient's conceptualization of illness)
  - Methods to assess patient's social context
  - Strategies for provider-patient negotiation and facilitation of participatory decision making
- Foundation to care for diverse populations through development of interviewing frameworks
- Practical approach for clinical years; taught in undergraduate, graduate, and continuing medical education

focuses on the patient, rather than theory, as the starting point for discovery (Shapiro and Lenahan, 1996). With the individual patient as teacher, providers are encouraged to adjust their practice style accordingly to meet their patients' specific needs. The cross-cultural approach has gained favor among educators who see its clinical applicability as a framework in caring for either diverse or targeted populations.

Teaching Methods and Opportunities

There have been a variety of teaching methodologies utilized for cross-cultural education at different levels of training (Table 6-6). In general, interactive, experiential, practical, case-based approaches that address cognitive, affective, and behavioral aspects of the learner are most effective (Welch, 1998). At the level of undergraduate and graduate medical education, strategies such as self-reflection (particularly for cultural sensitivity/awareness approach), focused didactics (especially for multicultural approach), and the use of vignettes, problem-based learning cases, medical encounter videos, and individual case-based discussion (usually for cross-cultural approach) are most common (Nunez, 2000; Carrillo et al., 1999; Louden et al., 1999; Culhane-Pera et al., 1997). Innovative educational strategies include learner community immersion (whereby students or residents rotate through community-based healthcare facilities), role-play (whereby students or residents practice interviewing techniques using scripted cases), patient narratives, video interviews of patients, and the use of patients or actors for faculty facilitated, simulated medical encounters (Gonzalez-Lee and Simon, 1987; Rubenstein et al., 1992). Continuing education for practicing providers has focused more on "culturally competent" approaches to treating specific clinical conditions in targeted populations (i.e. "Hypertension in African Americans," or "Managing Diabetes in Latinos"). In these instances, a knowledge-based approach is most commonly employed, in which disease incidence and prevalence of a specific condition in a target population is presented, along with focused strategies for managing said condition. These strategies may include evidence for the use of specific medications in certain populations or methods for incorporating community based resources for clinical support. Although other "provider-patient communication" continuing education courses focus more specifically on the process of improving understanding in the medical encounter, few have "cross-cultural communication" as a central theme.

There are various opportunities to incorporate cross-cultural issues in health professions education. In undergraduate and graduate medical education, courses have been taught during orientation, as part of established courses or electives, during retreats, as part of weekly conferences, or less frequently, as an optional or required stand-alone (see Table 6-5). Since there is currently no clear focus on cross-cultural issues within undergraduate and graduate health professions curricula, stand-alone courses are favored for the time being, although integration into the standard curricula would be optimal (Kai et al., 1999).

For practicing providers, integration of cross-cultural curricula as part of continuing education, or as part of the grand rounds series, or as part of faculty development, has been attempted. Certain states are considering requiring a standard number of continuing education credits in cross-cultural communication as part of professional licensure. Similarly, the Na-

TABLE 6-5 Methods and Opportunities for Cross-Cultural Education

Methods	Opportunities
Undergrad/Graduate Medical Education	*Undergrad/Graduate Medical Education*
• Facilitated reflection	• Orientation
• Didactics	• Electives
• Vignettes	• Retreats
• Individual Cases	• Rounds
• Problem-Based Learning	• Conferences
• Videos	• Introduction to Clinical Sciences
• Simulated Patients	• Stand Alone Course
• Community Immersion	
Continuing Education	**Practicing Providers**
• Didactics	• Continuing Education
• Problem-Based Learning	• Faculty Development
• Case-Based Discussion	• Licensure/Exams

tional Board of Medical Examiners is exploring methods of incorporating questions that address cross-cultural issues in medical care on licensing exams. Certain medical malpractice insurers are offering premium discounts to providers who complete provider-patient communication courses, and are now considering applying the same discounts to providers who complete cross-cultural communication courses. Regardless of the setting, it is felt that cross-cultural education should be linked to the level of the learner's training, with more theoretical approaches in the pre-clinical years and more practical approaches during the clinical years (Nunez, 2000).

Evaluation

To date, there has been limited evaluation published on the impact of cross-cultural education. Building on the three-legged stool model of attitudes, knowledge, and skills described above, we see some studies that have primarily shown improvements in cross-cultural knowledge (the type of knowledge has varied relative to the individual curricula taught). For example, Rubenstein et al. used pre- and post-test methodology to demonstrate that students who completed a "Culture, Communication, and Health" course displayed an increase in knowledge regarding:

1. The way in which a physician's ignorance of a patient's health beliefs and practices can adversely affect the clinical encounter;
2. The pervasiveness of non-conventional health beliefs and practices; and
3. The types of resources available for learning about patients' health beliefs and practices. (Rubenstein et al., 1992).

Similarly, Nora et al. used multiple-choice question methodology to show that an experimental group of students who completed a "Spanish Language and Cultural Competence Curriculum" had greater knowledge of Hispanic health and cultural issues, including disease prevalence, cultural perceptions of illness, and traditional health practices, compared with a control group (Nora, 1994). In addition, when compared with the control group, the experimental group was found to be less ethnocentric and more comfortable with others after the curricular intervention, based on the "Misanthropy Scale." In the area of graduate medical education, one published study found that family practice residents exposed to a three-year, multi-method cross-cultural curriculum displayed an increase in cultural knowledge and cross-cultural skills via self-report and faculty corroboration (Culhane-Pera et al., 1997). Research on continuing medical education courses for practicing providers targeted at improving communication skills (without a focus on cross-cultural communication) have shown mixed results (Haynes et al., 1984; Davis et al., 1992; Davis et al., 1995). Joos et al. showed no significant improvement in patient satisfaction for providers who had completed such courses versus those who hadn't (Joos et al., 1996). Levinson et al. did show a moderate increase in patient satisfaction and a significant increase in provider satisfaction for those who completed a course on improving doctor-patient communication (Levinson et al., 1993). It is difficult to know whether one can extrapolate these results to continuing medical education focusing on cross-cultural communication as there is yet no evaluative data in this area.

Cross-cultural education poses significant challenges for evaluation. For example, it's difficult to evaluate change in provider attitudes given the potential for social desirability bias on surveying, and the difficulty in observing encounters in real time. Assessing knowledge is perhaps easier, and can be assessed with standard evaluation tools such as pretest-posttests and essays (Louden et al., 1999; Nora et al., 1994; Rubenstein et al., 1992). Skills can be evaluated in undergraduate and graduate health professions education using techniques such as the objective structured clinical examination, or videotaping actual clinical encounters (Nunez, 2000; Robins et al., 1998a; Robins et al., 2001). For practicing providers, one might assess patient satisfaction improvements among those who have completed cross-cultural communication courses. All in all, we should be able to evaluate some dimensions of attitudes, knowledge, and skills.

Another approach to evaluation asks three questions about the impact of curricula, building towards the link to outcomes. First, do providers learn what is taught? Second, do they use what is taught? And third, does what is taught have an impact on care?

These questions can be assessed using mixed methodologies that include both quantitative and qualitative techniques (Table 6-6) (Nunez, 2000; Like et al., 1996). These include pre- and post-tests, unknown clinical cases, qualitative physician and patient interviews, medical chart review, audio or videotape of medical encounter, objective structured clinical exams, patient and provider satisfaction, and processes of care (i.e. completion of health promotion/disease prevention interventions). It's important that we not hold cross-cultural curricula to unfair evaluation standards, as detractors have asked for a direct link between curricula and the improvement of hard clinical outcomes Any assessment should match the educational objectives and be carried out in a careful, step-wise fashion, controlling for all possible confounders and focusing first on process measures (such as patient and provider satisfaction).

TABLE 6-6 Evaluation of Cross-Cultural Curricula

Key Question	Evaluation Strategy
Do providers learn what is taught?	Pre-, Post -Test Unknown Clinical Cases Objective Structured Clinical Exam
Do they use what is taught?	Qualitative physician and patient interviews Medical Chart Review Audio or Videotape of medical encounter Patient, Provider Satisfaction
Does what is taught have an impact on care?	Processes of Care (i.e., completion of health promotion/ disease prevention interventions)

Challenges and Opportunities

There are several challenges ahead for cross-cultural education (Table 6-7). First, given the biomedical focus of health professions education, there is significant resistance to curricula that are viewed as "soft" or lacking an evidence base (Culhane-Pera et al., 1997). Second, given that providers are accustomed to factual, practical learning, they are often disappointed when specific group cultural knowledge ("Hispanic patients believe . . . or behave . . .") is not presented (Kai et al., 1999). Third, providers feel that they don't have the time needed to explore and negotiate complex sociocultural issues with patients, due to the short length of today's medical encounter. Fourth, there is lack of consensus on fundamental, conceptual approaches and teaching methodologies, and lack of institutional support (both formal and informal) (Shapiro and Lenahan, 1996; Kai et al., 1999). Fifth and finally, although there is circumstantial

TABLE 6-7 Challenges for Cross-Cultural Education

Challenges: Provider Perspectives	Challenges: Developing the Field
• Provider resistance to curricula in this area • Limited awareness of impact of cross-cultural factors on healthcare and presence of health disparities • Desire for categorical approach to cross-cultural education • Time constraints for implementation of skills	• Varying fundamental approaches without consensus • Multiple teaching methodologies • Limited time, resources, faculty, and institutional support • Hypothetical link between cross-cultural education and the elimination of disparities that must be strengthened

evidence that would substantiate the claim that improving provider cross-cultural communication will help eliminate disparities in healthcare, there are yet to be published studies to support this hypothesis.

Despite these challenges, several opportunities exist for the field. First, since the government has realized the importance of educational initiatives in this area (U.S. DHHS, 1999), there are broadening funding streams for cross-cultural education and research. Given the evidence linking provider-patient communication to patient satisfaction, adherence, and outcomes, cross-cultural education holds promise as one effort of a multi-pronged approach towards eliminating racial/ethnic disparities in healthcare. Research that would help to solidify this link should be developed. Second, expanded cross-cultural curricula that include teaching specific data on racial/ethnic disparities in healthcare, in addition to exploration and discussion of potential causative factors, are being piloted. Given the limited awareness of disparities on the part of providers and the public (The Henry J. Kaiser Family Foundation, 1999), this seems to be a worthy strategy. Finally, with growing acknowledgement as to the impact of social cognitive factors (including stereotyping) on provider decision-making, cross-cultural curricula are now reviewing the normal processes by which clinical decisions are made, and what negative impact they might have on minority populations.

Ultimately, cross-cultural curricula should focus on securing provider buy-in by introducing evidence on how sociocultural barriers affect medical care and lead to racial/ethnic disparities in health, and how specific cross-cultural strategies can help ameliorate them. Curricula should balance their approaches between addressing attitudes, knowledge, and skills in a way that offers providers multiple approaches to address the problems they face.

SUMMARY

This chapter reviews evidence that sociocultural differences between patient and provider influence communication and clinical decision-making (Eisenberg, 1979). Evidence suggests that provider-patient communication is directly linked to patient satisfaction, adherence, and subsequently, health outcomes (Stewart et al., 1999). When sociocultural differences between patient and provider aren't appreciated, explored, understood, or communicated in the medical encounter, the result may be patient dissatisfaction, poor adherence, poorer health outcomes, and racial/ethnic disparities in care (Flores, 2000; Betancourt et al., 1999; Stewart et al., 1999; Morales et al., 1999; Cooper-Patrick et al., 1999; Langer, 1999).

There is a body of literature defining and supporting the importance of cross-cultural education in the training of health professionals. Despite this, curricula in this area have been implemented to a limited degree in health professions education. There are several theoretical approaches to cross-cultural education that vary in their relative emphasis on attitudes, knowledge, and skill building. Current published evaluations do not support conclusive statements about the effectiveness of particular approaches. However, the approaches that focus on skill building are likely more effective in providing clinicians with the clinical acumen to diagnose and treat diverse populations of patients.

There are various opportunities in which cross-cultural communication courses could be integrated into the health professional curricula, including during undergraduate, graduate, and continuing medical education. A set of core competencies for cross-cultural education should be developed. These should include achievement of certain attitudes, knowledge and skills from which learners will benefit and that they will utilize in the medical encounter. Improving quality of care and developing a strategy to eliminate racial/ethnic disparities in the medical encounter should be the goal. Research to date supports implementing a combination of each of the conceptual approaches presented here to develop efficient, solution-oriented ways of introducing cross-cultural principles to guide physician-patient interactions (Shapiro and Lenahan, 1996). Inductive frameworks should focus on individualized, patient-centered care (Donini-Lenhoff, 2000). While there is no one "right" way to teach cross-cultural medicine, and interventions should be tailored to the specific learning environment, there are some guiding principles that can be followed and disseminated—some of which exist in the literature today (Betancourt et al., 1999; Nunez 2000; Like et al., 1996; Carrillo et al., 1999; Kristal et al., 1983). There should be some determination as to how best to incorporate cross-cultural education into the health professional's curricula as part of a multipronged effort to eliminate racial/ethnic disparities in healthcare. Research suggests that required, full integration into the standard undergraduate and graduate medical curricula should be the gold standard. Yet in the absence of the capacity to do this, we should be including the teaching of cross-cultural medicine as a stand-alone (Flores, 2000; Nunez, 2000; Like et al., 1996; Bobo et al., 1991; Clinton, 1996). For practicing providers, continuing medical education—as part of licensure, as part of faculty development, and as part of obtaining medical malpractice insurance—all remain promising areas of integrating cross-cultural curricula and assessing cross-cultural communication skills.

Appropriate evaluation strategies and monitoring that directly assess the attitudes, knowledge and skills taught to providers should be devised. Careful attention should be given to the complexities of evaluation and measurement in these types of curricula, with a strategic, step-wise, mixed-method, process-driven approach as a starting point for future research.

Finding 6-1: Sociocultural differences between patient and provider influence communication and clinical decision making.
Evidence suggests that provider-patient communication is directly linked to patient satisfaction, adherence, and health outcomes. Ineffective communication in the medical encounter may lead to patient dissatisfaction, non-adherence, poorer health outcomes, and subsequently, racial and ethnic disparities in healthcare.

Finding 6-2: A significant body of literature defines and supports the importance of cross-cultural education in the training of health professionals.
Despite several approaches and various opportunities for integration, curricula in this area have been implemented to a limited degree in undergraduate, graduate, and continuing health professions education.

Finding 6-3: Cross-cultural education offers promise as a tool to improve healthcare professionals' ability to provide quality care to diverse patient populations and thereby reducing healthcare disparities.

Recommendation 6-1: Integrate cross-cultural education into the training of current and future health professionals.
Strategies should be developed to fully integrate cross-cultural curricula into undergraduate, graduate, and continuing education of health professionals. These curricula should be expanded to include modules documenting the existence of racial and ethnic disparities in healthcare, and the impact of social cognitive factors and stereotyping on clinical decision- making. Required, practical, case-based curricula based on a set of core competencies, amenable to evaluation, should be the desired standard of training.

7

Data Collection and Monitoring

The preceding chapters illustrate the complexity and variety of factors—including healthcare financing arrangements, institutional and organizational characteristics of healthcare settings, aspects of the clinical encounter, and the attitudes, perceptions, and beliefs of healthcare providers and their patients—that influence healthcare disparities. The complexity of these factors, coupled with the fact that disparities in care are not always apparent to patients or providers in clinical encounters, increases the need for data to better understand the extent of disparities and the circumstances under which disparities are likely to occur. Unfortunately, standardized data on racial and ethnic differences in care are generally unavailable. Federal, private, and state-supported data collection efforts are scattered and unsystematic, and many health plans, with a few notable exceptions, do not collect data on enrollees' race, ethnicity, or primary language, pointing to significant obstacles to the collection and analysis of such data (Perot and Youdelman, 2001).

Standardized data collection, however, is critically important in the effort to understand and eliminate racial and ethnic disparities in healthcare. Having data on patient and provider race and ethnicity would allow researchers to better disentangle factors that are associated with healthcare disparities. In addition, collecting appropriate data related to racial or ethnic differences in the process, structure and outcomes of care can help to identify discriminatory practices, whether they are the result of intentional behaviors and attitudes, or unintended—but no less harmful—biases or policies that result in racial or ethnic differences in care that cannot be justified by patient preferences or clinical need. Data collection and monitoring therefore provides critically needed information for civil rights enforcement. Further, collecting and analyzing patterns of care by patient race, ethnicity, and other demographic data can help health plans to monitor plan performance. Such monitoring can help to ensure accountability to enrolled members and payors, improve patient choice, and allow for evaluation of intervention programs. Such evaluations are likely to improve service delivery for racial and ethnic minority populations, and therefore may result in cost savings that would offset the costs of data collection.

The collection of racial and ethnic data in health systems poses special challenges, however. Traditionally, the practice of healthcare has been dominated by individual practitioners who delivered care in settings relatively unaffected by regulation, oversight, or government intervention. Hospitals enjoyed little external monitoring, and their professionally dominated and autonomous organizational structure was rarely challenged prior to the emergence of the federal government as the largest healthcare payor. Today's cost-conscious healthcare systems present an opportunity for greater healthcare practice accountability, but medicine's traditional autonomy and self-government presents little history of oversight, particularly with regard to civil rights, that can be expanded upon (Smith, 1998).

Specific recommendations regarding the types of healthcare data that should be collected, and how this information should be analyzed and reported has been the subject of intensive study and debate by governmental (U.S. DHHS, 1999) and private groups (National Quality Forum, 2001; Perot and Youdelman, 2001), and is beyond the scope of this report. Selecting indicators of healthcare disparities that can be readily measured, analyzed and reported, and developing methods to ensure reliable data collection will require careful consideration of costs, benefits, and other potential problems inherent in collecting and reporting patient care data (see discussion of obstacles to racial/ethnic data collection, below). These issues will be weighed by a forthcoming National Academies study committee that has been asked by Congress to assess the adequacy of racial and ethnic data within U.S. Department of Health and Human Services (DHHS) systems. Ideally, however, all patient encounters should be assessed for the quality of care and patient outcomes. This would enable the data to be aggregated to many different levels of the healthcare delivery system, including health plans, medical groups, and hospitals. Most of the information collected should be recorded as part of the patient's medical record, a task that in the future will be assisted greatly by the development of electronic patient records. These data should be stratified by race, ethnicity, as well as socioeconomic status and, where possible, primary language.

OBSTACLES TO RACIAL/ETHNIC DATA COLLECTION

The need for data on patients' race and ethnicity and quality of care must be balanced against other significant considerations. Foremost, patient privacy must be protected. The confidentiality and security of patient information and data transactions must, at minimum, conform with standards set forth in the Health Insurance Portability and Accountability Act of 1996 (HIPAA). Secondly, the costs of data collection must be weighed relative to its benefits. When and how such data are collected will have broad cost implications; collection of patient race and ethnicity data at the point of plan enrollment, for example, will likely be less expensive than data collection among members already enrolled in plans whose race or ethnicity is unknown. Similarly, administrative and paperwork burdens are likely to increase as the numbers of patient data elements are increased. Formal Congressional checks on such administrative burdens (e.g., the Paperwork Reduction Act) require that administrators of publicly-funded programs assess such costs and demonstrate the utility of additional data collection relative to costs.

Other legal constraints must be assessed, as well. While the vast majority of states do not prohibit collection of patients' race and ethnicity data, some may impose restraints on when and how such data may be collected (Perez and Satcher, 2001). The extent of these restraints must be assessed and this information provided to managed care organizations (MCOs) and payors to avoid confusion over what kinds of data collection are allowed, and under what circumstances.

Political concerns must be also addressed to ensure cooperation from all parties in data collection efforts. Resistance to data collection efforts may come from healthcare providers, institutions, plans, and patients, unless the purposes and benefits of data collection are clearly explicated. Providers, as noted earlier, may resent perceived intrusions on autonomy. Patients, particularly minority patients, may worry that racial or ethnic data collection will result in "redlining" of services, selection of enrollees, or rationing of services on the basis of race or ethnicity.

Efforts to enforce data collection from the federal level may also meet resistance from state authorities, who retain primary responsibility for determining data requirements of health plans with whom states contract for Medicaid MCO services. Federal efforts to require the collection of patients' racial and ethnic data would raise challenges from those who find federal reporting requirements already burdensome and the federal role in dictating the terms of managed care contracts too extensive. Finally, it should be noted that some individuals are broadly opposed to government involvement in monitoring race and ethnic trends among the U.S. population, and are mounting challenges to the notion that the government should collect any information about race or ethnicity. Ward Connerly, for example, the California businessman who led efforts to repeal affirmative action in that state, is spearheading a ballot initiative to prevent the state from collecting any information about race or ethnicity, except for a few limited circumstances (Jordan, 2001). This initiative would likely undercut efforts to assess racial and ethnic inequities in healthcare, as well as in other potentially discriminatory practices.

In addition, health plans have raised significant concerns regarding the collection of patient race and ethnicity information. Many plans, led by American Association of Health Plans (AAHP), increasingly see the collection of information on patient race and ethnicity as an important means to evaluate their own efforts to reduce disparities in care and develop better strategies to serve growing minority patient populations (Ignani and Bocchino, communication with Alan Nelson, M.D., March 19, 2001). However, some plans have operated under the erroneous assumption that federal and/or state law prohibits the collection of patient race and ethnicity information. Efforts by the U.S. Department of Health and Human Services Office for Civil Rights (OCR) and Office of Minority Health (OMH) to clarify federal law (Perez, 2000; Perez and Satcher, 2001) have helped to dismiss this assumption.

Many health plans, however, remain concerned that their ability to serve minority patients could be hampered should data collection efforts be seen by these populations as an effort to ration care. In addition, plans that serve disproportionately minority and lower-income populations could be hurt by the release of "report card" information that reveals their enrolled members to be less healthy or to require more services than the majority population. In such instances, information about the health status of plans' enrolled populations and case-mix may largely reflect conditions of poverty and the generally higher incidence of morbidity and mortality among lower-income and minority populations, and may not necessarily reflect poor service on the part of health plans. This kind of information might unfairly hurt health plans' efforts to expand their market share among minority populations, and should be taken into account (Fiscella et al., 2000).

Other challenges include the accuracy of racial and ethnic data. As noted earlier, "race" and "ethnicity" are fluid, socially defined concepts that are not consistently understood or applied in data collection efforts. Racial or ethnic identity is determined by multiple factors and may vary depending on the contexts in which these constructs are defined and the manner in which data are collected. Observers recording race and ethnicity data are notoriously inaccurate, particularly with regard to Hispanic or American-Indian populations (e.g., death certificates commonly misreport the race of American Indians). Further, a small but increasing proportion of individuals define themselves using two or more racial and ethnic categories, making simple classification difficult. Finally, efforts to address disparities in care must acknowledge the significant heterogeneity within each of the federally defined racial and ethnic groups (whites, African Americans, Native Americans, Asian Americans, Pacific Islanders, and Hispanics). Wide variations within each of these groups can be found in health status, health practices and behaviors, and healthcare resources. It is therefore important that data be collected on subgroups within these categories (e.g., Cuban American, Puerto Rican, Mexican American, Central American among the "Hispanic" ethnic group). Where possible and appropriate, data collected over several years can be combined to achieve sufficient analytic sample sizes (U.S. DHHS National Committee on Vital and Health Statistics, 1999).

These challenges underscore the need for consensus among health plans, providers, and consumers regarding data collection policies, and best practices regarding how data will be analyzed and to whom it will be presented. To this end, the committee believes that efforts by public and private groups, such as the National Quality Forum (NQF), the National Committee on Vital and Health Statistics (NCVHS), and the Agency for Healthcare Research and Quality (AHRQ), to convene experts and provide specific recommendations regarding the collection and analysis of data on patients' race and ethnicity will prove fruitful to help achieve broad consensus on best policies and practices. Development of a full, national database of healthcare quality that can be analyzed by race and ethnicity will take time, however, and it is clear that a sequence of steps must be undertaken to reach this goal. An important first step would involve an assessment of existing data sets within public and private plans that allows for an analysis of patient care by race and ethnicity.

THE FEDERAL ROLE IN RACIAL, ETHNIC, AND PRIMARY LANGUAGE HEALTH DATA

Several agencies of the DHHS, recognizing the importance of racial, ethnic, and primary language healthcare data, have attempted to promote data collection and monitoring efforts, particularly to address the challenges noted above. Despite these efforts, federal data collection remains unsystematic and lacks an overall guiding structure to ensure accountability and cooperation by HHS agencies, states, and private sector partners involved with federal health programs (Perot and Youdelman, 2001).

The Summit Health Institute for Research and Education, Inc. (SHIRE) and the National Health Law Program (NHeLP), with support from The Commonwealth Fund, analyzed an array of statutes, regulations, federal agency policies, practices, and data collection vehicles related to race, ethnicity, and primary language in healthcare settings. This analysis included an assessment of the extent to which federal policies mandate or encourage collection and reporting of race, ethnicity, and primary language data and an assessment of how current law is understood, interpreted, and implemented by federal officials. SHIRE and NHeLP analyzed 80 program-specific statutes and over 100 data collection vehicles, and developed 25 findings and 10 recommendations regarding federal data policies (Perot and Youdelman, 2001). These recommendations are listed in Box 7-1.

BOX 7-1
Recommendations, Racial, Ethnic, and Primary Language Data Collection in the Healthcare System: An Assessment of Federal Policies and Practices (Perot and Youdelman, 2001)

1. Ensure that Medicare data, as well as other data regarding individuals who are served by HHS programs or who participate in HHS research activities, are readily available and accurate by race, ethnicity, and primary language. Independent analysts have estimated that the Medicare beneficiary eligibility file compiled by the Social Security Administration is less than 60 percent accurate for all racial/ethnic classifications other than black or white.

2. Enforce state collection and reporting of data by race, ethnicity, and primary language for enrollees in Medicaid and the State Children's Health Insurance Program (SCHIP). Currently, data collection and reporting by states are often inconsistent and incomplete.

3. Revise the standards for implementation of the Health Insurance Portability and Accountability Act (HIPAA) to designate the code set for race and ethnicity data as mandatory for both claims and enrollment standards. Racial and ethnic categories used under HIPAA must be compliant with OMB standards.

4. Recommend that quality measurement and reporting tools such as the Health Plan Employer Data and Information Set (HEDIS) should collect and report health data by race, ethnicity, and primary language.

5. Ensure access to quality healthcare for people with limited English proficiency by effective monitoring of adherence to guidelines and collection of requisite data.

6. Include statutory conditions in new program initiatives, including block grants, stating that data must be collected and reported by race, ethnicity, and primary language, and that programs should allocate adequate resources to promote compliance, address technological dif-

SHIRE and NHeLP draw four principle conclusions regarding the federal role in racial, ethnic, and primary language data collection. First, the collection of such data is legal and authorized under Title VI of the Civil Rights Act of 1964. Second, a growing number of federal policies emphasizes the need for the collection of race, ethnicity, and primary language data. Third, such data is an indispensable tool for the assessment of progress toward federal goals of eliminating health disparities (U.S. Department of Health and Human Services, 1999). SHIRE and NHeLP found broad consensus within U.S. DHHS on this point, but a fourth conclusion of the investigators is that DHHS policies and practices fail to reflect this

ficulties, ensure privacy and confidentiality of data collected, and implement effective educational strategies to maximize beneficiary and provider cooperation with data gathering efforts.

7. Encourage public and private agencies to participate in the development and implementation of approaches to improve data availability and promote data collection and reporting. In support of agencies, HHS should:
   - create a "tool kit" containing information on effective data-related techniques, technologies, and privacy safeguards currently in use;
   - bolster the HHS Data Council's efforts to identify and document the benefits of collecting and reporting; and
   - support national policies to facility data-sharing among all federal and state agencies.

8. Expand or create public and private educational efforts to:
   - inform insurers, health plans, providers, private/public agencies, and the general public that data collection and reporting by race, ethnicity, and primary language are legal and in many instances required by federal law and regulations;
   - raise public awareness that the collection and reporting of these data are prerequisites for the achievement of Healthy People 2010 goals and essential to demonstrate compliance with the nondiscrimination requirements of Title VI; and
   - inform decision-makers that effective strategies exist for achieving compliance with data collection and reporting policies, including risk-adjustment, and make such compliance a condition for receiving government resources.

9. Provide states and healthcare providers with greater access to aggregated and disaggregated racial, ethnic, and primary language data acquired at the federal level, subject to privacy and confidentiality regulations.

10. Support research on existing best practices for data collection.

consensus, as data requirements and methods for collection and reporting vary across federal agencies, and no single HHS blueprint exists to provide a framework and rationale for the department's activities. Further, no department-wide mandate exists for racial, ethnic and primary language data collection and reporting, leaving only a patchwork of efforts across agencies to promote data collection and reporting (Perot and Youdelman, 2001).

The SHIRE-NHeLP report notes that two significant developments in early 2001 illustrate the "disconnect" between federal consensus and practice. In one instance, HHS finalized regulations regarding standard data elements for the electronic transmission of health information authorized under HIPAA, yet these rules failed to identify race or ethnicity as a required code, an omission that many HHS officials saw as a "lost opportunity." In another instance, HHS published regulations for Medicaid Managed Care and the State Child Health Insurance Program (SCHIP) that would require states to report the race, ethnicity, and primary language of enrollees on a quarterly basis, yet these regulations were suspended for further review following the change of presidential administrations in 2001 (Perot and Youdelman, 2001). Notably, the National Committee on Vital and Health Statistics (NCVHS), which serves to advise the federal government on health information and data policy, warned in a 1999 report that the limited data-collection practices of MCOs who serve Medicaid beneficiaries threatened to inhibit HHS's ability to monitor the quality of care provided by Medicaid MCOs. NCVHS urged that HHS develop more specific guidance about the manner and format in which Medicaid MCO data should be collected and reported by states (Mays, 2001).

Despite the lack of a framework or mandate for systematic data collection at the federal level, data on enrollee race and ethnicity is available to a limited degree for the two largest federal healthcare programs, Medicaid and Medicare. The Centers for Medicare and Medicaid Services (CMS—formerly the Healthcare Financing Administration [HCFA]) has generally required states to report patient encounter data for Medicaid enrollees, but has not required that states report data by race and ethnicity. Most states have voluntarily supplied CMS with data on Medicaid beneficiaries' race and ethnicity, and cumulative totals of beneficiaries' race and ethnicity are available from all states. As noted above, however, the proposed rule requiring all states to report the race and ethnicity of Medicaid and SCHIP recipients has yet to be implemented. Further, states would be expected, via CMS's proposed rule issued in August, 2001, to provide Medicaid MCOs with information regarding enrollees' race or ethnicity, but these data are often incomplete or inconsistent, and the rule did not require that this data be reported back to the agency (Perot and Youdelman, 2001). Medicare enrollees' race or ethnicity has been typically extracted from the Medicare Enrollee Database, which is based on Social Security Administration (SSA) information. Enrollment data is available for all Medicare beneficiaries, but SSA data are limited, particularly for data obtained prior to 1994, as SSA only identified beneficiaries' race or ethnicity as "white," "black," "other," and "unknown." Efforts by HCFA to reconstruct this data by surveying the 2.1 million beneficiaries whose race was listed as "other" or "unknown" reduced the number of unidentified race codes significantly, but accuracy of these data for beneficiaries identified as other than "black" or "white" is estimated to be less than 60% (Perot and Youdelman, 2001).

OTHER DATA SOURCES TO ASSESS
HEALTHCARE DISPARITIES

Several other federal, state, and private data sources currently exist or are planned that can be tapped to assess racial and ethnic disparities in care. As will be noted later in this chapter, data from these sources can be used to help identify sources of disparities in care and/or monitor changes in racial and ethnic disparities in care over time. The following summary of data collection systems is not intended as an exhaustive listing of federal, state, or privately funded data sets that may be used to assess racial and ethnic healthcare disparities. For a more exhaustive listing of federal data collection systems, see the HHS *Directory of Health and Human Services Data Resources* (U.S. DHHS, 2001).

Several relevant national-level data sources that can be used to assess aspects of racial and ethnic healthcare disparities include:

Consumer Assessment of Health Plans Survey (CAHPS)

The Consumer Assessment of Health Plans Survey (CAHPS), supported by the AHRQ, provides information to healthcare consumers, purchasers, health plans, and others regarding the quality of healthcare plans and services. CAHPS surveys ask consumers about their experiences with health plans, such as the quality of communication with providers, the provision of translation services for patients with limited English proficiency, and the timeliness and quality of care provided for a variety of medical conditions and procedures. CAHPS survey data can be analyzed by respondents' race or ethnicity to assess group differences in patient experiences.

Medical Expenditure Panel Survey (MEPS)

The Medical Expenditure Panel Survey (MEPS), the most recent of a series of federal surveys of medical care costs, was initiated by the AHRQ in 1996 for the purpose of assessing the types, frequency of use, and costs of healthcare services used in the United States. MEPS data yield information on health services expenditures and how they are paid for, as well as the extent of health insurance coverage among the U.S. population. MEPS consists of four components: the Household Component, which samples families and individuals to assess health status, insurance coverage, healthcare use and expenditures, and sources of payment for health services; the Nursing Home Component, which samples nursing homes and residents to assess characteristics of facilities and services offered, costs, and sources of payment of these services; the Medical Provider Component, which supplements information from the Household Component by surveying hospitals, physicians, and home healthcare providers; and the Insurance Component, which assesses the amount, types, and costs of health insurance available to employees. The Household Component collects data on respondents' race/ethnicity, and while the Nursing Home Component has racial and ethnic data available, only the African-American and white samples are large enough to permit analysis (U.S. DHHS, 2001). These data can be assessed by race and ethnicity, as well as other socio-demographic indicators, such as level of education, income and assets, and employment. Several of the studies summarized in Chapter 1 utilize MEPS data to assess patterns of disparities in care.

Medicare Beneficiary Enrollment Database

Medicare's Enrollment Database (EDB), supported by the CMS, is the principal database for Medicare beneficiary services, including access to and use of services covered under Medicare. The primary source for EDB beneficiary information, however, is the Social Security Administration's Master Beneficiary Record database. As noted above, these data are unreliable with respect to racial and ethnic populations other than black and white beneficiaries.

Medicare Current Beneficiary Survey

The Medicare Current Beneficiary Survey (MCBS), supported by CMS, is a continuing sample of Medicare beneficiaries to assess healthcare use, costs, and who pays for it. A variety of demographic data are collected from respondents during an initial interview, including race/ethnicity, health and insurance status, and education level. Data can be used to assess racial and ethnic differences in costs and utilization of care, and costs paid by Medicare as well as other public and private insurance sources.

Public and privately funded healthcare plans can take advantage of survey instruments developed as part of broader quality improvement initiatives, such as the Health Plan Employer Data and Information Set (HEDIS).

Health Plan Employer Data and Information Set (HEDIS)

The Health Plan Employer Data and Information Set (HEDIS), developed by the National Committee for Quality Assurance (NCQA) in conjunction with public and private purchasers, health plans, researchers, and consumer advocates, is a set of standardized performance measures that assesses the quality of healthcare and services provided by managed care plans. HEDIS was developed to ensure that purchasers and consumers have access to information to compare the performance of managed healthcare plans. HEDIS measures the effectiveness and availability of care in areas such as childhood immunization, breast cancer screening, cholesterol management, and treatment of heart attack. In addition, HEDIS offers information on structural attributes of health plans, such as practitioner turnover and rates of board certification and residency completion. HEDIS also includes a standardized survey of consumers' experiences that evaluates plan performance in areas such as customer service, access to care and claims processing.

At the state level, new data sets being developed, such as the California Health Interview Survey (CHIS), may allow researchers to explore regional and subpopulation variation in healthcare access and use.

California Health Interview Survey (CHIS)

The California Health Interview Survey (CHIS) is a collaboration of the UCLA Center for Health Policy Research, the California Department of Health Services, and the Public Health Institute to assess the health status, health behavior and risks, and healthcare access and utilization of the state's diverse population. Data from its survey of 55,000 California households will be available in early 2002 and will be made available through published reports, public-use files, and an Internet-based system that will allow requestors to gather information tailored to particular health topics, population groups, and geographic areas. In particular, CHIS asks respondents to provide information about their usual source of care, access to and use of specific services, experiences of discrimination in healthcare settings, and recall of provider advice, among other items. Results will be analyzed by respondents' race and ethnicity, with particular attention to racial and ethnic subgroups. Funding for CHIS has been provided by the California Department of Health Services, The California Endowment, the National Cancer Institute (NCI), California Children and Families Commission, the U.S. Centers for Disease Control and Prevention (CDC), and the Indian Health Service (IHS).

MODELS OF MEASURING DISPARITIES IN HEALTHCARE

Many models of healthcare "report cards" have been developed over the past few years, as healthcare consumers and purchasers of plans have expressed great interest in timely and accurate information about the quality of care delivered by plans, hospitals, and individual providers. Few such "report cards," however, have focused exclusively or in part on racial and ethnic disparities in care. This paucity of information on disparities in care is likely to change in the near future, as federal and private initiatives are increasing visibility and attention to the problem. In one instance, the Office of the Assistant Secretary for Planning and Evaluation of the U.S. Department of Health and Human Services (U.S. DHHS) has recently commissioned a review of measures of discrimination in healthcare settings. In another federal initiative, AHRQ has initiated plans to develop a national report on racial and ethnic disparities in healthcare, and plans to incorporate measures of racial and ethnic disparities in care in a national report of quality of care. Within the private sector, the National Quality Forum (NQF), with support from The Commonwealth Fund, has produced a report on measuring and reporting the quality of care for minority populations. These activities are likely to spur efforts to increase information available to consumers and purchasers of plans and promote greater choice when selecting plans, to promote accountability to consumers and purchasers, and to spark action on the part of plans, providers, and legal and regulatory bodies to reduce disparities in care.

Two models of "report cards" that specifically address racial and ethnic disparities in healthcare are reviewed below.

"Health Accountability 36"

Smith (1998) proposes a report card to assess racial and ethnic disparities consisting of 36 consensus indicators that have been developed and utilized in other settings by a range of public and private entities. The indicators were selected based on the availability of data, sensitivity of the indicators to key health conditions for vulnerable populations, and their amenability to public health and healthcare intervention. The first 12 indicators include measures adapted from the U.S. DHHS initiative *Healthy People 2000*, and are routinely collected and reported by the National Vital Statistics report system to evaluate the health of geographically defined populations. The second 12 indicators include measures of managed care plans to provide consumers and purchasers with information about plan performance. Of these, the first six were developed by the National Committee for Quality Assurance for HEDIS, while the subsequent six indicators were selected by the former Agency for Healthcare Policy and Research (now AHRQ). The third set of 12 indicators was developed by the Joint Committee on Accreditation of Health Care Organizations (JCAHO) as part of its accreditation process to measure hospital performance, and reflect measures of obstetrical, oncologic, and cardiovascular outcomes. Smith (1998) notes that data for these indicators are currently available and can be analyzed using the standard categories for race and ethnicity adapted by the Office of Management and Budget (see Chapter 1, Table 1). A goal for public health agencies and health systems, Smith suggests, would be to bring racial and ethnic disparities to within 80%. These measures are listed in Table 7-1.

Several of the measures proposed by Smith can be criticized on the grounds that as indicators of population health, they are influenced to a far greater extent by social and economic forces such as income inequality, residential segregation (and subsequent substandard living conditions, especially for lower-income minority groups), environmental risks, and other social problems. As such, they are less amenable to health system intervention. Further, health systems that disproportionately enroll lower-income and minority patients will have a greater challenge in improving the health of a generally sicker population with higher rates of co-morbidities, and thus, may not demonstrate improvement on many of the measures. Smith (1998) notes, however, that the impact of plans' case-mix can be adjusted statistically. In addition, he notes, some health plans, such as not-for-profit integrated delivery systems, recognize the impact of social and economic forces on the health of their enrolled populations and attempt to address these forces by improving screening and primary and preventive healthcare services, and by addressing housing and other social service needs of their patients.

Integrated Approaches

LaVeist and Gibbons (2001), in their report to U.S. DHHS[1] on poten-

---

[1]U.S. DHHS commissioned LaVeist to "summarize the literature on racial/ethnic discrimination within healthcare settings, with the primary goal of describing how discrimination has been measured" (LaVeist and Gibbons, 2001, p. 1). In this review, the authors note that the existence of racial and ethnic disparities in healthcare does not necessarily reflect discrimination, but focus their analysis on indicators that may detect patterns of discrimination apart from disparities that are not inherently discriminatory.

TABLE 7-1 "Health Accountability 36" Report Card Indicators

Unit of Analysis	Source	Indicators
Geographically Defined Population	Healthy People 2000	1. Total age-adjusted death rate 2. Automobile death rate 3. Suicide death rate 4. Lung cancer death rate 5. Breast cancer death rate 6. Cardiovascular death rate 7. Homicide death rate 8. Teen births 9. Inadequate prenatal care 10. % Low birthweight births 11. Infant death rate 12. Children in poverty
Health Plan Covered Lives	HEDIS AHCPR	1. % Women for whom prenatal care began in the first trimester 2. % Children receiving all childhood immunizations by 24 months 3. Cholesterol screening age 40-64 once in 5-year period 4. % Women 51-64 continuously enrolled for 2 years who received mammogram breast cancer screening 5. % Women 21-64 continuously enrolled for 3 years who received a Pap test 6. % Members 2-19 with one or more asthma admissions 7. % Diabetics 31-64 who had retinal exam during the preceding calendar year 8. % Members 23-39 who visited a health practitioner in the past year 9. % Rating how well the doctor listened as excellent 10. % For whom last visit to doctor fully met their needs 11. % Choice of doctors not a problem 12. % Satisfied with overall plan
Hospital Patient Clinical Population	JCAHO	Obstetrical Indicators: 1. % Low birthweight infants 2. % Term infants admitted to NICU within one day of delivery 3. % Neonates with an Apgar of 3 or less at 5 minutes and a birthweight > 1,500 grams 4. % Neonates with a discharge diagnosis of significant birth trauma Oncology Indicators: 5. Survival of patient with primary cancer of the lung, colon/rectum, by state and histologic type 6. Use of test critical to diagnosis, prognosis, and treatment 7. Use of treatment approaches that have an impact on quality of life 8. Interdisciplinary treatment and follow-up Cardiovascular Indicators: 9. Intrahospital mortality as a means of assessing multiple aspects of CABG care 10. Extended postoperative stay as a means of assessing multiple aspects of CABG care 11. Intrahospital mortality as a means of assessing multiple aspects of PTCA care 12. Intrahospital mortality as a means of assessing multiple aspects of acute MI care

SOURCE: Smith (1998).

tial measures of discrimination in healthcare settings, note that such measures must not only address structural differences in receipt of care (e.g., the proportion of women receiving prenatal care in the first trimester, as suggested by Smith [1998]), but should also assess the quality of interpersonal interactions in healthcare settings. Structural differences shape the parameters of care provided to different populations, they note, but individual, subjective factors affect the quality of care in clinical interactions. They argue for an integrated approach that includes multiple measures, and meets the following criteria:

1. *Applicable to multiple racial/ethnic groups*—the indicators must be applicable to all racial and ethnic groups that make up the U.S. population.
2. *Produce unique scores for individual healthcare facilities*—the report card must be producible for individual healthcare facilities and not merely produce scores for the nation or a particular region.
3. *Data sources must be accessible*—the report card must be easily understandable to a broad audience of healthcare consumers and the indicators must have high "face validity."
4. *No confounding*—indicators must not be confounded with other variables such as health insurance, patient preferences or larger societal factors. If there is confounding, there must be a way to adjust for it.
5. *Longitudinality*—the indicators must have the ability to be replicated over time (LaVeist and Gibbons, 2001, p. 7).

LaVeist and Gibbons weigh the merits of four potential approaches to measuring discrimination in care, including Smith's (1998) "Health Accountability 36," patient assessments, administrative claims audits, and assessments of substandard care. The "Health Accountability 36" measures draw largely upon existing data, and can be applied to geographically defined populations, individuals in health plans, and hospital and clinic patients. LaVeist and Gibbons note, however, that many of the measures, particularly those assessing racial differences in health status, are confounded with larger social and economic factors.

Several measures of patient satisfaction have been extensively evaluated, according to LaVeist and Gibbons, and several studies have assessed racial and ethnic differences in patients' perceptions of the quality of care they receive (reviewed earlier). Few of these measures, however, have explicitly assessed patients' perceptions of racial discrimination in care settings (the Seattle-King County survey of patient perceptions of discrimination in care, reviewed earlier, is a notable exception). Such measures have the potential of providing unique scores for individual healthcare facilities and can be used to assess changes over time. Patient perceptions of care, however, can be influenced by a wide range of factors, and may not reflect whether patients are receiving care appropriate to their needs. Nonetheless, such perceptions form an important component of a multi-pronged assessment profile, particularly if measures can assess the degree of patient participation in treatment decisions and understanding of their diagnosis and course of treatment.

Administrative claims data have been used extensively in prior research to audit care and demonstrate racial disparities in access to diagnostic and therapeutic procedures (much of this research is reviewed in Chapter 1). Well-controlled studies using claims data have adjusted for many potentially confounding factors, such as co-morbid conditions and insurance status, to isolate the influence of patient race on receipt of care. LaVeist and Gibbons (2001) suggest that administrative audits can produce unique scores for individual hospitals and healthcare facilities. Such data often fail, however, to illuminate process-of-care variables, such as referral patterns or participation in treatment decisions (e.g., whether providers present all treatment options and whether patients accept or refuse them). Prospective studies are therefore needed to supplement typically retrospective analyses of administrative claims data (see Chapter on "Research Needs").

Measures of adverse events due to practitioner or healthcare setting error are also an important component of assessing disparities in care, according to LaVeist and Gibbons (2001). Increasingly, healthcare providers and consumers have focused on the problem of medical errors and patient safety, and at least two methodologies have been developed to evaluate adverse events. Both involve an initial screening of potentially problematic cases, typically by two trained healthcare professionals, but screening methods differ in that one approach utilizes actual medical records, while the other uses administrative claims data. Such analysis could indicate whether minority patients are differentially more or less likely to face substandard care. This method has the advantage of yielding objective data on the quality of care provided, relative to standard criteria. Data are free of confounding, and the accuracy and validity of these methods has been demonstrated, the authors note.

LaVeist and Gibbons (2001) conclude that a two-tiered, multi-assessment approach may be useful to assess discrimination in healthcare settings. In the first tier, routine monitoring of healthcare facilities can be accomplished by audits of administrative data and analyses of data on substandard care. This initial "screen" could identify facilities that should be investigated more closely. In the second assessment tier, facilities are informed of the disparities and are given a period of time to address them. If progress has not been made, LaVeist and Gibbons suggest, a method used more commonly to assess housing and employment discrimination—paired testing—may be used to further assess the possibility of racial or ethnic discrimination. In this strategy, individuals are trained to present the same needs and background information to targeted healthcare facilities, but vary only in race or ethnicity (see Chapter on "Racial Attitudes and Discrimination"). The purpose of such testing, according to the authors, is to enhance awareness and to facilitate voluntary efforts to address racial disparities in care. Should these efforts fail, judicial remedies could be explored if clear violations of civil rights laws are found (LaViest and Gibbons, 2001). Unlike paired testing in housing and employment, however, the use of such strategies in healthcare settings poses unique legal and ethical challenges that should be addressed before such strategies are adopted.

Reporting of Racial and Ethnic Disparities Using Existing Data Sets

As noted earlier, the HEDIS data sets developed by NCQA offer a ready set of measures of plan performance that are widely used and accepted by health plans, purchasers, and consumers. Health plans voluntarily report this information to NCQA, which then disseminates data as part of its Quality Compass database in regular publications such as the NCQA *State of Managed Care Quality* report. Quality Compass 2000 contains measures of plan performance in several clinical areas, such as cancer screening, childhood and adult immunization, timely outpatient care, and evidence-based treatments for hypertension, cardiovascular disease, asthma, diabetes, and depression. Approximately half of the nation's HMOs participate in Quality Compass, with another 90% participating in NCQA's Accreditation and HEDIS programs.

Some researchers and plan administrators have raised concerns that health plan performance on these or other quality measures is affected by the sociodemographic mix of plan enrollees. According to this view, plans that enroll a high percentage of low-income or racial and ethnic minorities (who tend to be sicker, face a greater number of barriers to accessing care, and are less likely to utilize preventive and primary care services) may tend to face poorer health plan performance scores as a result of factors exogenous to the health system (Zaslavsky et al., 2000). Zaslavsky et al. (2000) tested this hypothesis by studying the relationship between plan performance on HEDIS measures and sociodemographic mix, including enrollee age, gender, and area of residence as an indicator of race/ethnicity and household income. The authors found that plan performance was negatively associated with the percentage of individuals receiving public assistance and the percentage of African Americans and Hispanics in enrollees' area of residence, and positively associated with the percentage of college-educated and Asian-American residents. Adjusting for these demographic variables, however, had a limited effect on plan performance, as most plans changed by less than 5% in performance measures.

Romano (2000) argues that even if case-mix differences could be adequately adjusted statistically, such adjustment does not necessarily improve analysis of the quality of care that plans deliver. To the contrary, he argues that statistical adjustment may hamper accurate assessment of plan performance by failing to identify the direction of the relationship between case-mix and plan performance—in other words, does the plan's case-mix result in poor performance, or does poor performance lead to the observed case-mix? In addition, statistical adjustment may "excuse" health plans for failing to address socioeconomic and racial/ethnic health disparities. Adjustment for case-mix may inadvertently remove plans' incentive to reduce disparities, according to Romano, by masking differences in the level of care provided to racial and ethnic minorities and low-income enrollees. He argues for reporting of data stratified by race, ethnicity, and socioeconomic status, which would offer the advantage of highlighting, rather than masking, sociodemographic disparities, and would allow consumers to make better informed choices about plans based on their own sociodemographic profile. In addition, by presenting performance data stratified by race, ethnicity, and socioeconomic status, plans could be rewarded for efforts to reduce disparities (Romano, 2000; Fiscella et al., 2000).

DATA NEEDS AND RECOMMENDATIONS

The preceding discussion illustrates that despite the many challenges inherent in efforts to collect data on patients' race and ethnicity and monitor the quality of their care, data collection and monitoring are a feasible, critically important step in understanding and eliminating disparities in care. As Tom Perez (this volume) notes, "Effective data collection is the linchpin of any comprehensive strategy to eliminate racial and ethnic disparities in health."

Currently, data collection efforts are unsystematic and inadequate to monitor the quality of care provided to racial and ethnic minorities. These efforts must be improved to ensure accountability of plans and providers to healthcare payors and consumers, to track disparities and assess the impact of quality improvement efforts, and to identify best practices that may be replicated by other plans and health systems. Federal leadership is needed to spearhead data collection efforts; for this reason, the committee advocates that the Secretary of the U.S. Department of Health and Human Services produce periodic studies to assess progress in eliminating racial and ethnic disparities in healthcare. The private sector, however, also shares a role in encouraging data collection and reporting of patient care data by race, ethnicity, and where possible, primary language. Accreditation bodies, such as JACHO and NCQA, should require the inclusion of data on patient race, ethnicity, and highest level of education attained (in case of children, highest level of education attained by mother) in performance reports of public and private providers as part of healthcare performance measurement. Such an emphasis would help to ensure that addressing healthcare disparities is seen by plans, providers, and purchasers as central to broader healthcare quality improvement efforts.

Data collection should be accomplished using a standard racial/ethnic classification scheme. Current OMB standards can be used, but data categories must go beyond the existing minimum standards to reflect the diversity within racial and ethnic populations, particularly at the local level (e.g., subgroups of Hispanics, African Americans, Asian Americans, etc.). In addition, information is needed on patients' socioeconomic status and primary language. These data should be stratified, where possible, to better understand the relative contributions of race/ethnicity, socioeconomic status, and other demographic variables to variations in care.

In the future, a standardized, central database is needed, with safeguards for privacy and confidentiality, which can be merged with other data systems. This database should be consistent with efforts to develop electronic patient medical records, and should be compatible to merge with other data systems. Such a long-term goal will require federal leadership and financial support.

Recommendation 7-1: Collect and report data on healthcare access and utilization by patients' race, ethnicity, socioeconomic status, and where possible, primary language.
Standardized data should be collected on the race, ethnicity, and highest level of education (in case of children, highest level of education attained by mother) of all patients enrolled in publicly funded health programs and reported to Congress. Collection of data on patients' primary language should be encouraged, where feasible, as part of this effort. Data on healthcare access, use, and outcomes should be reported by race, ethnicity (including subgroups, and primary language where possible), and adjusted for highest level of education.

Recommendation 7-2: Include measures of racial and ethnic disparities in performance measurement.
JCAHO and NCQA should require the inclusion of data on patient race, ethnicity, and highest level of education attained (in case of children, highest level of education attained by mother) in performance reports of public and private providers as part of health care perfor-

mance measurement, such as NCQA's HEDIS indicators. The collection of data on patients' primary language should be encouraged. These performance reports should make elimination of healthcare disparities a focus of quality improvement efforts.

Recommendation 7-3: Monitor progress toward the elimination of healthcare disparities.
The secretary of HHS should conduct periodic studies to monitor the nation's progress toward eliminating racial and ethnic healthcare disparities, to provide insight into the root causes of these disparities, and to assess opportunities for intervention and improvement.

Recommendation 7-4: Report racial and ethnic data by OMB categories, but use subpopulation groups where possible.
Current OMB categories for race and ethnicity should be used in all reporting and monitoring efforts, but data categories must go beyond the existing minimum standards to reflect the diversity within racial and ethnic populations (e.g., subpopulations), particularly at the local level.

8

Needed Research

In previous chapters, the committee has reviewed extensive evidence of racial and ethnic disparities in care, and has assessed potential sources of these disparities, as well as promising strategies to eliminate them. In the process, the committee notes that the evidence base to better understand and eliminate disparities in care remains less than clear. In this chapter, several broad areas of research needs are outlined. Some of this research is already underway or planned as a result of leadership and support from the federal Agency for Healthcare Research and Quality (AHRQ) and several private foundations (for a more thorough description of ongoing federal and private research and intervention efforts to address racial and ethnic disparities in care, see *Federal and Private Initiatives to Reduce Healthcare Disparities* in the appendix of this volume). The committee urges greater support from a range of federal and private sources, however, for a more ambitious research agenda aimed at disentangling the many influences on the process, structure, and outcomes of care for minority Americans.

This chapter is divided into several sections. The first three sections highlight research opportunities that should better illuminate the ways in which race and ethnicity influence the delivery of healthcare. To date, far greater research attention has been directed to documenting racial and ethnic disparities in care than in understanding how these disparities emerge in the structure and process of care, as these recommendations illustrate. The latter sections discuss areas where research has been minimal or notably absent. This includes intervention research; research on disparities in care among non-African-American racial and ethnic minority populations, such as Native Americans, Asian Americans, Pacific Islanders, Hispanics, and subgroups of these populations; and research on the role of non-physician healthcare professionals, such as nurses, physician assistants, occupational and rehabilitation therapists, mental heath care providers, and others in eliminating racial and ethnic disparities in care. Finally, the last section offers suggestions for strategies to carry out this research.

UNDERSTANDING CLINICAL DECISION-MAKING AND THE ROLES OF STEREOTYPING, UNCERTAINTY, AND BIAS

Much of the research cited in previous chapters relies on retrospective analyses of administrative claims or hospital discharge data. While these data sets have proven useful in identifying racial and ethnic disparities in a range of hospital and clinic-based services (from relatively routine diagnostic and treatment services through specialized surgical procedures), they pose a number of inherent limitations. Hospital discharge records yield only limited data regarding patients' interactions with the range of healthcare professionals with whom they come into contact and the race or ethnicity of these providers. Further, such data are often limited with regard to clinical decision-making processes and the information that clinicians must consider when recommending a course of treatment. For example, administrative data sets often contain only crude information regarding co-morbid conditions, diagnostic test data, and specific treatments.

Prospective studies are needed to focus on decision-making by patients and providers, to assess care management at different points along the continuum of care, and to assess the impact of patient-provider interactions on diagnosis and treatment. More complete records of patients' co-morbid conditions, as well as results of diagnostic tests, will help in the context of prospective research to assess the appropriateness of treatment. Such data will also assist in determining if physicians experience greater uncertainty in assessing presenting complaints of cultural or linguistic minority patients, or if their treatment decisions for these patients fail to correspond to accepted standards of care.

Beyond prospective studies of healthcare service delivery, additional research is needed on provider decision-making, heuristics employed in diagnostic evaluation, and how patients' race, ethnicity, gender, and social class may influence these decisions. As noted in earlier chapters, some experimental research has been conducted to assess the extent to which physicians' treatment recommendations differ by patient race and gender (e.g., Schulman et al., 1999). This research should be expanded to both replicate these findings and explore how social cognitive processes may operate to influence patients' and providers' conscious and unconscious perceptions of each other and affect the structure, processes, and outcomes of care.

As noted in Chapters 3 and 4, it is likely that clinical uncertainty and discretion with regard to diagnostic and treatment options may play a role in healthcare disparities. When clinicians are uncertain about a patient's presenting symptoms, or when multiple treatment options are available but "best" practices among racial and ethnic minorities are unclear, treatment may be less well matched to patients' needs, because such conditions increase the likelihood that biases and implicit stereotypes may affect clinicians' decisions. Alternatively, when empirically-based practice guidelines offer evidence of the effectiveness of specific interventions among minority patients, uncertainty may be lessened. Future research should therefore assess whether disparities are reduced when clinicians are provided with and make use of evidence of treatment efficacy.

UNDERSTANDING PATIENT-LEVEL INFLUENCES ON CARE

As noted earlier, patient mistrust of providers may affect decisions to seek care, and may negatively influence the quality of the patient-provider relationship. Investigators should assess patients' attitudes and preferences toward healthcare providers and services, and examine the extent of these influences on the quality of care and treatment decisions. Research should also evaluate appropriate means of addressing and modifying negative cultural beliefs about care-seeking and mistrust of healthcare systems. Further, strategies to increase minority patients' ability to participate in treatment decisions and empower them as self-advocates within healthcare systems should be evaluated. It is important that these research efforts be conducted in active collaboration with racial and ethnic minority communities, both to avoid the perception that patients are to blame for unequal or poor treatment in healthcare settings, as well as to tap into cultural knowledge and traditions that may serve as sources of strength in the effort to "activate" patients.

UNDERSTANDING THE INFLUENCE OF HEALTHCARE SYSTEMS AND SETTINGS ON CARE FOR MINORITY PATIENTS

Studies Within Healthcare Plans

There is considerable variation across healthcare plans in the type and extent of coverage that beneficiaries receive. Even among those insured by public programs such as Medicare, some beneficiaries may hold a variety of types of supplemental insurance that enhances coverage for specific services, thereby increasing their access to care. Many studies of racial and ethnic differences in healthcare, however, fail to account for these differences, often collapsing the privately-insured or publicly-insured into broad categories that mask differences in coverage. Future research should better account for these differences by assessing racial and ethnic disparities in care among similarly-insured patients within the same plan.

Studies of DoD and VA Systems

The committee's analysis revealed that for some healthcare services and under some conditions, racial and ethnic disparities in care are less pronounced. These findings are somewhat more consistent in studies of healthcare provided to active-duty personnel and their families through the U.S. Department of Defense healthcare system, which provides universal access to care, and are inconsistent among studies of the "equal-access" Veterans Administration healthcare system. Future research should seek to illuminate the conditions of health systems, including factors such as co-payment and accessibility that may be associated with racial and ethnic disparities in care.

Type of Hospital or Clinic and Racial and Ethnic Disparities in Care

Several studies find differences as to where racial and ethnic minorities receive care, even when holding insurance status constant. Lillie-Blanton, Martinez, and Salganicoff (2001) found that independent of sociodemographic factors, health status, and insurance status, African-American and Latino patients are more likely than white patients to have a hospital-based provider and are less likely to have an office-based provider as a usual source of care. Lillie-Blanton et al. (2001) note that these differences could reflect geographic or sociocultural barriers to care, patient preferences, or some combination of these factors. Structural, institutional, and organizational aspects of healthcare settings can affect the cost, content, and quality of care, as well as patient satisfaction. The contribution of these factors to healthcare disparities must be more thoroughly assessed. In addition, research should determine whether structural, institutional and organizational factors of healthcare settings affect the content of care or quality of communication for racial and ethnic minority patients.

Similarly, little is known about the healthcare providers that tend to serve racial and ethnic minority patients. Research indicates that racial and ethnic minority physicians, particularly those who are African American and Hispanic, disproportionately serve poor, underserved and minority patients (Komaromy et al., 1996). However, these providers remain a small fraction of the overall healthcare workforce. More must be understood about the racial and ethnic composition of providers who tend to serve minority patients, and the impact of racial concordance/discordance on care. In particular, little is known about the impact of international medical graduates working in minority communities. As noted earlier in this report, these providers disproportionately serve racial and ethnic minority patients, yet little is known about the quality of their interactions with minority patients, despite the apparent greater likelihood of cultural and linguistic misunderstanding. To better understand sources of racial and ethnic disparities in care, future research should analyze the experience, qualifications, specialties, and other attributes of providers who disproportionately serve racial and ethnic minority patients and to assess whether these factors may in part explain racial and ethnic disparities in care.

UNDERSTANDING THE ROLES OF
NON-PHYSICIAN HEALTH PROFESSIONALS

The vast majority of research that documents racial and ethnic disparities in care and patient-provider communication in racially concordant and discordant dyads has focused on the role of the physician. This research has been important in illuminating key processes and decision points that may contribute to healthcare disparities. The disproportionate focus of research on physicians, however, unfairly places the locus of attention regarding disparities primarily on physicians. This fails to reflect the reality that much of healthcare is provided by non-physician professionals, including nurses, physician assistants, occupational and rehabilitation therapists, mental health professionals (including psychologists, social workers, and marital and family therapists), pharmacists, and allied health professionals. Further, with a few exceptions, research on racial and ethnic disparities in care has failed to consider the roles of other hospital and clinic staff—such as receptionists, admitting clerks, translators, and others—in contributing to the "climate" in which care is delivered. These individuals play at least as significant a role as physicians (if not more so) in conveying messages of respect and dignity to patients and in influencing how patients feel about the healthcare setting. Research is critically needed to assess how these individuals communicate with racial and ethnic minority patients, and in turn, how patients respond to them. Further, research should assess how educational programs can best improve these staffs' attitudes, behaviors, and communication with racial and ethnic minority patients. In this regard, the committee notes that many corporations and organizations (and indeed, some health plans) have developed extensive training programs to assist their workforce in better serving and addressing needs of culturally and linguistically diverse customers; these training programs offer potentially valuable models for healthcare institutions wishing to become more "customer-friendly" and improve service.

ASSESSING HEALTHCARE DISPARITIES AMONG NON-AFRICAN AMERICAN MINORITY GROUPS

A central concern throughout the committee's review of the literature on racial and ethnic disparities in healthcare has been the relative paucity of research on non-African-American racial and ethnic minority groups. While a number of important studies have sought to assess the extent of disparities among diverse racial and ethnic populations (e.g., Carlisle et al., 1995), the extent of disparities in care faced by Asian-American, Pacific Islander, Native American, and Hispanic populations remains unclear. Furthermore, barriers to care experienced by various subgroups of these populations must be better assessed. As noted earlier, focus group data and other information gathered by the committee suggest that linguistic and cultural mismatches pose greater challenges for recent immigrant minorities than for African Americans. There is tremendous cultural, linguistic, and socioeconomic variation within the "racial" populations noted above, and their historic and contemporary experiences in the United States—as noted by Byrd and Clayton (see appendix)—vary considerably, all of which significantly influence the context by which care is delivered to these populations.

ASSESSING THE EFFECTIVENESS OF INTERVENTION STRATEGIES

The committee's analysis suggests several promising avenues for interventions to eliminate racial and ethnic disparities in healthcare. To date, however, relatively less research attention has been devoted to assessing intervention efforts than to understanding the extent and sources of disparities in care. Several promising strategies have been identified that should continue to be the focus of research efforts, such as comprehensive cross-cultural education and communication training for healthcare providers. Research should assess not only the effectiveness of these interventions in reducing racial and ethnic gaps in appropriate care, but also their cost-effectiveness and the extent to which these interventions result in organizational and institution-level changes to improve care for minority patients. Research should also assess the benefits of other intervention strategies described earlier in this report, including language translation and interpretation services, lay health navigators, patient education and "activation" strategies, and efforts to make healthcare services more culturally and linguistically accessible.

DEVELOPING METHODS FOR MONITORING HEALTHCARE DISPARITIES

As discussed in the chapter on data collection and monitoring, the collection and reporting of healthcare information by patient race and ethnicity is an important step in monitoring the nation's progress in eliminating racial and ethnic disparities in healthcare. Such efforts will assist consumers and purchasers in making better-informed choices about health plans, will help plans and providers to identify effective intervention strategies, and will identify practice settings where disparities occur and assist efforts to monitor compliance with civil rights laws. Data collection and monitoring efforts, however, will face several significant challenges to implementation, as noted earlier. Among these challenges are the need to ensure the privacy of medical records, problems posed in analyzing data from small population groups, the inconsistent use of and understanding of the federally-defined "race" and "ethnicity" categories, and the effect of differences in enrollee case-mix among plans on plan performance. Future research must address these challenges and identify efficient means for such data to be collected that do not pose undue bureaucratic burdens on healthcare providers, consumers, and plans.

UNDERSTANDING THE CONTRIBUTION OF HEALTHCARE TO HEALTH OUTCOMES AND THE HEALTH GAP BETWEEN MINORITY AND NON-MINORITY AMERICANS

As noted earlier in this report, health status disparities observed between many minority and non-minority populations in the United States likely reflect a complex interplay of social, economic, biologic, and environmental factors. While some evidence suggests that preventive and primary care services can have a greater impact on improving health status for low-income than middle- and higher-income individuals, the contribution of healthcare disparities to health status differences between minority and non-minority populations remains unknown. Future research must assess this contribution, and identify how and why healthcare disparities play a role in poorer health outcomes for minorities relative to non-minorities. In addition, future research is needed to determine whether new medical services and technologies are implemented among minority patient populations at the same rates as the general patient population. New medical breakthroughs are occurring at staggering rates, and promise to improve the quality of life and mitigate disease in ways never previously imagined. To the extent that these new technologies are made available and are within economic reach, research must assure that racial and ethnic minorities who have the ability to pay for such care are not disadvantaged in their efforts to receive it.

MECHANISMS TO IMPROVE RESEARCH ON HEALTHCARE DISPARITIES

Research on racial and ethnic disparities in healthcare has grown significantly over the past two decades, and continues to offer new insights into the causes of and possible solutions to care disparities. To strengthen this research, however, and stimulate new insights and perspectives that may lead to innovative intervention strategies, the research enterprise may be strengthened in a number of ways. Much of the research reviewed earlier in this report has been conducted in specific departments of academic or research institutions, and has not taken full advantage of opportunities for interdisciplinary collaboration. Such collaboration will be necessary to address the complexities and multiple causal dimensions of healthcare disparities, as discussed earlier. Therefore, rather than dispersing research throughout the various departments of academic hospitals or other research institutions, researchers may seek to establish multidisciplinary units that encourage collaboration between departments as well as institutions (e.g., law, public health, sociology). In addition, federal and private research sponsors should encourage the conduct of research in a variety of settings (inner city; other urban; community health centers; etc.), and should encourage the participation of researchers from ethnic and racial minority groups.

Recommendation 8-1: Conduct further research to identify sources of racial and ethnic disparities and assess promising intervention strategies.
Research is needed to illuminate how and why racial and ethnic disparities in care occur and to test intervention strategies to eliminate them. Specifically, research is needed to:
• **Better understand the relative contribution of patient, provider, and institutional characteristics to healthcare disparities;**
• **Further illuminate provider decision-making, heuristics employed in diagnostic evaluation, and how patients' race, ethnicity, gender, and social class may influence these decisions;**
• **Assess the relative contributions of provider biases, stereotyping, prejudice, and uncertainty in producing racial and ethnic disparities in diagnosis, treatment, and outcomes of care;**

- Understand the role of non-physician healthcare professionals, including nurses, physician assistants, occupational and rehabilitation therapists, mental health professionals (including psychologists, social workers, and marital and family therapists), pharmacists, allied health professionals, as well as non-professional staff in contributing to healthcare disparities;
- Assess healthcare disparities among non-African-American minority groups and subgroups;
- Assess the impact of international medical graduates (IMGs) on healthcare service delivery in racial and ethnic minority communities;
- Develop and test the utility for healthcare improvement of patient-based measures of (1) trust in providers and systems and (2) exposure to discriminatory practices by providers or systems;
- Develop methods for monitoring progress toward eliminating racial and ethnic disparities in healthcare; and
- Understand the relationship between healthcare disparities and the health gap between minority and non-minority Americans.

Finally, it is apparent that efforts to eliminate healthcare disparities will benefit from efforts to better address barriers to research and intervention. As noted earlier, these include ethical issues and data-related concerns, such as the need to protect patient privacy. At minimum, research and intervention efforts must conform to the Health Insurance Portability and Accountability Act of 1996 (HIPAA) regulations regarding the protection of patients' medical records and other confidential data. The Agency for Healthcare Research and Quality (AHRQ), the Centers for Disease Control and Prevention (CDC), and the National Institutes of Health (NIH) have already begun to address some of these concerns through ongoing research and data management, and should be encouraged to continue addressing barriers to data collection and research.

Recommendation 8-2: Conduct research on ethical issues and other barriers to eliminating disparities.
AHRQ, CDC, and NIH should conduct research on barriers to eliminating racial and ethnic disparities in care, including data-related concerns (especially those related to HIPAA privacy regulations) and ethical issues.

References

Abreu JM. (1999). Conscious and nonconscious African American stereotypes: Impact on first impression and diagnostic ratings by therapists. *Journal of Consulting and Clinical Psychology* 67(3):387–393.

Accreditation Council for Graduate Medical Education. *ACGME Outcomes Project: General Competencies.* [Online]. Available: http://www.acgme.org/outcomes/comptv13.htm [accessed March 15, 2001].

Alexander GC, Sehgal AR. (1998). Barriers to cadaveric renal transplantation among blacks, women, and the poor. *The Journal of the American Medical Association* 280(13):1148–1152.

Allison JJ, Kiefe CI, Centor RM, Box JB, Farmer RM. (1996). Racial differences in the medical treatment of elderly medicare patients with acute myocardial infarction. *Journal of General Internal Medicine* 11:736–743.

American Medical Association Council on Ethical and Judicial Affairs. (1990). Black-white disparities in health care. *Journal of the American Medical Association*, 263(17):2344–2346.

Andrews RM, Elixhauser A. (2000). Use of Major Therapeutic Procedures: Are Hispanics Treated Differently than Non-Hispanic Whites? *Ethnicity & Disease* (10):384–394.

Aron DC, Gordon HS, DiGiuseppe DL, Harper DL, Rosenthal GE. (2000). Variations in risk-adjusted cesarean delivery rates according to race and health insurance. *Medical Care* 38(1):35–44.

Arozullah AM, Ferreira MR, Bennett RL, Gilman S, Henderson WG, Daley J, Khuri S, Bennett CL. (1999). Racial variation in the use of laparoscopic cholecystectomy in the Department of Veterans Affairs Medical System. *Journal of the American College of Surgeons* 188(6):604–622.

Arrow KJ. (1963). Uncertainty and the welfare economics of medical care. *American Economic Review* 53:941–973.

Association of American Medical Colleges. (1998). *Minority Graduates of U.S. Medical Schools: Trends, 1950-1998.* Washington, DC: Association of American Medical Colleges.

Association of American Medical Colleges. (2000). *Minority Graduates of U.S. Medical Schools: Trends, 1950-1998.* Washington, DC: Association of American Medical Colleges.

Ayanian JZ, Cleary PD, Weissman JS, Epstein AM. (1999). The effect of patients' preferences on racial differences in access to renal transplantation. *The New England Journal of Medicine* 341(22):1661–1669.

Ayanian JZ, Udvarhelyi IS, Gatsonis CA, Pashos CL, Epstein AM. (1993). Racial differences in the use of revascularization procedures after coronary angiography. *Journal of the American Medical Association* 269:2642–2646.

Ayanian JZ, Weissman JS, Chasan-Taber S, Epstein AM. (1999). Quality of care by race and gender for congestive heart failure and pneumonia. *Medical Care* 37:1260–1269.

Bach PB, Cramer LD, Warren JL, Begg CB. (1999). Racial differences in the treatment of early-stage lung cancer. *New England Journal of Medicine* 341:1198–1205.

Baker DW, Stevens CD, Brook R H. (1996). Determinants of emergency department use: Are race and ethnicity important? *Annals of Emergency Medicine* 28(6):677–682.

Baker EA, Bouldin N, Durham B, Lowell ME, Gonzalez M, Jodaitis N, Cruz LN, Torres I, Adams, ST. (1997). The Latino Health Advocacy Program: A collaborative lay health advisor approach. *Health Education & Behavior* 24(4):495–509.

Baker DW, Hayes R, Fortier JP. (1998). Interpreter use and satisfaction with interpersonal aspects of care for Spanish-speaking patients. *Medical Care* 36(10):1461–1470.

Ball JD, Elixhauser A. (1996). Treatment differences between blacks and whites with colorectal cancer. *Medical Care* 34:970–984.

Balsa A, McGuire TG. (2001a). *Prejudice, Uncertainty and Stereotypes as Sources of Health Care Disparities.* Boston University, unpublished manuscript.

Balsa A, McGuire TG. (2001b). Statistical discrimination in health care, *Journal of Health Economics* 20:881–907.

Barfield WD, Wise PH, Rust FP, Rust KJ, Gould JB, Gortmaker SL. (1996). Racial disparities in outcomes of military and civilian births in California. *Archives of Pediatrics & Adolescent Medicine* 150:1062–1067.

Barker-Cummings C, McClellan W, Soucie JM, Krisher J. (1995). Ethnic differences in the use of peritoneal dialysis as initial treatment for end-stage renal disease. *Journal of the American Medical Association* 274(23):1858–1862.

Barnes M, Weiner W. (1999). Evidence of race-based discrimination triggers new legal and ethical scrutiny. 8 *BNA Health Law Reporter*, 1984.

Bauchner H, Simpson L, Chessare J. (2001). Changing physician behaviour. *Archives of Disease in Childhood* 84:459–462.

Bell PD, Huson, S. (2001). Equity in the diagnosis of chest pain: Race and gender. *American Journal of Health Behavior* 25(1):60–71.

Bellochs C, Carter AB. (1990). *Building Primary Health Care in New York City's Low-income Communities.* New York: Community Health Service Society of New York.

Bennett CL, Horner RD, Weinstein RA, Dickinson GM, Dehovitz JA, Cohn SE, Kessler HA, Jacobson J, Goetz MB, Simberkoff M, Pitrak D, George WL, Gilman SC, Shapiro MF. (1995). Racial differences in care among hospitalized patients with pneumocystis carinii pneumonia in Chicago, New York, Los Angeles, Miami, and Raleigh-Durham. *Archives of Internal Medicine* 155(15):1586–1592.

Berger JT. (1998). Culture and ethnicity in clinical care. *Archives of Internal Medicine* 158:2085–2090.

Berlin EA, Fowkes WC, Jr. (1998). A teaching framework for cross-cultural health care. Application in family practice. *Western Journal of Medicine* 139(6):934–938.

Bernabei R, Gambassi G, Lapane K, Landi F, Gatsonis C, Dunlop R, Lipsiz L, Steel K, Mor V. (1998). Management of pain in elderly patients with cancer. SAGE Study Group. Systematic assessment of geriatric drug use via epidemiology. *Journal of the American Medical Association* 279:1877–1882.

Betancourt JR, Carrillo JE, Green AR. (1999). Hypertension in multicultural and minority populations: Linking communication to compliance. *Current Hypertension Reports* 1:482–488.

Biernat M, Dovidio JF. (2000). Stigma and stereotypes. [chapter] Heatherton TF, Kleck RE, et al., eds. *The Social Psychology of Stigma.* (pp. 88–125). New York, NY: The Guilford Press.

Bindman AB, Grumbach K, Vranizan K, Jaffe D, Osmond D. (1998). Selection and exclusion of primary care physicians by managed care organizations. *Journal of the American Medical Association* 279(9):675–679.

Bird JA, McPhee SJ, HA N-T, Le, B, Davis T, Jenkins CNH. (1998). Opening pathways to cancer screening for Vietnamese-American women: Lay health workers hold a key. *Preventive Medicine* 27:821–829.

Blackwell JE. (1977). *In Support of Preferential Admissions and Affirmative Action in Medical Education: Pre-and Post-Bakke Considerations.* University of Massachusetts at Boston, unpublished document.

Blixen CE, Tilley B, Havstad S, Zoratti E. (1997). Quality of life, medication use, and health care utilization of urban African Americans with asthma treated in emergency departments. *Nursing Research* 46(6):338–341.

Bloche MG. (2001). Race and discretion in American medicine. *Yale Journal of Health Policy, Law, and Ethics* 1:95–131.

Bloche MG. (1999). Clinical loyalties and the social purposes of medicine. *Journal of the American Medical Association* 281(3):268–274.

Blumenthal D. (1996). Part 1:Quality of care—what is it? *New England Journal of Medicine* 335(12):891–894.

Blustein J, Arons RR, Shea, S. (1995). Sequential events contributing to variations in cardiac revascularization rates. *Medical Care* 33:864–880.

Bobo LD. (2001). Racial Attitudes and Relations at the Close of the Twentieth Century. In: Smelser NJ, Wilson WJ, Mitchell F., eds. *America Becoming: Racial Trends and Their Consequences.*Vol.1. Washington, DC: National Academy Press. Pp. 264–301.

Bobo L, Schuman H, Steeh. (1986). Changing Racial Attitudes Toward Residential Integration. In J. Goering, ed. *Housing Desegregation and Federal Policy* 152–169. Chapel Hill: University of North Carolina Press.

Bobo L, Womeodu RJ, Knox AL, Jr. (1991). Principles of intercultural medicine in an internal medicine program. *American Journal of Medical Science* 302(4):244–248.

Bonham VL. (2001). Race, ethnicity, and pain treatment: Striving to understand the causes and solutions to the disparities in pain treatment. *Journal of Law, Medicine, and Ethics* 29:52–68.

Brach C, Fraser I. (2000). Can cultural competency reduce racial and ethnic disparities? A review and conceptual model. *Medical Care Research and Review* 1:181–217.

Braveman P, Egerter S, Edmonston F, Verdon M. (1995). Racial/ethnic differences in the likelihood of cesarean delivery, California. *American Journal of Public Health* 85(5):625–630.

Brett KM, Schoendorf KC, Kiley JL. (1994). Differences between black and white women in the use of prenatal care technologies. *American Journal of Obstetrics and Gynecology* 170(1):41–46.

Brewer MB. (1996). When Stereotypes Lead to Stereotyping: The Use of Stereotypes in Person Perception. In N. Macrae, C. Stangor, M. Hewstone (Eds.), *Stereotypes and Stereotyping* (254–275). New York: Guilford Press.

Brogan D, Tuttle EP. (1988). Transplantation and the Medicare end-stage renal disease program [Letter]. *New England Journal of Medicine* 319:55.

Brown RE, Ojeda VD, Wyn R, Levan R. (2000). *Racial and Ethnic Disparities in Access to Health Insurance and Health Care.* Los Angeles, CA:UCLA Center for Health Policy Research.

Brown AF, Perez-Stable EJ, Whitaker EE, Psner SF, Alexander M, Gathe J, Washington AE. (1999). Ethnic differences in hormone replacement prescribing patterns. *Journal of General Internal Medicine* 14(11):663–669.

Brownstein JN, Cheal H, Ackermann SP, Bassford TL, Campos-Outcalt D. (1992). Breast and cervical cancer screening in minority populations: A model for using lay health educators. *Journal of Cancer Education* 7(4):321–326.

Burns RB, McCarthy EP, Freund KM, Marwill SL, Shwarz M, Ash A, Moskowitz MA. (1996). Variability in mammography use among older women. *Journal of the American Geriatrics Society* 44(8):922–926.

Burns RB, McCarthy EP, Freund KM, Marwill SL, Shwarz M, Ash A, Moskowitz MA. (1996). Black women receive less mammography even with similar use of primary care. *Annals of Internal Medicine* 125(3):173–182.

Burstin HR. (1993). Do the poor sue more? A case-control study of malpractice claims and socioeconomic status. *Journal of the American Medical Association* 270:1697.

Bursztajn HJ. (1990). *Medical Choices, Medical Changes.* New York: Routledge.

Byrd WM, Clayton LA. (this volume). Racial and Ethnic Disparities in Health Care: A Background and History.

Byrd WM, Clayton LA. (2001). *An American Health Dilemma, Volume 1, A Medical History of African Americans and the Problem of Race: Beginnings to 1900.* New York: Routledge.

Byrd WM, Clayton LA, Kinchen K, Richardson D, Lawrence L, Butcher R, Davidson E. (1994). African-American physicians' views on health reform: Results of a survey. *Journal of the National Medical Association* 86(3):191-9.

Canto JG, Allison JJ, Kiefe CI, Fincher C, Farmer R, Sekar P, Person S, Weissman NW. (2000). Relation of race and sex to the use of reperfusion therapy in medicare beneficiaries with acute myocardial infarction. *New England Journal of Medicine* 342:1094–1100.

Cantor JD, Miles EL, Baker LC, Barker DC. (1996). Physician service to the underserved: Implications for affirmative action in medical education. *Inquiry* 33:167–180.

Carlisle DM, Gardner JE. (1998). The entry of African-American students into US medical schools: An evaluation of recent trends. *Journal of the National Medical Association* 90:466-73.

Carlisle DM, Leake BD, Shapiro MF. (1995). Racial and ethnic differences in the use of invasive cardiac procedures among cardiac patients in Los Angeles County, 1986 through 1988. *American Journal of Public Health* 85:352–356.

Carlisle DM, Leape LL, Bickel S, Bell R, Kamberg C, Genovese B, French WJ, Kaushik VS, Mahrer PR, Ellestad MH, Brook RH, Shapiro MF. (1999). Underuse and overuse of diagnostic testing for coronary artery disease in patients presenting with new-onset chest pain. *American Journal of Medicine* 106(4):391–398.

Carrasquillo O, Orav EJ, Brennan TA, Burstin HR. (1999). Impact of language barriers on patient satisfaction in an emergency department. *Journal of General Internal Medicine* 4(2):82–87.

Carrasquillo O, Lantigua RA, Shea S. (2001). Preventive services among Medicare beneficiaries with supplemental coverage versus HMO enrollees, Medicaid recipients, and elders with no additional coverage. *Medical Care* 39(6):616-26.

Carrillo JE, Green AR, Betancourt JR. (1999). Cross-cultural primary care: A patient-based approach. *Annals of Internal Medicine* 130(10):829–834.

Chen J, Rathore SS, Radford MJ, Wang Y, Krumholz HM. (2001). Racial differences in the use of cardiac catheterization after acute myocardial infarction. *New England Journal of Medicine* 344:1443–1449.

Chin JL. (2000). Culturally competent health care. *Public Health Reports* 115:25–33.

Chin MH, Zhang JX, Merrell K. (1998). Diabetes in the African-American Medicare population: Morbidity, quality of care, and resource utilization. *Diabetes Care* 21(7):1090–1095.

Cho J, Solis BM. (2001). *Healthy Families Culture and Linguistics Resources Survey: A Physician Perspective on their Diverse Member Population.* Los Angeles: LA Care Health Plan.

Chung H, Mahler JC, Kakuma T. (1995). Racial differences in treatment of psychiatric inpatients. *Psychiatric Services* 46(6):586–591.

Cleeland CS, Gonin R, Baez L, Loehrer P, Pandya KJ. (1997). Pain and treatment of pain in minority patients with cancer: The Eastern Cooperative Oncology Group Minority Outpatient Pain Study. *Annals of Internal Medicine* 127(9):813–816.

Clinton JF. (1996). Cultural diversity and health care in America: Knowledge fundamental to cultural competence in baccalaureate nursing students. *Journal of Cultural Diversity* 3(1): 4–8.

Cobb WM. (1981). The Black American in medicine. *Journal of the National Medical Association* 73(Suppl):1185-244.

Coleman-Miller B. (2000). A physician's perspective on minority health. *Health Care Financing Review* (Health Care Financing Administration) 21:45–56.

Collins KS, Hall A, Neuhaus C. (1999). *U.S. Minority Health: A Chartbook.* New York: The Commonwealth Fund.

Collins TC, Johnson M, Henderson W, Khuri SF, Daley J. (2002). Lower extremity nontraumatic amputation among veterans with peripheral arterial disease: Is race an independent factor? *Medical Care* 40(1 Supp):I-106-I-116.

Committee on the Future of Primary Care. (1994). *Institute of Medicine: Defining primary care: An interim report.* Washington, DC: National Academy Press.

The Commonwealth Fund. 1995. National Comparative Survey of Minority Health Care. Washington DC: The Commonwealth Fund.

Conigliaro J, Whittle J, Good CB, Hanusa BH, Passman LJ, Lofgren RP, Allman R, Ubel PA, O'Connor M, Macpherson DS. (2000). Understanding racial variation in the use of coronary revascularization procedures. *Archive of Internal Medicine* 160:1329–1335.

Cooper LA, and Roter DL. (this volume). Patient-Provider Communication: The Effect of Race and Ethnicity on Process and Outcomes of Health Care.

Cooper CP, Roter DL, Langlieb AM. (2000). Using entertainment televeision to build a context for prevention news stories. *Preventive Medicine* 31(3):225–231.

Cooper-Patrick L, Gallo JJ, Gonzales JJ, Vu HT, Powe NR, Nelson C, Ford DE. (1999). Race, gender, and partnership in the patient-physician relationship. *Journal of the American Medical Association* 282(6):583–589.

Corkery E, Palmer C, Foley ME. (1997). Effect of a bicultural community health worker on completion of diabetes education in a Hispanic population. *Diabetes Care* 20(3):254–257.

Council on Ethical and Judicial Affairs, AMA. (1990). Black-white disparities in health care. *Journal of the American Medical Association* 23:2344–2346.

Council on Graduate Medical Education. (1996). *Eighth report: Patient Care Physician Supply and Requirements: Testing COGME Recommendations.* Washington, DC: Government Printing Office. Downloaded from web site (http://www.cogme.gov/rpt8.htm).

Council on Graduate Medical Education. (1998). *Tenth report: Physician distribution and health care challenges in rural and inner-city areas.* Washington, DC: Government Printing Office. Downloaded from web site (http://www.cogme.gov/rpt10.htm).

Council on Graduate Medical Education. (1999). *Twelfth report: Minorities in Medicine.* Washington, DC: Government Printing Office. Downloaded from web site (http://www.cogme.gov/rpt12.htm).

Cowie CC, Harris MI. (1997). Ambulatory medical care for Non-Hispanic Whites, African-Americans, and Mexican-Americans with NIDDM in the U.S. *Diabetes Care* 20(2):142–147.

Cross TL, Bazron BJ, Dennis KW, Isaacs MR. (1989). Towards a Culturally Competent System of Care: A Monograph on Effective Services for Minority Children Who are Severely Emotionally Disturbed. Washington DC: CASSP Technical Assistance Center, Georgetown University Child Development Center.

Culhane-Pera KA, Like RC, Lebensohn-Chialvo P, Loewe R. (2000). Multicultural curricula in family practice residencies. *Family Medicine* 32(3):167–173.

Culhane-Pera KA, Relf C, Egil E, Baker NJ, Kassekert R. (1997). A curriculum for multicultural education in family medicine. *Educational Research Methods* 29:719–723.

Cunningham WE, Mosen DM, Morales LS. (2000). Ethnic and racial differences in long-term survival from hospitalization for HIV infection. *Journal of Health Care for the Poor and Underserved* 11(2):163–178.

Daumit GL, Hermann JA, Coresh J, Powe NR. (1999). Use of Cardiovascular Procedures among Black Persons and White Persons: A 7-Year Nationwide Study in Patients with Renal Disease *Annals of Internal Medicine* 173–182.

David RA, Rhee M. (1998). The impact of language as a barrier to effective health care in an underserved urban Hispanic community. *Mount Sinai Journal of Medicine* 65(5-6):393–397.

Davidson RC, Lewis EL. (1997). Affirmative action and other special consideration admissions at the University of California, Davis, School of Medicine. *Journal of the American Medical Association* 278(14):1153–1158.

Davis DA, Thomson MA, Oxman AD, Haynes RB. (1992). Evidence for the effectiveness of CME: A review of 50 randomized controlled trials. *Journal of the American Medical Association* 268:1111–1117.

Davis DA, Thomson MA, Oxman AD, Haynes RB. (1995). Changing physician performance: A systematic review of the effect of continuing medical education strategies. *Journal of the American Medical Association* 274:700–705.

Denoba DL, Bragdon JL, Epstein LG, Garthright K, Goldman TM. (1998). Reducing health disparities through cultural competence. *Journal of Health Education* 29(5 Suppl.):S47-S58.

Derose KP, Baker DW. (2000). Limited English proficiency and Latinos' use of physician services. *Medical Care Research and Review* 57(1):76–91.

Devgan U, Yu F, Kim E, Coleman A. (2000). Surgical undertreatment of glaucoma in black beneficiaries of medicare. *Archives of Ophthalmology* 118:253–256.

Devine PG. (1989). Stereotypes and prejudice: Their automatic and controlled components. *Journal of Personality and Social Psychology* 56:5–18.

Diehr P, Yergan J, Chu J, Feigl P, Glaefke G, Moe R, Bergner M, Rodenbaugh J. (1989). Treatment modality and quality differences for black and white breast-cancer patients treated in community hospitals. *Medical Care* 27(10): 942–959.

Dignan MB, Michielutte R, Wells HB, Sharp P, Blinson K, Case LD, Bell R, Konen J, Davis St., McQuellon RP. (1998). Health education to increase screening for cervical cancer among Lumbee Indian Women in North Carolina. *Health Education Research Theory & Practice* 13(4):545–556.

Doescher MP, Saver BG, Franks P, Fiscela K. (2000). Racial and ethnic disparities in perceptions of physician style and trust. *Archives of Family Medicine* 9(10):1156–1163.

Dominitz JA, Samsa GP, Landsman P, Provenzale D. (1998). Race, treatment, and survival among colorectal carcinoma patients in an equal-access medical system. *Cancer* 82:2312–2320.

Dominitz JA, Maynard C, Billingsley KG, Boyko EJ. (2002). Race, Treatment, and Survival of Veterans With Cancer of the Distal Esophagus and Gastric Cardia. *Medical Care* 40 (1 Supp):14-26.

Donini-Lenhoff FG, Hedrick HL. (2000). Increasing awareness and implementation of cultural competence principles in health professions education. *Journal of Allied Health* 29(4):241–245.

Dovidio JF. (1999). Stereotyping. In Wilson RA and Keil FC, eds. *The MIT Encyclopedia of the Cognitive Sciences*. Cambridge, MA: MIT Press.

Dovidio JF, Brigham JC, Johnson BT, Gaertner SL. (1996). Stereotyping, Prejudice, and Discrimination: Another Look. In N Macrae, C Stangor, and M Hewstone, eds. *Stereotypes and Stereotyping* 276–319. New York: Guilford.

Dovidio JF, Gaertner SL. (1998). On the nature of contemporary prejudice: The causes, consequences, and challenges of aversive racism. In JL Eberhardt and ST Fiske, eds. *Confronting racism: The problem and the response*, 3–32. Thousand Oaks, CA: Sage Publications, Inc.

Dovidio JF, Kawakami K, Gaertner SL. (2002). Implicit and explicit prejudice and interracial interaction. *Journal of Personality & Social Psychology* 82(1):62–68.

D'Souza D. (1996). *The End of Racism: Principles for a Multiracial Society*. New York: The Free Press.

Dudley RA, Landon BE, Rubin HR, Keating NL, Medlin CA, Luft HS. (2000). Assessing the relationship between quality of care and the characteristics of health care organizations. *Medial Care Research and Review* 57(2):116–135.

Dudley RA, Miller RH, Korenbrot TY, Luft HS. (1998). The impact of financial incentives on quality of health care. *Milbank Quarterly* 76(4):649–686.

Duke University Medical Center. (1999). *Black History Month: A Medical Perspective*. Downloaded from web site (http//:www.mclibrary.duke.edu/hot/blkhist.html).

Earp JL, Flax VL. (1999). What lay health advisors do: An evaluation of advisors' activities. *Cancer Practice* 7(1):16–21.

Ebell MH, Smith M, Kruse JA, Drader-Wilcox J, Novak J. (1995). Effect of race on survival following in-hospital cardiopulmonary resuscitation. *The Journal of Family Practice* 40(6):571-7.

Ebden P, Carey OJ, Bhatt A, Harrison B. (1988). The bilingual consultation. *Lancet* 1(8581):347.

Eddy DM. (1996). Clinical decision making: From theory to practice. Benefit language: Criteria that will improve quality while reducing costs. *Journal of the American Medical Association* 275(8):650–657.

Edsall TB. (2001). 25% of U.S. View Chinese Americans Negatively. The *Washington Post*, April 26, 2001.

Educational Commission for Foreign Medical Graduates. (1992). *Educational Commission for Foreign Medical Graduates: Annual Report*.

Einbinder LC, Schulman KA. (2000). The effect of race on the referral process for invasive cardiac procedures. *Medical Care Research and Review* 1:162–177.

Eisenberg JM. (1979). Sociologic influences on medical decision making by clinicians. *Annals of Internal Medicine* 90(6):957–964.

Eisenberg JM. (1986). *Doctors' Decisions and the Costs of Medical Care*. Ann Arbor, Michigan: Health Administration Press.

Eliason MJ. (1998). Correlates of prejudice in nursing students. *Journal of Nursing Education* 37:(1)27–29.

Elston Lafata J, Cole Johnson C, Ben-Menachem T, Morlock RJ. (2001). Sociodemographic differences in the receipt of colorectal cancer surveillance care following treatment with curative intent. *Medical Care* 39(4):361–72.

Epstein AJ. (2001). The role of public clinics in preventable hospitalizations among vulnerable populations. *Health Services Research* 32(2):405–420.

Epstein AM, Zyanian JZ, Keogh JH, Noonan SJ, Armistead N, Cleary PD, Weissman JS, David-Kasdan JA, Carlson D, Fuller J, March D, Conti R. (2000). Racial disparities in access to renal transplantation. *The New England Journal of Medicine* 343(21):1537–1544.

Escarce JJ, Epstein KR, Colby DC, Schwartz JS. (1993). Racial differences in the elderly's use of medical procedures and diagnostic tests. *American Journal of Public Health* 83(7):948–954.

Exner DV, Dries DL, Domanski MJ, Cohn JN. (2001). Lesser response to angiotensin-converting–enzyme inhibitor therapy in black as compared with white patients with left ventricular dysfunction. *New England Journal of Medicine* 344:1351–1357.

Farley J, Hines JF, Taylor RR, Carlson JW, Parker MF, Kost ER, Rogers SJ, Harrison TA, Macri CI, Parham GP. (2001). Equal care ensures equal survival for African-American women with cervical carcinoma. *Cancer* 91(4):869–873.

Farley R, Steeh C, Krysan M, Jackson T, Reeves K. (1994). Stereotypes and segregation: Neighborhoods in the Detroit area. *American Journal of Sociology* 100:750–780.

Fendrick AM, Chernew ME, Hirth RA, Bloom BS. (1995). Alternative management strategies for patients with suspected peptic ulcer disease. *Annals of Internal Medicine* 123:260-268.

Finucane TE, Carrese JA. (1990). Racial bias in presentation of cases. *Journal of General Internal Medicine* 5:120-1.

Fiscella K, Franks P, Gold MR, Clancy CM. (2000). Inequality in quality: Addressing socioeconomic, racial, and ethnic disparities in health care. *Journal of the American Medical Association* 283:2579–2584.

Fiske ST. (1998). Stereotyping, prejudice, and discrimination. [chapter] Gilbert DT, Fiske ST, et al., eds. *The handbook of social psychology, Vol. 2* (4th ed.). (pp. 357-411). New York: McGraw-Hill.

Fix M, Galster G, Struyk R. (1993). An Overview of Auditing for Discrimination. In M Fix, R Struyk, eds. *Clear and Convincing Evidence: Measurement of Discrimination in America*, 1-68. Washington, DC: The Urban Institute Press.

Flores G, Gee D, Kastner B. (2000). The teaching of cultural issues in the U.S. and Canadian medical schools. *Academic Medicine* 75(5):451–455.

Flores G. 2000. Culture and the patient-physician relationship: Achieving cultural competency in health care. *Journal of Pediatrics* 136:14–23.

Ford ES, Cooper RS. (1995). Racial/ethnic differences in health care utilization of cardiovascular procedures: A review of the evidence. *Health Services Research* 30:237–252.

Ford E, Cooper R, Castaner A, Simmons B, Mar, M. (1989). Coronary arteriography and coronary bypass among whites and other racial groups relative to hospital-based incidence rates for coronary artery disease: Findings from NHDS. *American Journal of Public Health* 79(4):437–440.

Forrest CB, Whelan E. (2000). Primary care safety-net delivery sites in the United States: A comparison of community health centers, hospital outpatient departments, and physicians' offices. *Journal of the American Medical Association* 284(16):2077–2083.

Fossett JW, Peroff JD, Peterson JA, Kletke PR. (1990). Medicaid in the inner city: The case of maternity care in Chicago. *Milbank Quarterly* 68:111–141.

Fronstin P. (2000). *Sources of Health Insurance and Characteristics of the Uninsured: Analysis of the March 2000 Current Population Survey.* Issue Brief No. 228, Washington, DC: Employee Benefit Research Institute.

Furth SL, Garg PP, Neu AM, Hwang W, Fivush BA, Powe NR. (2000). Racial differences in access to the kidney transplant waiting list for children and adolescents with end-stage renal disease. *Pediatrics* 106(4):756–761.

Galster G. (1990). Racial steering by real estate agents: Mechanisms and motives. *The Review of Black Political Economy* 19:39–63.

Gamble VN. (1997). Under the shadow of Tuskegee: African-Americans and health care. *American Journal of Public Health* 87(11):1773–1778.

Garg PP, Diener-West M, Powe NE. (2001). Reducing racial disparities in transplant activation: Whom should we target? *American Journal of Kidney Diseases* 37(5):921–931.

Gaskin DJ. (1999). The hospital safety net: A study of inpatient care for non-elderly vulnerable populations. In M Lillie-Blanton, R Martinez, D Rowland, eds. *Access to Health Care: Promises and Prospects for Low-Income Americans,* 123. Washington DC: Kaiser Commission on Medicaid and the Uninsured.

Gaskin DJ, Hoffman C. (2000). Racial and ethnic differences in preventable hospitalizations across 10 states. *Medical Care Research & Review* 57(1):85–107.

Gaylin DS, Held PJ, Port FK, Hunsicker LG, Wolfe RA, Kahan BD, Jones CA, Agoda LY. (1993). The impact of comorbid and sociodemographic factors on access to renal transplantation. *Journal of the American Medical Association* 269:603-8.

Geiger HJ. (this volume). Racial and Ethnic Disparities in Diagnosis and Treatment: A Review of the Evidence and a Consideration of Causes.

Geiger HJ. (2000). Understanding and Eliminating Racial and Ethnic Disparities in Health Care—What Is Known and What Needs to Be Known? Presentation to IOM Committee on Understanding and Eliminating Racial and Ethnic Disparities in Health Care, December 19, 2000, Washington, DC.

Geoffrey W, Deci EL. (2001). Activating patients for smoking cessation through physician autonomy support. *Medical Care* 39(8):813–823.

Gerrish, K. (1999). Inequalities in service provision: An examination of institutional influences on the provision of district nursing care to minority ethnic communities. *Journal of Advanced Nursing* 30(6):1263–1271.

Giacomini, MK. (1996). Gender and ethnic differences in hospital-based procedure utilization in California. *Archives of Internal Medicine* 156:1217–1224.

Giblin, PT. (1989). Effective utilization and evaluation of indigenous health care workers. *Public Health Reports* 104(8):361–368.

Giles WH, Anda RF, Casper ML, Escobedo LG, Taylor HA. (1995). Race and sex differences in rates of invasive cardiac procedures in U.S. hospitals. *Archives of Internal Medicine,* 155:318-324.

Ginzberg E. (1994). Improving health care for the poor. Lessons from the 1980s. *Journal of the American Medical Association* 271(6):464-7.

Goff DC Jr, Sellers DE, McGovern PG, Meischke H, Goldberg RJ, Bittner V, Hedges JR, Allender PS, Nichaman MZ. (1998). Knowledge of heart attack symptoms in a population survey in the United States: The REACT Trial. Rapid Early Action for Coronary Treatment. *Archives of Internal Medicine* 158(21):2329–2338.

Goldberg KC, Hartz AH, Jacobsen SJ, Krakauer H, Rimm AA. (1992). Racial and community factors influencing coronary artery bypass graft surgery rates for all 1986 Medicare patients. *Journal of the American Medical Association* 267:1473-1477.

Gomes C, McGuire TG. (2001). Identifying the sources of racial and ethnic disparities in health care use. Unpublished manuscript.

Gonzalez-Klayman N, Barnhart, JM. (1998). Racial differences in the utilization of coronary revascularization: A review of the literature. *CVD Prevention* 1:114–122.

Gonzalez-Lee T, Simon HJ. (1991). Teaching Spanish and cross-cultural sensitivity to medical students. *Western Journal of Medicine* 146(4):502–504.

Good MJD, James C, Good BJ, and Becker AE. (this volume). The Culture of Medicine and Racial, Ethnic and Class Disparities in Health Care.

Gornick ME. (2000). Disparities in medicare services: Potential causes, plausible explanations and recommendations. *Health Care Financing Review* (Health Care Financing Administration) 21:23–43.

Gornick ME, Egers PW, Reilly TW, Mentnech RM, Fitterman LK, Kucken LE, Vladeck BC. (1996). Effects of race and income on mortality and use of services among Medicare beneficiaries. *New England Journal of Medicine* 335(11):791–799.

Gregory PM, Rhoads GG, Wilson AC, O'Dowd KJ, Kostis JB. (1999). Impact of availability of hospital-based invasive cardiac services on racial differences in the use of these services. *American Heart Journal* 138:507-17.

Grumbach K, Coffman J, Rosenoff E, and Munoz C. (2001). Trends in Underrepresented Minority Participation in Health Professions Schools. In Smedley BD, Stith AY, Colburn L, and Evans C, eds. *The Right Thing to Do, The Smart Thing to Do: Enhancing Diversity in Health Professions.* Washington, DC: National Academy Press.

Guadagnoli E, Ayanian JZ, Gibbons G, McNeil BJ, LoGerfo, FW. (1995). The Influence of Race on the Use of Surgical Procedures for Treatment of Peripheral Vascular Disease of the Lower Extremities. *Archieves of Surgery* 130:381–387.

Gurin P. (1999). Expert testimony of Patricia Gurin, Gratz, et al. v, Bollinger, et al., No. 97-75321 (E.D. Mich.). [www document] URL http://www.umich.edu/~newsinfo/Admission/Expert/gurintoc.html (accessed March 3, 1999).

Hahn, BA. (1995). Children's health: Racial and ethnic differences in the use of prescription medications. *American Academy of Pediatrics* 95(5):727–732.

Hampers LC, Cha S, Gutglass, DJ, Binns HJ, Krug SE. (1999). Language barriers and resource utilization in a pediatric emergency department. *Pediatrics* 103(6):1253–1256.

Hannan EL, van Ryn M, Burke J, Stone D, Kumar D, Arani D, Pierce W, Rafii S, Sanborn TA, Sharma S, Slater J, DeBuono BA. (1999). Access to coronary artery bypass surgery by race/ethnicity and gender among patients who are appropriate for surgery. *Medical Care* 37:68–77.

Harada ND, Chun A, Chiu V, Pakalniskis A. (2000). Patterns of rehabilitation utilization after hip fracture in acute hospitals and skilled nursing facilities. *Medical Care* 38(11): 1119-1130.

Hargraves JL, Stoddard JJ, Trude S. (2001). Minority physicians' experiences obtaining referrals to specialists and hospital admissions. *Medscape General Medicine* 3(4):10.

Harlan L, Brawley O, Pommerenke F, Wali P, Kramer B. (1995). Geographic, age, and racial variation in the treatment of local/regional carcinoma of the prostate. *Journal of Clinical Oncology* 13:93–100.

Harris DR, Andrews R, Elixhauser A. (1997). Racial and gender differences in use of procedures for black and white hospitalized adults. *Ethnicity & Disease* 7:91–105.

Harris JE. (1979). Pricing rules for hospitals. *Bell Journal of Economics* 10:224–243.

Harris MI, Eastman RC, Cowie CC, Flegal KM, Eberhardt MS. (1999). Racial and ethnic differences in glycemic control of adults with type 2 diabetes. *Diabetes Care* 22(3):403–408.

Hashimoto DM. (2001). The proposed Patients' Bill of Rights: The case of the missing equal protection clause. *Yale Journal of Health Policy, Law, and Ethics* 1:77–93.

Haynes RB, Davis DA, McKibbon A, Tugwell P. (1984). A critical appraisal of the efficacy of continuing medical education. *Journal of the American Medical Association* 251:61–64.

Health Centers Consolidation Act of 1996. Pub. L. No. 104-299. 110 Stat. 3626-3645 (1996).

Health Resources and Services Administration. (1996). *The Registered Nurse Population March 1996: Findings from the National Sample Survey of Registered Nurses.* U.S. Department of Health and Human Services, HRSA, Bureau of Health Professions, Division of Nursing. Downloaded from HRSA web site (ftp://ftp.hrsa.gov/bhpr/nursing/samplesurveys/1996sampsurv.pdf).

Health Resources and Services Administration. (2001). *The Registered Nurse Population: National Sample Survey of Registered Nurses, March 2000, Preliminary Findings.* U.S. Department of Health and Human Services, HRSA, Bureau of Health Professions, Division of Nursing; Downloaded from HRSA web site (ftp://ftp.hrsa.gov//bhpr/nursing/sampsurvpre.pdf).

Heinrich J. (2000). *Health Care Access: Programs for Underserved Populations could be Improved,* testimony, GAO/T-HEHS-00-81.

Hemingway H, Crook AM, Feder G, Banerjee S, Dawson JR, Magee P, Philpott S, Sanders J, Wood A, Timmis AD. (2001). Underuse of coronary revascularization procedures in patients considered appropriate candidates for revascularization. *New England Journal of Medicine* 344(9):645–654.

Herholz H, Goff DC, Ramsey DJ, Chan FA, Ortiz C, Labarthe DR, Nichaman MZ. (1996). Women and Mexican Americans receive fewer cardiovascular drugs following myocardial infarction than men and non-Hispanic whites: The Corpus Christi Heart Project, 1988-1990. *Journal of Clinical Epidemiology* 49(3):279–287.

Hill RF, Fortenberry JD, Stein HF. (1990). Culture in clinical medicine. *Southern Medical Journal* 83:1071-1080.

Hill MN, Miller NH. (1996). Compliance enhancement: A call for multidisciplinary team approaches. *Circulation* 93(1):4–6.

Hobson WD. (2001). *Racial Discrimination in Health Care Interview Project—A Special Report.* Seattle, WA: Seattle and King County Department of Public Health.

Hoenig H, Rubenstein L, Kahn K. (1996). Rehabilitation and hip fracture—equal opportunity for all? *Archives of Physical Medicine and Rehabilitation* 77:58–63.

Hoffman C, Pohl M. (2000). *Health Insurance Coverage in America: 1999 Data Update.* Washington, DC: The Kaiser Commission on Medicaid and the Uninsured.

Hornberger JC, Gibson CD, Wood W, Dequeldre C, Corso I., Palla B, Bloch, DA. (1996). Eliminating language barriers for non-English-speaking patients. *Medical Care* 34(8):845–856.

Horner RD, Hoenig H, Sloane R, Rubenstein LV, Kahn KL. (1997). Racial differences in the utilization of inpatient rehabilitation services among elderly stroke patients. *Stroke* 28(1):19–25.

Horner RD, Lawler FH, Hainer BL. (1991). Relationship between patient race and survival following admission to intensive care among patients of primary care physicians. *Health Services Research* 26(4):531–542.

House JS, Williams D. (2000). Understanding and reducing socioeconomic and racial/ethnic disparities in health. In BD Smedley and SL Syme, eds. *Promoting Health: Intervention Strategies from Social and Behavioral Research.* Washington, DC: National Academy Press.

Howard DL, Penchansky R, Brown MB. (1998). Disaggregating the effects of race on breast cancer survival. *Family Medicine* 30(3):228–235.

Hypertension Detection and Follow-up Program Cooperative Group. (1979). Five-year findings of the Hypertension Detection and Follow-up Program I: Reduction of mortality of persons with high blood pressure, including mild hypertension. *Journal of the American Medical Association* 242:2562–2571.

Immigration Statistics: Populations and Change. Available at http://www.prcdc.org. [Accessed March 15, 2001].

Imperato PJ, Nenner RP, Will TO. (1996). Radical prostatectomy: Lower rates among African American men. *Journal of the National Medical Association* 88(9):589–594.

Institute of Medicine (2001a). *Crossing the Quality Chasm.* Washington, DC: National Academy Press.

Institute of Medicine. (2001b). *Coverage Matters: Insurance and Health Care.* Washington, DC: National Academy Press.

Institute of Medicine. (1999a). *Measuring the Quality of Health Care*. MS Donaldson, ed. Washington, DC: National Academy Press.

Institute of Medicine. (1999b). *The Unequal Burden of Cancer: An Assessment of NIH Programs and Research for Minorities and the Medically Underserved*. MA Haynes and BD Smedley, eds. Washington, DC: National Academy Press.

Institute of Medicine. (1999c). *Toward Environmental Justice: Research, Education, and Health Policy Needs*. Washington, DC: National Academy Press.

Jackson EJ, Parks CP. (1997). Recruitment and training issues from selected lay health advisor programs among African Americans: A 20-year perspective. *Health Education & Behavior* 24(4):418–431.

Janes S, Hobson K. (1998). An innovative approach to affirming cultural diversity among baccalaureate nursing students and faculty. *Journal of Cultural Diversity* 5(4):132–137.

Jha AK, Shlipak MG, Hosmer W, Frances CD, Browner WS. (2001). Racial differences in mortality among men hospitalized in the Veterans Affairs health care system. *Journal of the American Medical Association* 285(3):297–303.

Joe JR. (this volume). The Rationing of Healthcare and Health Disparity for the American Indians/Alask Natives.

Johnson PA, Lee TH, Cook EF, Rouan GW, Goldman L. (1993). Effect of race on the presentation and management of patients with acute chest pain. *Annals of Internal Medicine* 118:593–601.

Joos SK, Hickam DH, Gordon GH, Baker LH. (1996). Effects of a physician communication intervention on patient care outcomes. *Journal of General Internal Medicine* 11:147–155.

Jordan H. (2001). Ward Connerly plans to prohibit state from gathering racial data. *Mercury News Sacramento Bureau*, April 11, 2001.

Joskow PL. (1981). Certificate-of-need regulation. *Controlling Hospital Costs: The Role of Government Regulation*, 76. Cambridge, Mass: MIT Press.

Jussim L. (1991). Social perception and social reality: A reflection-construction model. *Psychological Review* 98:54–73.

Kahn KL, Pearson ML, Harrison ER, Desmond KA, Rogers WH, Rubenstein LV, Brook RH, Keeler EB. (1994). Health care for black and poor hospitalized Medicare patients. *Journal of the American Medical Association* 271:1169–1174.

Kai J, Spencer J, Wilkes M, Gill P. (1999). Learning to value ethnic diversity—what, why and how? *Medical Education* 33(8):616–623.

The Henry J. Kaiser Family Foundation. (1999). *Perceptions of How Race and Ethnic Background Affect Medical Care: Highlights from Focus Groups*. Washington, DC: The Henry J. Kaiser Family Foundation.

The Henry J. Kaiser Family Foundation. (2000a). *Key Facts: Kaiser Commission on Medicaid and the Uninsured*. Accessed from internet site www.kff.org, June 18, 2001.

The Henry J. Kaiser Family Foundation. (2000b). *Health Insurance Coverage in America—1999 Data Update*. Washington, DC: The Kaiser Commission on Medicaid and the Uninsured.

Kales HC, Blow FC, Bingham CR, Roberts JC, Copeland LA, Mellow AM. (2000). Race, psychiatric diagnosis, and mental health care utilization in older patients. *American Journal of Geriatric Psychiatry* 8(4):301–309.

Kaplan GA, Everson SA, Lynch JW. (2000). The contribution of social and behavioral research to an understanding of the distribution of disease: A multilevel approach. In BD Smedley and SL Syme, eds. *Promoting Health: Intervention Strategies from Social and Behavioral Research*. Washington, DC: National Academy Press.

Kasiske B, London W, Ellison MD. (1998). Race and socioeconomic factors influencing early placement on the kidney transplant waiting list. *Journal of the American Society of Nephrology* 9(11):2142–2147.

Khandker KR, Simoni-Wastila LJ. (1998). Differences in prescription drug utilization and expenditures between blacks and whites in the Georgia Medicaid population. *Inquiry* 35:78–87.

Kjellstrand CM. (1988). Age, sex and race inequality in renal transplantation. *Archives of Internal Medicine* 148:1305–1309.

Kleinman A, Eisenberg L, Good B. (1978). Culture, illness and care: Clinical lessons from anthropologic and cross-cultural research. *Annals of Internal Medicine* 88(2):251–258.

Kogan MD, Kotelchuck M, Alexander GR, Johnson WE. (1994). Racial Disparities in Reported Prenatal Care Advice from Health Care Providers. *American Journal of Public Health* 84(1):82–88.

Komaromy M, Grumbach K, Drake M, Vranizan K, Lurie N, Keane D, Bindman AB. (1996). The role of black and Hispanic physicians in providing health care for underserved populations. *New England Journal of Medicine* 334:1305–1310.

Korenbrot CC, Moss NE. (2000). Preconception, prenatal, perinatal, and postnatal influences on health. In Institute of Medicine (2000), *Promoting Health: Intervention Strategies from Social and Behavioral Research.* BD Smedley and SL Syme, eds. Washington, DC: National Academy Press.

Korsch BM. (1994). Patient-physician communication: more research needed. *Clinical Pediatrics* 33(4):202–203.

Korsch BM, Harding C. (1998). *The Intelligent Patient's Guide to the Doctor-Patient Relationship: Learning how to Talk so Your Doctor Will Listen.* New York: Oxford University Press.

Korsch BM. (1984). What do patients and parents want to know? What do they need to know? *Pediatrics* 74(5 Pt 2):917–919.

Kravitz RL. (1999). Ethnic differences in use of cardiovascular procedures: New insights and new challenges. *Annals of Internal Medicine* 130(3):231–233.

Kreps D. (1990). *A Course in Microeconomic Theory.* Princeton, NJ: Princeton University Press.

Kressin NR, Petersen LA. (2001). Racial differences in the use of invasive cardiovascular procedures: Review of the literature and prescription for future research. *Annals of Internal Medicine* 135(5):352–366.

Krishnan JA, Diette GB, Skinner EA, Clark BD, Steinwachs D, Wu AW. (2001). Race and sex differences in consistency of care with national asthma guidelines in managed care organizations. *Archives of Internal Medicine* 161(13):1660–1668.

Kristal L, Pennock PW, Foote SM, Trygstad CW. (1983). Cross-cultural family medicine residency training. *Journal of Family Practice* 17(4):683–687.

Krumholz HM, Fendrick AM, Williams C, Hynes WM. (1997). Differences in physician compensation for cardiovascular services by age, sex, and race. *American Journal of Managed Care* 3:557–563.

Langer N. (1999). Culturally competent professionals in therapeutic alliances enhance patient compliance. *Journal of Health Care for the Poor and Underserved* Feb10(1):19–26.

Laouri M, Kravitz RL, French WJ, Yang I, Milliken JC, Hilborne L, Wachsner R, Brook RH. (1997). Underuse of coronary revascularization procedures: Application of a clinical method. *Journal of the American College of Cardiology* 29:891–897.

LaVeist TA, Gibbons MC. (2001). *Measuring racial and ethnic discrimination in the U.S. healthcare setting: A review of the literature and suggestions for a monitoring program.* Final report to U.S. DHHS, April 12, 2001.

LaVeist TA, Nickerson KJ, Bowie JV. (2000). Attitudes about racism, medical mistrust, and satisfaction with care among African American and white cardiac patients. *Medical Care Research and Review* 57(Supplement 1):146–161.

LaVeist TA, Nuru-Jeter A. (In press). Is doctor-patient race concordance associated with greater satisfaction with care? Forthcoming, *Journal of Health and Social Behavior.*

Lavizzo-Mourey R, Mackenzie E. (1996). Cultural Competence—An essential hybrid for delivering high quality care in the 1990's and beyond. *Transactions of the American Clinical Climatological Association* 1996 (VII, 226-238).

Leape LL, Hilborne LH, Bell R, Kamberg C, Brook RH. (1999). Underuse of cardiac procedures: Do women, ethnic minorities, and the uninsured fail to receive needed revascularization? *Annals of Internal Medicine* 130:183–192.

Leigh WA, Lillie-Blanton M, Martinez RM, Collins KS. (1999). Managed care in three states: Experiences of low-income African-Americans and Hispanics. *Inquiry*,36(3):318–331.

Levine DM, Becker D, Bone LR, Hill MN, Tuggle MB, Zeger SL. (1994). Community-academic health center partnerships for underserved minority populations: One solution to a national crisis. *Journal of the American Medical Association* 272:309–311.

Levinson W, Roter D. (1993). The effects of two continuing medical education programs on communication skills of practicing primary care physicians. *Journal of General Internal Medicine* 8:318–324.

Levision W, Roter DL, Mullooly JP, Dull VT, Frankel RM. (1997). Physician-patient communication: The relationship with malpractice claims among primary care physicians and surgeons. *Journal of the American Medical Association* 277(7):553–559.

Liaison Committee on Medical Education. *Accreditation Standards.* [Online]. Available: http://www.lcme.org/standard.htm#culturaldiversity [accessed March 15, 2001].

Light DW. (1997). From Managed Competition to Managed Cooperation: Theory and Lessons from the British Experience. *The Milbank Quarterly* 75:297–341.

Like RC, Steiner RP, Rubel AJ. (1996). Recommended core curriculum guidelines on culturally sensitive and competent health care. *Family Medicine* 28(4):291–297.

Lillie-Blanton M, Martinez RM, Salganicoff, A. (2001). Site of medical care: Do racial and ethnic differences persist? *Yale Journal of Health Policy, Law, and Ethics* 1(1):1–17.

Lillie-Blanton M, Felt S, Redmon P, Renn S, Machlin S, Wennar E. (1992). Rural and urban hospital closures, 1985-1988: Operating and environmental characteristics that affect risk. *Inquiry* 29:332–344.

Lillie-Blanton M, Brodie M, Rowland D, Altman D, McIntosh M. (2000). Race, ethnicity, and the health care system: Public perceptions and experiences. *Medical Care Research and Review* 57(Suppl 1):218-35.

Louden RF, Anderson PM, Paranjit S, Greenfield SM. (1999). Educating medical students for work in culturally diverse societies. *Journal of the American Medical Association* 282(9):875–880.

Lowe RA, Chhaya S, Nasci K, Gavin LJ, Shaw K, Zwanger ML, Zeccardi JA, Dalsey WC, Abbuhl SB, Feldman H, Berlin JA. (2001). Effect of ethnicity on denial of authorization for emergency department care by managed care gatekeepers. *Academic Emergency Medicine* 8(3):259–66.

Lum CK, Korenman SG. (1994). Cultural-sensitivity training in U.S. medical schools. *Academic Medicine* 69(3):239–241.

Mackenzie ER, Taylor LS, Lavizzo-Mourey R. (1999). Experiences of ethnic minority primary care physicians with managed care: A National survey. *American Journal of Managed Care* 5:1251–1264.

Mackie DM, Devos T, Smith, ER. (2000). Intergroup emotions: Explaining offensive action tendencies in an intergroup context. *Journal of Personality & Social Psychology* 79(4):602–616.

Mackie DM, Hamilton DL, Susskind J, Rosselli F. (1996). Social psychological foundations of stereotype formation. In N Macrae, C Stangor, M Hewstone, eds. *Stereotypes and Stereotyping* (pp. 41-78). New York: Guilford Press.

Manson A. (1988). Language concordance as a determinant of patient compliance and emergency room use in patients with asthma. *Medical Care* 26:1119.

Marsh JV, Brett KM, Miller LC. (1999). Racial differences in hormone replacement therapy prescriptions. *Obstetrics & Gynecology* 93(6):999–1003.

Martensen R. (1995). Sundown medical education: Top-down reform and its social displacemements. *Journal of the American Medical Association* 273 (4):271 .

Massey D.G. (2001). Residential segregation and neighborhood conditions in U.S. metropolitan areas. In: Smelser NJ, Wilson WJ, Mitchell F, eds. *America Becoming: Racial Trends and Their Consequences.* Vol.1. Washington, DC: National Academy Press. Pp. 391–434.

Mayberry RM, Mili F, Ofili E. (2000). Racial and ethnic differences in access to medical care. *Medical Care Research and Review* 57(1):108–145.

Mays V. (2001). Presentation to the IOM Committee on Understanding and Eliminating Racial and Ethnic Disparities in Health Care, May 15, 2001, Washington, D.C.

McBean AM, Warren JL, Babish JD. (1994). Continuing differences in the rates of percutaneous transluminal coronary angioplasty and coronary artery bypass graft surgery between elderly black and white Medicare beneficiaries. *American Heart Journal* 127(2): 287–295.

McBean AM, Gornick MD. (1994). Differences by race in the rates of procedures performed in hospitals for Medicare beneficiaries. *Health Care Financing Review* 15(4):77–90.

McMahon LF, Wolfe RA, Huang S, Tedeschi P, Manning W, Edlund MJ. (1999). Racial and gender variation in use of diagnostic colonic procedures in the Michigan Medicare population. *Medical Care* 37(7):712–717.

McRoy SW, Liu-Perez A, Ali SS. (1998). Interactive computerized health care education. *Journal of the American Medical Informatics Association* 5(4):347–356.

MedPAC (Medicare Payment Advisory Commission). (1998). Physician Workforce Issues: International Medical Graduates. Presentation by Susanne Weinrauch, December 15, 1998, on Capitol Hill. Washington, DC.

Meister JS, Warrick LH, de Zapien JG, Wood AH. (1992). Using lay health workers: Case study of a community-based prenatal intervention. *Journal of Community Health* 17(1):37–51.

Melfi CA, Croghan TW, Hanna MP, Robinson RL. (2000). Racial variation in antidepressant treatment in a Medicaid population. *Journal of Clinical Psychiatry* 61(1):16–21.

Merrill RM, Merrill AV, Mayer LS. (2000). Factors associated with no surgery or radiation therapy for invasive cervical cancer in black and white women. *Ethnicity and Disease* 10:248–256.

Mickelson JK, Blum CM, Geraci JM. (1997). Acute myocardial infarction: Clinical characteristics, management and outcomes in a metropolitan Veterans Affairs medical center teach hospital. *Journal of the American College of Cardiology* 29:915–925.

Milewa T, Calnan M, Almond S, Hunter A. (2000). Patient education literature and help seeking behaviour: Perspectives from an evaluation in the United Kingdom. *Social Science and Medicine* 51:463-75.

Miller RH, Luft HS. (1997). Does managed care lead to better or worse quality of care? *Health Affairs* 16 (5):7–25.

Ming T-S, Freund D, LoSasso A. (2001). Racial disparities in service use among Medicaid beneficiaries after mandatory enrollment in managed care: A Difference-in-Differences approach. *Inquiry* 38:49–59.

Minority Health and Health Disparities Research and Education Act of 2000. (2000). *Federal Register* S-1880.

Mirvis DM, Burns R, Gaschen L, Cloar FT, Graney M. (1994). Variation in utilization of cardiac procedures in the Department of Veterans Affairs health care system: Effect of race. *Journal of the American College of Cardiology* 24:1297–1304.

Mirvis DM, Graney MJ. (1998). Impact of race and age on the effects of regionalization of cardiac procedures in the Department of Veterans Affairs Health Care System. *The American Journal of Cardiology* 18:982–987.

Mitchell JB, Ballard DJ, Matchar DB, Whisnant JP, Samsa GP. (2000). Racial variation in treatment for transient ischemic attacks: Impact of participation by neurologists. *Health Services Research* 34:1413–1428.

Mitchell JB, McCormack LA. (1997). Time trends in late-stage diagnosis of cervical cancer: Differences by race/ethnicity and income. *Medical Care* 35(12):1220–1224.

Mitchell JB. (1991). Physician participation in Medicaid revisited. *Medical Care* 29:645–653.

Mitchell JB, Cromwell J. (1980). Large Medicaid practices and Medicaid mills. *Journal of the American Medical Association* 244:2433–2437.

Mock KD. (2001). Keep lawsuits at bay with compassionate care. *RN* 64(5):83–84.

Moore RD, Stanton D, Gopalan R, Chaisson RE. (1994). Racial differences in the use of drug therapy for HIV disease in an urban community. *The New England Journal of Medicine* 330(11):763–768.

Morales LS, Cunningham WE, Brown JA, Liu H, Hays RD. (1999). Are Latinos less satisfied with communication by health care providers? *Journal of General Internal Medicine* 14:409–417.

Morin R. (2001). Misperceptions cloud whites' view of blacks. *The Washington Post*, July 11, 2001.

Morrison RS, Wallenstein S, Natale DK, Senzel RS, Huang L. (2000). "We don't carry that"—Failure of pharmacies in predominantly nonwhite neighborhoods to stock opioid analgesics. *The New England Journal of Medicine* 342(14):1023–1026.

Moy E, Bartman BA. (1995). Physician race and care of minority and medically indigent patients. *Journal of the American Medical Association* 273(19):1515–1520.

Multiple Risk Factor Intervention Trial Research Group. (1982). Multiple risk factor intervention trial risk factor changes and mortality results. *Journal of the American Medical Association* 248:1465–1477.

Murphy J, Chang H, Montgomery JE, Rogers WH, Safran DG. (2001). The quality of physician-patient relationships: Patients' experiences 1996-1999. *Journal of Family Practice* 50(2):123–129.

Mushlin AI. (1997). Uncertain decision making in primary care. In Grady, ML., ed. *Primary Care Research: Theory and Methods*. AHCPR Publication No. 91-0011. Washington, DC: U.S. Department of Health and Human Services, p. 153–158.

Nallamothu BK, Saint S, Saha S, Fendrick AM, Kelly K, Ramsey S. (2001). Coronary artery bypass grafting in Native Americans: A higher risk of death compared to other ethnic group? *Journal of General Internal Medicine* 16(8):554–559.

National Center for Health Statistics. (2000). *Health, United States, 1999, With Socioeconomic Status and Health Chartbook*. Hyattsville, MD: National Center for Health Statistics.

National Indian Health Board. (2001). *IHS Per Capita Appropriations Compared to U.S. Medicaid Per Capita Expenditure*. Accessed from internet site www.nihb.org/ihsvsmed.htm, July 3, 2001.

National Quality Forum. 2001 (June 28-29). Workshop on Measuring and Reporting the Quality of Healthcare for Minority Populations. Crystal City, VA.

Navarro AM, Senn KL, McNicholas LJ, Kaplan RM, Roppe B, Campo MC. (1998). Por La Vida model intervention enhances use of cancer screening tests among Latinas. *American Journal of Preventive Medicine* 15:32–41.

Ng B, Dimsdale JE, Rollnik JD, Shapiro H. (1996). The effect of ethnicity on prescriptions for patient-controlled analgesia for post-operative pain. *Pain* 66:9–12.

Nickens HW, Cohen JJ. (1996). On affirmative action. *Journal of the American Medical Association* 275(7):572–574.

Nickens HW, Ready T. (1999). A strategy to tame the "savage inequalities." *Academic Medicine* 74:310-1.

Nora LM, Daugherty SR, Mattis-Peterson A, Stevenson L, Goodman LJ. (1994). Improving cross-cultural skills of medical students through medical school-community partnerships. *Western Journal of Medicine* 161(2):144–147.

Nunez AE. (2000). Transforming cultural competence into cross-cultural efficacy in women's health education. *Academic Medicine* 75:1071–080.

Oddone EZ, Horner RD, Sloane R, McIntyre L, Ward A, Whittle J, Passman LJ, Kroupa L, Heaney R, Diem S, Matchar D. (1999). Race, presenting signs and symptoms: Use of carotid artery imaging, and appropriateness of carotid endarterectomy. *Stroke* 30:1350–1356.

Oddone EZ, Horner RD, Diers T, Lipscomb J, McIntyre L, Cauffman C, Whittle J, Passman LJ, Kroupa L, Heaney R, Matchar D. (1998). Understanding racial variation in the use of carotid endarterectomy: The role of aversion to surgery. *Journal of the National Medical Association* 90(1):25–33.

Office for Civil Rights, U.S. Department of Health and Human Services. (2000). Title VI of the Civil Rights Act of 1964; Policy Guidance on the Prohibition Against National Origin Discrimination as it Affects Persons With Limited English Proficiency. *Federal Register* 65(169):2762–2774.

Office of Juvenile Justice and Delinquency Prevention. (1999). *Minorities in the Juvenile Justice System. 1999 National Report Series.* Washington, DC: U.S. Department of Justice.

Office of Management and Budget. (2001). Provisional Guidance on the Implementation of the 1997 Standards for Federal Data on Race and Ethnicity. *Federal Register* 66(10):3829–3831, January 16, 2001.

Okelo S, Taylor AL, Wright, Jr. JT, Gordon N, Mohan G, Lesnefsky E. (2001). Race and the decision to refer for coronary revascularization: The effect of physician awareness of patient ethnicity. *Journal of the American College of Cardiology* 38(3):698–704.

Omi, MA. (2001). The Changing Meaning of Race. In: Smelser NJ, Wilson WJ, Mitchell F, eds. *America Becoming: Racial Trends and Their Consequences.* Vol. 1. Washington, DC: National Academy Press. Pp. 243–263.

Operario D, Fiske S T. (2001). Stereotypes: Processes, Structures, Content, and Context. In R Brown, S Gaertner, eds. *Blackwell Handbook in Social Psychology,* (Vol. 4: Intergroup Processes, pp. 22–44). Cambridge MA: Blackwell.

Optenberg SA, Thompson IM, Friedrichs P, Wojcik B, Stein CR, Kramer B. (1995). Race, treatment, and long-term survival from prostate cancer in an equal-access medical care delivery system. *Journal of the American Medical Association* 274:1599–1606.

Ozminkowski RJ, White AJ, Hassol A, Murphy M. (1997). Minimizing racial disparity regarding receipt of a cadaver kidney transplant. *American Journal of Kidney* 30(6):749–759.

Padget DK, Patrick C, Burns BJ, Schlesinger HJ. (1994). Ethnic differences in use of inpatient mental health services by Blacks, Whites, and Hispanics in a national insured population. *Health Services Research* 29(2):135–153.

Paniagua FA. (1994). *Assessing and Treating Culturally Diverse Clients: A Practical Guide.* Thousand Oaks, CA: Sage Publications.

Pederson TR, Kjekshus J, Berg K, Haghfelt T, Paegeman O, Thongeirsson G, Pyorala K, Miettinen T, Wilhelmsen L, Olsson AG, Wedel H. (1994). Randomized trial of cholesterol lowering in 4444 patients with coronary heart disease: The Scandinavian Simvasltatin Survival Study. *Lancet* 344:1383–1389.

Perez, TE. (this volume). The Civil Rights Dimension of Racial and Ethnic Disparities in Health Status.

Perez TE. (2000). Letter to Mr. Dennis Oakes, Executive Director, The Academic Medicine and Managed Care Forum, from TE Perez, Director, Office for Civil Rights, U.S. DHHS, June 7, 2000.

Perez TE, Satcher D. (2001). Letter to Dr. Bruce R. Zimmerman, President, American Diabetes Association, from TE Perez, Director, Office for Civil Rights, U.S. DHHS, and D. Satcher, Assistant Secretary for Health and Surgeon General, U.S. DHHS, January 19, 2001.

Perez-Stable EJ, Napoles-Springer A, Miramontes JM. (1997). The effects of ethnicity and language on medical outcomes of patients with hypertension or diabetes. *Medical Care* 35(12):1212–1219.

Perloff JD, Kletke PR, Neckerman KM. (1986a). Recent trends in pediatrician participation in Medicaid. *Medical Care* 24:749–760.

Perloff JD, Neckerman K, Kletke PR. (1986b). Pediatrician participation in Medicaid—findings of a five-year follow-up study in California. *Western Journal of Medicine* 145(4):546–550.

Perot RT, Youdelman M. (2001). *Racial, Ethnic, and Primary Language Data Collection in the Health Care System: An Assessment of Federal Policies and Practices.* The Commonwealth Fund.

Petersen LA, Wright SM, Peterson ED, Daley J. (2002). Impact of Race on Cardiac Care and Outcomes in Veterans With Acute Myocardial Infarction. *Medical Care* 40(1 Supp):86-96.

Peterson ED, Shaw LK, DeLong ER, Pryor DB, Califf RM, Mark DB. (1997). Racial variation in the use of coronary-revascularization procedures: Are the differences real? Do they matter? *New England Journal of Medicine* 336:480–486.

Peterson ED, Wright SM, Daley J, Thibault GE. (1994). Racial variation in cardiac procedure use and survival following acute myocardial infarction in the Department of Veterans Affairs. *Journal of the American Medical Association* 271(15):1175–1180.

Pew Health Professions Commission. (1995). *Critical challenges: Revitalizing the health professions for the twenty-first century.* San Francisco: UCSF Center for the Health Professions.

Phelps CE. (2000). "Information Diffusion and Best Practice Adoption," in Culyer and Newhouse, eds. *Handbook of Health Economics.* North Holland Publishing.

Philbin EF, DiSalvo TG. (1998). Influence of race and gender on care process, resource use, and hospital-based outcomes in congestive heart failure. *American Journal of Cardiology* 82:76–81.

Phillips KA, Mayer ML, Aday LA. (2000). Barriers to care among racial/ethnic groups under managed care. *Health Affairs* 19:65–75.

Phillips RS, Hamel MB, Teno JM, Bellamy P, Broste SK, Califf, RM,Vidaillet H., Davis RB, Muhlbaier LH, Connors AF, Jr. (1996). Race, resource use, and survival in seriously ill hospitalized adults. The support Investigators. *Journal of General Internal Medicine* 11(7):387–396.

Ramsey DJ, Goff DC, Wear ML, Labarthe DR, Nichaman MZ. (1997). Sex and ethnic difference in use of myocardial revascularization procedures in Mexican Americans and non-Hispanic whites: The Corpus Christi Heart Project. *Journal of Clinical Epidemiology* 50(5):603–609.

Rathore SS, Lenert LA, Weinfurt KP, Tinoco A, Taleghani CK, Harless W, Schulman KA. (2000). The effects of patient sex and race on medical students' ratings of quality of life. *American Journal of Medicine* 108(7):561–566.

Raup RM, Williams E. (1964). Negro students in medical schools in the United States. *Journal of Medical Education* 39:444–450.

Reitzes DC. (1958). *Negroes and Medicine.* Harvard University Press: Cambridge, MA.

Ren XS, Amick BC, Williams DR. (1999). Racial/ethnic disparities in health: The interplay between discrimination and socioeconomic status. *Ethnicity and Disease* 9:151–165.

Rice T. (1997). Physician payment policies: Impacts and implications. *Annual Review of Public Health* 18:549-65.

Rice T. (this volume). The impact of cost containment efforts on racial and ethnic disparities in health care: A conceptualization.

Richardson LD. (1999). Patients' rights and professional responsibilities: The moral case for cultural competence. *The Mount Sinai Journal of Medicine* 66:267–770.

Richter RW, Bengen B, Alsup PA, Bruun B, Kilcoyne MM, Challenor BD. (1974). The community health worker: A resource for improved health care delivery. *American Journal of Public Health* 64(11):1056–1061.

Rios EV, Simpson CE. (1998). Curriculum enhancement in medical education: Teaching cultural competence and women's health for a changing society. *Journal of the American Medical Women's Association* 53(3):114–120.

Robins LS, Alexander GL,Wolf FM, Fantone JC, Davis WK. (1998a). Development and evaluation of an instrument to assess medical students' cultural attitudes. *Journal of the American Medical Women's Association* 53(3 Suppl.):124–129.

Robins LS, Fantone JC, Hermann J, Alexander GL, Zweifler AJ. (1998b). Improving cultural awareness and sensitivity training in medical school. *Academic Medicine* 73(10 Suppl.): S31–S34.

Robins LS, White CB, Alexander GL, Gruppen LD, Grum CM. (2001). Assessing medical students' awareness of and sensitivity to diverse health beliefs using a standardized patient station. *Academic Medicine* 76(1):76–80.

Rodney M, Clasen C, Goldman G, Markert R, Deane D. (1998). Three evaluation methods of a community health advocate program. *Journal of Community Health* 23:371-81.

Roland D, Lyons B. (1987). Mandatory HMO care for Milwaukee's poor. *Health Affairs* (Millwood) 6:87–100.

Romano PS. (2000). Should health plan quality measures be adjusted for case mix? *Medical Care* 38(10):977–980.

Rosenbaum S, Dievler A. (1992). A literature review of the community and migrant health center programs. Unpublished.

Rosenbaum S, Markus AR, Darnell J. (2000). U.S. civil rights policy and access to health care by minority Americans: Implications for a changing health care system. *Medical Care Research and Review* 57 Suppl. 1:236–259.

Rosenbaum (this volume). Racial and Ethnic Disparities in Healthcare: Issues in the Design, Structure and Administration of Federal Healthcare Financing Programs Supported Through Direct Public Funding.

Rosenblatt RE, Law SA, Rosenbaum S. (1997). *Law and the American Health Care System,* 60–61. Westbury, NY: Foundation Press.

Roter D. (1977). Patient participation in the patient-provider interaction: The effects of patient question asking on the quality of interaction, satisfaction, and compliance. *Health Education Monographs* 5(4):281–315.

Roter DL, Hall JA, Merisca R, Nordstrom B, Cretin D, Svarstad B. (1998). Effectiveness of interventions to improve patient compliance: a meta-analysis. *Medical Care* 36:1138–61.

Roter DL, Hall JA. (1994). Strategies for enhancing patient adherence to medical recommendations. *Journal of the American Medical Association* 271(1):80.

Roter DL, Hall J, Kern D, Barker LR, Karan A, Robert R. (1995). Improving physicians' interviewing skills and reducing patients' emotional distress: A randomized clinical trial. *Archives Internal Medicine* 155(7):1877–1884.

Roter DL, Hernandez O, deNegri B, DiPrete-Brown L, Rosenberg J. (1996). Communication skills training in Honduras and Trinidad. *Journal of General Internal Medicine* 11(1):108.

Roter DL, Rudd RE, Coming J. 1998 Patient literacy. A barrier to quality of care. *Journal of General Internal Medicine* 13(12):850–851.

Rubenstein HL, O'Connon BB, Nieman LZ, Gracely EJ. (1992). Introducing students to the role of folk and population health belief-systems in patient care. *Academic Medicine* 67:566–568.

Sacco RL, Boden-Albala B, Abel G, Lin I-F, Elkind M, Hauser WA, Paik MC, Shea S. (2001). Race-ethnic disparities in the impact of stroke risk factors. The Northern Manhattan Stroke Study. *Stroke* 32:1725–1731.

Safran DG, Rogers WH, Tarlov AR, Inui T, Taira DA, Montgomery JE, Ware JE, Slavin CP. (2000). Organizational and financial characteristics of health plans: Are they related to primary care performance? *Archives of Internal Medicine* 160(1): 69–76.

Safran DG, Taira DA, Rogers,WH, Kosinski MA, Ware JE, Tarlov AR. (1998). Linking primary care performance outcomes of care. *The Journal of Family Practice* 47(3):213–220.

Safran DG, Tarlov AR, Rogers WH. (1994). Primary care performance in fee-for-service and prepaid health systems: Results from the medical outcomes study. *Journal of the American Medical Association* 271(20):1579–1586.

Saha S, Komaromy M, Koepsell TD, Bindman AB. (1999). Patient-physician racial concordance and the perceived quality and use of health care. *Archives of Internal Medicine* 159:997–1004.

Schecter AD, Goldschmidt-Clermont PJ, McKee G, Hoffeld D, Myers M, Velez R, Duran J, Schulman SP, Candra NG, Ford D.E. (1996). Influence of gender, race, and education on patient preferences and receipt of cardiac catheterizations among coronary care unit patients. *American Journal of Cardiology* 78(9):996–1001.

Schneider EC, Clearly PD, Zaslavsky AM, Epstein AM. (2001a). Racial disparity in influenza vaccination: Does managed care narrow the gap between African Americans and Whites? *Journal of the American Medical Association* 286(12):1455–1460.

Schneider EC, Leape LL, Weissman JS, Piana RN, Gatsonis C, Epstein AM. (2001b). Racial differences in cardiac revascularization rates: Does "overuse" explain higher rates among White patients? *Annals of Internal Medicine* 135(5):328–337.

Schulman KA, Berlin JA, Harless W, Kerner JF, Sistrunk S, Gersh BJ, Dube R, Taleghani CK, Burke JE, Williams S, Eisenberg J, Escarce JJ, Ayers W. (1999). The effect of race and sex on physicians' recommendations for cardiac cathetrization. *New England Journal of Medicine* 340:618–626.

Schuman H, Steeh C, Bobo L, Krysan M. (1997). *Racial Attitudes in America: Trends and Interpretations.* Revised edition. Cambridge, MA: Harvard University Press.

Schwartz LM, Woloshin S, Welch HG. (1999). Misunderstanding about the effects of race and sex on physicians' referrals for cardiac catheterization. *New England Journal of Medicine* 341(4):279–283.

Scirica BM, Moliterno DJ, Every NR, Anderson HV, Aguirre FV, Granger CB, Lambrew CT, Rabbani LE, Sapp SK, Booth JE, Ferguson JJ, Cannon CP. (1999). Racial differences in the management of unstable angina: Results from the multicenter GUARANTEE registry. *American Heart Journal* 138 (6 Pt 1):1065-72.

Sedlis SP, Fisher VJ, Tice D, Esposito R, Madmon L, Steinberg EH. (1997). Racial differences in performance of invasive cardiac procedures in a Department of Veterans Affairs Medical Center. *Journal of Clinical Epidemiology* 50(8):899–901.

Segal SP, Bola RJ, Watson MA. (1996). Race, quality of care, and antipsychotic prescribing practices in psychiatric emergency services. *Psychiatric Services* 47(3):282–286.

Selim AJ, Fincke G, Ren XS, Deyo RA, Lee A, Skinner K, Kazis L. (2001). Racial Differences in the Use of Lumbar Spine Radiographs. *Spine* 26(12):1364–1339.

Shapiro J, Lenahan P. (1996). Family medicine in a culturally diverse world: A solution-oriented approach to common cross-cultural problems in medical encounters. *Family Medicine* 28(4):249–255.

Shapiro MF, Morton SC, McCaffrey DF, Senterfitt JW, Fleishman JA, Perlman JF, Athey LA, Keesey JW, Goldman DP, Berry SH, Bozette SA. (1999). Variations in the care of HIV-infected adults in the United States: Results from the HIV Cost and Services Utilization Study. *Journal of the American Medical Association* 281:2305–2375.

Sheifer SE, Escarce JJ, Schulman KA. (2000). Race and sex differences in the management of coronary artery disease. *American Heart Journal* 139(5):848–857.

SHEP Cooperative Research Group. (1991). Prevention of stroke by anti-hypertensive drug treatment in older persons with isolated systolic hypertension. *Journal of the American Medical Association* 265:3255–3264.

Shi L. (1999). Experience of primary care by racial and ethnic groups in the United States. *Medical Care* 37:1068–1077.

Shi L, Frick K, Lefkowitz B, Tillman J. (2000). Managed care and community health centers. *Journal of Ambulatory Care Management* 23(1):1–22.

Shi L, Politzer RM, Regan J, Lewis-Idema D, Falik M. (2001). The impact of managed care on the mix of vulnerable populations served by community health centers. *Journal of Ambulatory Care Management* 224(1):51–66.

Sibicky ME, Dovidio JF. (1986). Stigma of psychological therapy: Stereotypes, interpersonal reactions, and the self-fulfilling prophecy. *Journal of Counseling Psychology* 33:148–154.

Slater JS, Ha CN, Malone ME, McGovern P, Madigan SD, Finnegan JR, Casey-Paal AL, Margolis KL, Lurie N. (1998). A randomized community trial to increase mammography utilization among low-income women living in public housing. *Preventive Medicine* 27(6):862–870.

Smedley BD, Stith AY, Colburn L, Evans CH. (2001). *The Right Thing To Do, The Smart Thing To Do: Enhancing Diversity in the Health Professions. Summary of the Symposium on Diversity in the Health Professions in Honor of Herbert W. Nickens, M.D.* Washington, DC: National Academy Press.

Smith DB. (1998). Addressing racial inequities in health care: Civil rights monitoring and report cards. *Journal of Health Politics, Policy, and the Law* 23:75–105.

Smith DB. (1999). *Health Care Divided: Race and Healing a Nation.* Ann Arbor: The University of Michigan Press.

Stevens R, Goodman LW, Mick SS. (1978). *The Alien Doctors: Foreign Medical Graduates in American Hospitals.* New York: Wiley-Interscience.

Stewart M, Brown JB, Boon H, Galajda J, Meredith L, Sangster M. (1999). Evidence on patient-doctor communication. *Cancer Prevention and Control* 3(1):25–30.

Sullivan P, Adelson J. (1954). Ethnocentrism and misanthropy. *Journal Abnormal Social Psychology* 49:246–250.

Summit Health Institute for Research and Education. (2001). *Racial, Ethnic, and Primary Language Health Data Collection: An Assessment of Federal Policies, Practices and Perceptions.* Washington, DC, May 2001.

Sun BC, Adams J, Orav EJ, Rucker DW, Brennan TA, and Burstin HR. (2000). Determinants of patient satisfaction and willingness to return with emergency care. *Annals of Emergency Medicine* 35(5):426–434.

Svenson JE, Spurlock CW. (2001). Insurance status and admission to hospital for head injuries: Are we part of a two-tiered medical system? *American Journal of Emergency Medicine* 19(1):19–24.

Swanson GM, Ward AJ. (1995). Recruiting minorities into clinical trials: Toward a participant-friendly system. *Journal of the National Cancer Institute* 87:1747–1759.

Swift EK. (2001). *An Overview of Major Federal Health Care Quality Programs: A Technical Report for the Institute of Medicine Committee on Enhancing Federal Healthcare Quality Programs.* Washington, DC: Institute of Medicine.

Tai-Seale M, LoSasso AT, Freund DA, Gerber SE. (2001). The long-term effects of Medicaid managed care on obstetrics care in three California counties. *Health Services Research* 36(4):751–771.

Tai-Seale M, Freund D, LoSasso A. (2001). Racial disparities in service use among Medicaid beneficiaries after mandatory enrollment in managed care: A difference-in-differences approach. *Inquiry* 38:49–59.

Tajfel H, Turner JC. (1979). An integrative theory of intergroup conflict. In WG Austin, S Worchel, eds. *The Social Psychology of Intergroup Relations.* Monterey, CA: Brooks/Cole.

Taylor AJ, Meyer GS, Morse RW, Pearson CE. (1997). Can characteristics of a health care system mitigate ethnic bias in access to cardiovascular procedures? Experience from the military health services system. *Journal of the American College of Cardiology* 30:901–907.

Tervalon M, Murray-Garcia J. (1998). Cultural humility versus cultural competence: a critical distinction in defining physician training outcomes in multicultural education. *Journal of Health Care for the Poor and Underserved* 9(2):117–125.

Thamer M, Hwang W, Fink NE, Sadler JH, Bass EB, Levey A, Brookmeyer R, Powe NR. (2001). U.S. nephrologists' attitudes towards renal transplantation: Results from a national survey. *Transplantation* 71(2):281–288.

The impact of managed care on doctors who serve poor and minority patients (1995). *Harvard Law Review* 108:1625–1642.

Thernstrom S, Thernstrom A. (1997). *America in Black and White: One Nation Indivisible.* New York: Simon and Schuster.

Tocher TM, Larson E. (1998). Quality of diabetes care for non-English speaking patients: A comparative study. *Western Journal of Medicine* 168:504–511.

Todd KH, Deaton C, D'Adamo AP, Goe L. (2000). Ethnicity and analgesic practice. *Annals of Emergency Medicine* 35(1):11–16.

Todd KH, Lee T, Hoffman JR. (1994). The effect of ethnicity on physician estimates of pain severity in patients with isolated trauma. *Journal of the American Medical Association* 271(12):925–928.

Todd KH, Samaroo N, Hoffman JR. (1993). Ethnicity as a risk factor for inadequate emergency department analgesia. *Journal of the American Medical Association* 269:1537–1539.

Treatment of Mild Hypertension Study Research Group. (1993). Treatment of mild hypertension study: Final results. *Journal of the American Medical Association* 270:713–724.

Turner JC, Hogg MA, Oakes PJ, Reicher SD, Wetherell MS. (1987). *Rediscovering the Social Group: A Self-Categorization Theory.* Oxford, UK: Blackwell.

Turner MA, Skidmore F. (1999). *Mortgage Lending Discrimination: A Review of Existing Evidence.* From Urban Institute website, http://www.urban.org/housing/mortgage_lending.html, September 1999.

U.S. Bureau of the Census. (2000). Available at http://www.census.gov [Accessed March 15, 2001].

U.S. Bureau of the Census. (1993). 1990 Census of the Population: Social and Economic Characteristics. Washington, DC: U.S. Department of Commerce.

U.S. Bureau of the Census. (1996). Current Population Reports, Series P25-1130: Population Projections of the United States by Sex, Race, and Hispanic Origin, 1995 to 2050. Washington, DC: U.S. Bureau of the Census.

U.S. Commission on Civil Rights. (1999). The Health Care Challenge: Acknowledging Disparity, Confronting Discrimination, and Ensuring Equality, Vols. I and II. Washington, DC: U.S. Government Printing Office.

U.S. Commission on Civil Rights. (2001). *Funding Federal Civil Rights Enforcement, 2000 and Beyond: A Report of the United States Commission on Civil Rights.* Washington, DC: U.S. Commission on Civil Rights.

U.S. DHHS (U.S. Department of Health and Human Services) (1980). Health for the Disadvantaged. Washington, DC: U.S. DHHS.

U.S. Department of Health and Human Services, Agency for Health Care Policy and Research. (1995). *Directory of Minority Health and Human Services Data Resources.* Washington, DC: U.S. DHHS.

U.S. Department of Health and Human Services, National Committee on Vital and Health Statistics. (1999). *Improving the Collection and Use of Racial and Ethnic Data in HHS.* Washington, DC: U.S. DHHS, internet address: http://www.aspe.hhs.gov/datacncl/racerpt.index.htm.

U.S. Department of Health and Human Services. (1999). Call for comments on draft standards on culturally and linguistically appropriate health care and announcement of regional informational meetings on draft standards. *Federal Register* 64(240):70042–70044.

U.S. Department of Health and Human Services. (2000a). *Healthy People 2010: Understanding and Improving Health.* 2nd ed. Washington, DC: U.S. Government Printing Office.

U.S. Department of Health and Human Services, Office of Minority Health. (2000b). Culturally and linguistically appropriate services (CLAS) in health care. Final Report. *Federal Register* 65(247):80865-80879.

U.S. Department of Health and Human Services. (2001). HHS Directory of Health and Human Services Data Resources. Accessed from internet site http://aspe/hhs/gov/datacncl/datadir on November 7, 2001.

U.S. Department of Health and Human Services. (2001a). *Mental Health: Culture, Race, and Ethnicity—A Supplement to Mental Health: A Report of the Surgeon General.* MD: U.S. Department of Health and Human Services, Substance Abuse and Mental Health Services Administration, Center for Mental Health Services.

U.S. Department of Health and Human Services. (2001b). *The Registered Nurse Population. National Sample Survey of Registered Nurses.* MD: U.S. Department of Health and Human Services, Health Resources and Services Administration, Bureau of Health Professions, Division of Nursing.

U.S. Department of Housing and Urban Development. (1999). *What we know about mortgage lending discrimination in America.* Accessed from Internet Site http://www.hud.gov/library/bookshelf18/pressrel/newsconf/menu.html.

U.S. Department of Justice, Office of Justice Programs, Office of Juvenile Justice and Delinquency Prevention. *Juvenile Offenders and Victims. 1999 National Report Series. Minorities in the Juvenile Justice System.*

U.S. General Accounting Office. (1995). *Community health centers: Challenges in transitioning to prepaid managed care* (GAO/HEHS-95-143).

U.S. General Accounting Office (1990). *Rural Hospitals: Factors that Affect Risk of Closure* (GAO/HRD-90-134).

U.S. Health Resources and Services Administration. (2001). *The Registered Nurse Population. Preliminary Findings from the National Sample Survey of Registered Nurses—March 2000.* Accessed from Internet Site http://bhpr.hrsa.gov/healthworkforce/rnsurvey/.

van Ryn, M. (2002). Research on the Provider Contribution to Race/Ethnicity Disparities in Medical Care. *Medical Care* 40(1) (Supplement):I-140-I-151.

van Ryn M, Burke J. (2000). The effect of patient race and socio-economic status on physician's perceptions of patients. *Social Science and Medicine* 50:813-828.

Verghese A. (1994). *My Own Country: A Doctor's Story.* Vintage Books: New York, NY.

Wang F, Javit JC, Tielsch JM. (1997). Racial variations in treatment for glaucoma and cataract among Medicare recipients. *Ophthalmic Epidemiology* 4(2):89–100.

Ware JE, Jr., Bayliss MS, Rogers WH, Kosinski M, Tarlov AR. (1996). Differences in 4-year health outcomes for elderly and poor, chronically ill patients treated in HMO and fee-for-service systems. Results from the Medical Outcomes Study. *Journal of the American Medical Association* 276(13):1039–1047.

Washington Business Group on Health. (2001). *Promoting Health for a Culturally Diverse Workforce: The Impact of Racial and Ethnic Health Disparities on Employee Health and Productivity.* Proceedings of a WBGH Employer Leadership Forum. Washington, DC: Washington Business Group on Health.

Watson RE, Stein AD, Dwamena FC, Kroll J, Mitra R, McIntosh BA, Vasilenko P, Holmes-Rovner MM., Chen Q, Kupersmith J. (2001). Do race and gender influence the use of invasive procedures? *Journal of General Internal Medicine* 16(4):227–234.

Watson SD. (1995). Medicaid physician participation: patients, poverty, and physician self-interest. *American Journal of Law and Medicine* 21:191.

W.K. Kellogg Foundation. (2001). *The Big Cavity: Decreasing Enrollment of Minorities in Dental Schools.* Battle Creek, MI: W.K. Kellogg Foundation.

Weech-Maldonado R, Morales LS, Spritzer K, Elliott M, Hays RD. (2001). Racial and ethnic differences in parents' assessments of pediatric in Medicaid managed care. *Health Services Research* 36(3):575–595.

Weiler PC. (1993). *A Measure of Malpractice: Medical Injury, Malpractice, Litigation, and Patient Compensation* 69–70. Cambridge, MA: Harvard University Press.

Weinick R M, Zuvekas SH, Cohen JW. (2000). Racial and ethnic differences in access to and use of health care services, 1977 to 1996. *Medical Care Research and Review* 57(1):36–54.

Weinstein M, Fineberg H, Elstein A, Frazier H, Neuhauser D, Neutra R, McNeil B. (1980). *Clinical Decision Analysis*, W.B. Saunders Company: Philadelphia.

Weisse CS, Sorum PC, Sanders KN, Syat BL. (2001). Do gender and race affect decisions about pain management? *Journal of General Internal Medicine* 16(4):211–217.

Weitzman S, Cooper L, Chambless L, Rosamond W, Clegg L, Marcucci G, Romm F, White A. (1997). Gender, racial, and geographic differences in the performance of cardiac diagnostic and therapeutic procedures for hospitalized acute myocardial infarction in four states. *The American Journal of Cardiology* 79:722–726.

Welch M. 1998. Required curricula in diversity and cross-cultural medicine: the time is now. *Journal of the American Medical Women's Association* 53(Suppl.):121–123.

Wells KB, Sturm R, Sherbourne CD, Meredith L. (1996). *Caring for Depression.* Cambridge, MA: Harvard University Press.

Wennberg, J.E. (1999). Understanding geographic variations in health care delivery. *New England Journal of Medicine* 340(1):32-39.

Wennberg JE. (1985). On patient need, equity, supplier-induced demand, and the need to assess the outcome of common medical practices. *Medical Care* 23:512–520.

Wenneker MB, Epstein, AM. (1989). Racial inequalities in the use of procedures for patients with ischemic heart disease in Massachusetts. *Journal of the American Medical Association* 261:253-257.

White O. (1993). This could end the rural doctor shortage. *Medical Economics* 70(23):42-4, 47-9.

White-Means, SI. (2000). Racial patterns in disabled elderly persons' use of medical services. *Journal of Gerontology* 55B(2):S76–S89.

Whittle J, Conigliaro J, Good CB, Lofgren RP. (1993). Racial differences in the use of invasive cardiovascular procedures in the Department of Veterans Affairs medical system. *The New England Journal of Medicine* 329(9):621–627.

Williams GC, Deci EL. (2001). Activating patients for smoking cessation through physician autonomy support. *Medical Care* 39:813-23.

Williams DR. (1999). Race, socioeconomic status, and health: The added effects of racism and discrimination. *Annals of the New York Academy of Sciences* 896:173–188.

Williams DR, Rucker TD. (2000). Understanding and addressing racial disparities in health care. *Health Care Financing Review* (Health Care Financing Administration) 21:75–90.

Williams DR. (2001). Racial variations in adult health status: Patterns, paradoxes, and prospects. In: Smelser NJ, Wilson WJ, and Mitchell F., eds. *America Becoming: Racial Trends and Their Consequences*. Vol. 2. Washington, DC: National Academy Press. Pp. 371-410.

Williams JF, Zimmerman JE, Wagner DP, Hawkins M, Knaus WA. (1995). African-American and white patients admitted to the intensive care unit: Is there a difference in therapy and outcome? *Critical Care Medicine* 23(4):626–636.

Wilson MG, May DS, Kelly JJ. (1994). Racial differences in the use of total knee arthroplasty for osteoarthritis among older Americans. *Ethnicity and Disease* 4:57-67.

Witmer A, Seifer SD, Finocchio L, Leslie J, O'Neil, J. (1995). Community health workers: Integral members of the health care work. *American Journal of Public Health* 85(8):1055-1058.

Woloshin S, Bickell NA., Schwartz LM, Gany T, Welch HG. (1995). Language barriers in medicine in the United States. *Journal of the American Medical Association* 273(9):724–728.

Wood AJ. (2001). Racial differences in the response to drugs—pointers to genetic differences. *New England Journal of Medicine* 344:1393-1395.

Wright Charles H. (1995). *The National Medical Association Demands Equal Opportunity: Nothing More, Nothing Less.* Southfield, MI: Charro Book Company, Inc.

Wyatt GE, Bass BA, Powell, GJ. (1978). A survey of ethnic and sociocultural issues in medical school education. *Journal of Medical Education* 53(8):627–632.

Yergan J, Flood AB, LoGerfo, JP, Diher, P. (1987). Relationship between patient race and the intensity of hospital services. *Medical Care* 25(7):592–603.

Yinger J. (1995). *Closed Doors, Opportunities Lost: The continuing Costs of Housing Discrimination.* New York: Russell Sage.

Young CJ, Gaston, RS. (2000). Renal transplantation in Black Americans. *New England Journal of Medicine* 343(21):1545–1552.

Zaslavsky AM, Hochheimer JN, Schneider ED, Cleary PD, Seidman JJ, McGlynn EA, Thomspon JW, Sennett C, Epstein AM. (2000). Impact of sociodemographic case mix on the HEDIS measures of health plan quality. *Medical Care* 38(10):981–982.

Ziem G. (1977). Medical Education Since Flexner: A Seventy-Year Tracking Record. *Health-PAC Bulletin* 76: 8-14.

Zito JM, Safer DJ, dosReis S, Riddle MA. (1998). Racial disparity in psychotropic medications prescribed for youth with Medicaid insurance in Maryland. *Journal of the American Academy of Child & Adolescent Psychiatry* 37(2):179–184.

Zoratti EM, Havstad S, Rodriguez J, Robens-Paradise Y, LaFata JE, McCarthy, B. (1998). Health service use by African Americans and Caucasians with asthma in a managed care setting. *American Journal of Respiratory and Critical Care Medicine* 158:371–377.

Zweifler J, Gonzalez AM. (1998). Teaching residents to care for culturally diverse populations. *Academic Medicine* 73(10):1056–1061.

Appendixes

A

Data Sources and Methods

In an effort to provide a comprehensive response to the study charge, the study committee examined various sources of data to assess the scope of disparities in healthcare, explore sources of these disparities, and generate strategies to eliminate them. These data sources included a review of recent scientific literature, commissioned papers, public input from professional societies and organizations, input from technical liaison panels, and focus group/roundtable input. The committee received these data over the course of the 17-month study period. The study timeline is depicted in Figure A-1.

Study Committee

A 15-member study committee was convened to assess these data. Membership of the committee included individuals with expertise in clinical medicine, economics, healthcare services research, health policy, health professions education, minority health, psychology, anthropology and related fields. The committee was convened for five two-day meetings held in December 2000, February 2001, May 2001, July 2001, and September 2001.

Literature Review

The literature review included, but was not limited to, seminal articles published in peer-reviewed journals within the last ten years, with an emphasis on the most recent publications. In selecting literature to re-

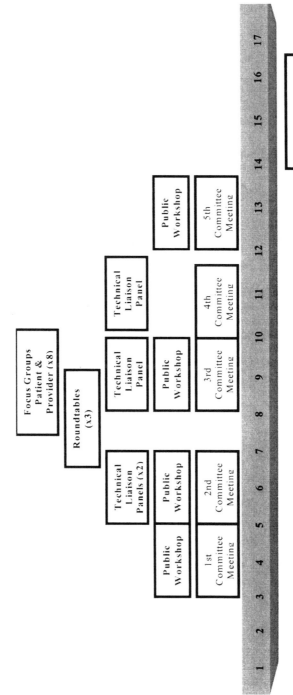

FIGURE A-1 Study components and timeline.

view, the committee identified only peer-reviewed studies that assessed racial and ethnic variation in healthcare while controlling for differences in access to healthcare (either by studying similarly insured patients or by statistically adjusting for differences in insurance status) and socioeconomic differences. This body of literature, however, represents only a fraction of the published studies that investigate racial and ethnic differences in access to and use of healthcare services.

Commissioned Papers

The study committee commissioned seven papers. These papers were intended to provide in-depth information on selected topic areas (e.g., legal aspects of healthcare discrimination, studies on patient-provider interaction, extensive literature review). Topics and paper authors were determined by the study committee. It should be noted that the commissioned paper contributions do not serve to substitute for the committee's own review and analysis of the literature, as described above and in Chapter 1. Much of the committee's own analysis was conducted independently, prior to receiving the draft commissioned papers.

Public Workshops

The study committee hosted four workshops to gain additional information from the public on aspects of the study charge. These workshops occurred during open portions of the committee's scheduled meetings. The topics and nature of the workshops were determined by the study committee. They were intended to allow the committee to gain additional perspectives on potential sources of bias in clinical settings; institutional or system-based obstacles that may differentially affect service provision to racial and ethnic minority patients; other potential sources of healthcare disparities; and explore potential interventions to eliminate disparities in health service delivery. Content included the perspectives of racial and ethnic minority and non-minority health professions organizations (e.g., American Medical Association), and government agencies, as well as programs and strategies employed by organizations to address disparities. In addition, at the fourth workshop selected commissioned papers served as topic areas for a discussion of legal and ethical perspectives. At each public workshop meeting, individuals and groups were invited to present information to the study committee in a roundtable setting to facilitate discussion and interaction. Agendas from public workshops and lists of participants are listed in Boxes A-1 through A-4.

BOX A-1

INSTITUTE OF MEDICINE
COMMITTEE ON UNDERSTANDING AND ELIMINATING
RACIAL AND ETHNIC DISPARITIES IN HEALTHCARE

NATIONAL ACADEMY OF SCIENCES,
2101 CONSTITUTION AVENUE, NW
ROOM 150

AGENDA
TUESDAY, DECEMBER 19, 2000

1:00 p.m.   **WELCOME AND INTRODUCTIONS**
Alan Nelson, M.D.
Chair
IOM Committee on Understanding and Eliminating Racial
and Ethnic Disparities in Healthcare

1:15 p.m.   **OVERVIEW FROM STUDY SPONSOR**
Nathan Stinson Ph.D., M.D., M.P.H.
Deputy Assistant Secretary for Minority Health,
U.S. Department of Health and Human Services

1:35 p.m.   **CONGRESSIONAL PERSPECTIVE**
Charles Dujon
Legislative Assistant, Office of the Honorable Jessie Jack-
son, Jr. U.S. House of Representatives

2:00 p.m.   **PRESENTATIONS FROM OTHER INTEREST GROUPS**
AND STAKEHOLDERS

Rodney Hood, M.D., National Medical Association

Adolph Falcon, M.P.P., National Alliance for Hispanic Health

Jeanette Noltenius, Ph.D., Latino Council on Alcohol and
Tobacco, Representing the Multicultural Action Agenda for
Eliminating Health Disparities

Yvonne Bushyhead, J.D., & Beverly Little Thunder, R.N.
Indian Health Board

3:00 p.m.   **UNDERSTANDING AND ELIMINATING RACIAL AND**
ETHNIC DISPARITIES IN HEALTHCARE — WHAT IS
KNOWN AND WHAT NEEDS TO BE KNOWN?
H. Jack Geiger, M.D.
City University of New York

4:00 p.m.   **ADJOURN**

BOX A-2

INSTITUTE OF MEDICINE
COMMITTEE ON UNDERSTANDING AND ELIMINATING
RACIAL AND ETHNIC DISPARITIES IN HEALTHCARE

NATIONAL ACADEMY OF SCIENCES
CECIL AND IDA GREEN BUILDING, 2001 WISCONSIN AVENUE, NW
ROOM 126

AGENDA
TUESDAY, FEBRUARY 20, 2001

9:00 a.m.   **WELCOME AND INTRODUCTIONS**
Alan Nelson, M.D.
Chair
IOM Committee on Understanding and Eliminating Racial
and Ethnic Disparities in Healthcare

9:15 a.m.   *Deborah Danoff, M.D.*
Assistant Vice President, Division of Medical Education
American Association of Medical Colleges

9:45 a.m.   *Paul M. Schyve, M.D.*
Senior Vice President
Joint Commission on Accreditation of Healthcare
Organizations

10:15 p.m.   *Sindhu Srinivas, M.D.*
President
American Medical Student Association

10:45 a.m.   *Mary E. Foley, R.N., M.S.*
President
American Nurses Association

11:15 a.m.   *Randolph D. Smoak, Jr., M.D.*
President
American Medical Association

11:45 a.m.   *Terri Dickerson*
Assistant Staff Director
U.S. Commission on Civil Rights

12:15 p.m.   **PUBLIC WORKSHOP ADJOURNS**

BOX A-3

INSTITUTE OF MEDICINE
COMMITTEE ON UNDERSTANDING AND ELIMINATING
RACIAL AND ETHNIC DISPARITIES IN HEALTHCARE

NATIONAL ACADEMY OF SCIENCES
CECIL AND IDA GREEN BUILDING, 2001 WISCONSIN AVENUE, NW
ROOM 126

AGENDA
TUESDAY, MAY 15, 2001

1:00 p.m.   *Carolyn Clancy, M.D.*
              Agency for Healthcare Research and Quality

1:45 p.m.   *James Youker, M.D.*
              President, American Board of Medical Specialties

2:15 p.m.   *Ray Werntz*
              Consumer Health Education Council

2:45 p.m.   *Vickie Mays, Ph.D., Chair*
              National Committee on Vital and Health Statistics
              Subcommittee on Populations

3:15 p.m.   QUESTIONS AND COMMENTS

3:30 p.m.   PUBLIC WORKSHOP ADJOURNS

WEDNESDAY, MAY 16, 2001

9:00 a.m.   *Robyn Nishimi, Ph.D.*
              Chief Operating Officer, National Quality Forum

9:30 a.m.   *Lovell Jones, Ph.D.*
              Intercultural Cancer Council

10:00 a.m.   PUBLIC WORKSHOP ADJOURNS

BOX A-4

INSTITUTE OF MEDICINE
COMMITTEE ON UNDERSTANDING AND ELIMINATING
RACIAL AND ETHNIC DISPARITIES IN HEALTHCARE

NATIONAL ACADEMY OF SCIENCES,
2101 CONSTITUTION AVENUE, NW
MAIN BUILDING—LECTURE ROOM

PUBLIC WORKSHOP
"RACE, THE MEDICAL MARKETPLACE, AND HEALTHCARE DISPARITIES"

AGENDA
THURSDAY, SEPTEMBER 6, 2001

8:30 a.m. **WELCOME AND INTRODUCTIONS**
Alan Nelson, M.D.
Chair, IOM Committee on Understanding and Eliminating Racial
and Ethnic Disparities in Healthcare

8:35 a.m. **OPENING REMARKS**
David Satcher, M.D., Ph.D.
U.S. Surgeon General

8:55 a.m. **PANEL DISCUSSION**
M. Gregg Bloche, J.D., M.D.
Moderator, IOM Committee on Understanding and Eliminating
Racial and Ethnic Disparities in Healthcare

PARTICIPANTS:

Richard Epstein, J.D.
James Parker Hall Distinguished Service, Professor of Law,
University of Chicago Law School

Clark C. Havighurst, J.D.
Wm. Neal Reynolds Professor of Law, Duke University School of Law

Marsha Lillie-Blanton, Dr. P.H.
Vice President in Health Policy, The Henry J. Kaiser Family Foundation

June O'Neill, Ph.D.
Director, Center for the Study of Business and Government,
Baruch College of Public Affairs

Thomas Perez, J.D., M.P.P.
Assistant Professor and Director of Clinical Law Programs,
University of Maryland Law School

Thomas Rice, Ph.D.
Professor and Vice-Chair, Department of Health Services, UCLA
School of Public Health

11:00 a.m. **ADJOURN**

Technical Liaison Panels

Four liaison panels were assembled to serve as a resource to the committee, to provide advice and guidance in identifying key information sources, to provide recommendations to the study committee regarding intervention strategies, and to ensure that relevant consumer and professional perspectives were represented. Liaison panels were composed of individuals with relevant experience or expertise on the study charge. Nominations for individuals invited to the panels were sought from over 100 stakeholder groups. Panel members included patient advocates, providers of healthcare services, payer groups, as well as representatives from ethnic minority professional organizations and federal agencies. Each liaison panel was convened by study staff in Washington, D.C. for a half-day meeting. Panelists were asked to provide recommendations regarding potential sources of data, intervention strategies, and other recommendations relevant to the study charge. Discussion content and recommendations from the liaison panels were presented by staff to the study committee at its meetings. The agenda for panel meetings is presented in Box A-5. Lists of participants for each of the four panels are presented in Boxes A-6 through A-9.

Focus Groups and Roundtable Discussions

A series of focus groups were conducted by the Westat Corporation, Rockville, MD, for the study committee (see Appendix E). Information gathered at focus group discussions was intended to afford the study committee greater insight into the experiences and perceptions of patients and providers, supplementing data from the empirical literature, and providing a richer context for data interpretation. Qualitative data gathered during focus group discussions were used to illustrate and expand upon findings and recommendations provided in the committee report.

Six groups, composed of 8-10 individuals each, were conduced with healthcare consumers with participants from various racial and ethnic backgrounds. Two groups were conducted with African Americans: one in Los Angeles, CA, and the other in Rockville, MD. The third group was conducted in Los Angeles with Hispanics who were fluent in English, and the fourth was conducted in Washington, DC, with Hispanics who identified themselves as primary Spanish-speaking with little or no English fluency. The fifth group was conducted with American Indians in Albuquerque, New Mexico. The final group was conducted in Los Angeles with Chinese Americans who identified themselves as primarily Mandarin-speaking with little or no English fluency. Participants were asked to comment on the quality of healthcare they received and experiences encountered when seeking medical care in a variety of public and private

BOX A-5

INSTITUTE OF MEDICINE
COMMITTEE ON UNDERSTANDING AND ELIMINATING
RACIAL AND ETHNIC DISPARITIES IN HEALTHCARE

AGENDA—LIAISON PANEL

12:00 p.m. LUNCH

12:15 p.m. INTRODUCTIONS
Daniel J. Wooten, M.D.
IOM Scholar in Residence
Panel Chair

12:30 p.m. OVERVIEW OF IOM STUDY
Brian Smedley, Ph.D.
Adrienne Stith, Ph.D.
IOM study staff

12:45 p.m. CURRENT INITIATIVES AND RESOURCES FOCUSED ON
REDUCING HEALTHCARE DISPARITIES

1:30 p.m. BREAK

1:45 p.m. DISCUSSION OF FACTORS THAT CONTRIBUTE TO
INEQUITIES IN HEALTHCARE

2:30 p.m. PANEL INPUT—RECOMMENDATIONS TO STUDY
COMMITTEE
• Recommendations for Intervention Strategies
• Policy Recommendations
• Research Recommendations

4:00 p.m. ADJOURN

BOX A-6

INSTITUTE OF MEDICINE
COMMITTEE ON UNDERSTANDING AND ELIMINATING
RACIAL AND ETHNIC DISPARITIES IN HEALTHCARE

TECHNICAL LIAISON
FEDERAL PANEL

FEBRUARY 12, 2001

Jonca Bull, M.D., Food and Drug Administration

Denice Cora-Bramble, M.D., Health Resources and Services
Administration

Marsha Davenport, M.D., Center for Medicare and Medicaid Services

Carole Brown, Office for Civil Rights, Office of the Secretary of Health
and Human Services

LTC Willie L. Hensley, Department of Veterans Affairs

*Joan Jacobs, Office of Minority Health, Office of the Secretary of Health
and Human Services

Camara Phyllis Jones, M.D., M.P.H., Ph.D., Centers for Disease Control
and Prevention

Raynard Kington, M.D., Ph.D., National Institutes of Health

Yvonne T. Maddox, Ph.D., National Institutes of Health

Beverly Malone, Ph.D., Office of Public Health and Science, Office of
the Secretary of Health and Human Services

George A. Mensah, M.D., Centers for Disease Control and Prevention

Leo J. Nolan III, Indian Health Service

Delores L. Parron, M.D., Planning and Evaluation Program, Department
of Health and Human Services

Capt. Adam M. Robinson, Jr., M.D., Department of Defense

Craig Vanderwagen, M.D., Indian Health Service

*observer from sponsoring office

BOX A-7

INSTITUTE OF MEDICINE
COMMITTEE ON UNDERSTANDING AND ELIMINATING
RACIAL AND ETHNIC DISPARITIES IN HEALTHCARE

TECHNICAL LIAISON PANEL

FEBRUARY 14, 2001

Joseph A. Berry, M.D., United Healthcare

Zora Brown, Breast Cancer Resource Committee

Gina Gregory-Burns, M.D., Kaiser Permanente

Mary Lou de Leon Siantz, R.N., Ph.D., National Association of Hispanic Nurses

Gary C. Dennis, M.D., Howard University Hospital

Richard Levinson, M.D., DPA, American Public Health Association

Joseph Quash, M.D., Association of Black Cardiologists

Rene F Rodriguez, M.D., Interamerican College of Physicians and Surgeons

Cynthia A. Warrick, Ph.D., Howard University

Donald A. Young, M.D., Health Insurance Association of America

BOX A-8

INSTITUTE OF MEDICINE
COMMITTEE ON UNDERSTANDING AND ELIMINATING
RACIAL AND ETHNIC DISPARITIES IN HEALTHCARE

LIAISON PANEL

MAY 4, 2001

David Baines, M.D., Seattle Indian Health Board

Henry Chung, M.D., Pfizer Pharmaceuticals Groups

Tom Chung, Ph.D., Commonwealth of Massachusetts, Executive Office of Elder Affairs

Carolyn M. Clancy, M.D., Agency for Health Research & Quality

Gem P. Daus, M.A., Asian and Pacific Islander American Health Forum

Lucille Davis, Ph.D., R.N., Southern University School of Nursing, Baton Rouge, LA

Pete Duarte, M.D., Thomason Hospital, El Paso, TX

Alicia C. Georges, Ed.D., Department of Nursing, Herbert H. Lehman College, Bronx, NY

Robert D. Gibson, Pharm.D., Sc.D., American Pharmaceutical Association

Miya Iwataki, Los Angeles County Department of Health Services

Anita Moncrease, M.D., M.P.H., Health Resources and Service Administration

Tom Perez, J.D., Maryland University School of Law

Elena Rios, M.D., M.S.P.H., National Hispanic Medical Association

Richard Allen Williams, M.D., University of California at Los Angeles and Minority Health Institute

*Violet Ryo-Hwa Woo, M.S., M.P.H., Office of Minority Health

* observer from sponsoring office

BOX A-9

INSTITUTE OF MEDICINE
COMMITTEE ON UNDERSTANDING AND ELIMINATING
RACIAL AND ETHNIC DISPARITIES IN HEALTHCARE

LIAISON PANEL

JUNE 21, 2001

Dennis Andrulis, Ph.D., M.P.H., State University of New York Downstate Medical Center
Deborah Bohr, M.P.H., Health Research and Educational Trust
Cindy Brach, M.P.P., Agency for Healthcare Research and Quality
Deborah Danoff, M.D., Association of American Medical Colleges
Leonard G. Epstein., M.S.W., Bureau of Primary Health Care, Health Resources Services Administration
George Flouty, M.D., Pfizer, Inc.
Candice Mathew Healy, M.P.A., State University of New York Downstate Medical Center
Laura Hernandez, M.P.I.A., Centers for Medicare and Medicaid Services (formerly the Health Care Financing Administration)
Charlene Landis, M.A., Pfizer, Inc.
Ed Martinez, M.S., National Association of Public Hospitals
*Guadalupe Pacheco, M.S.W., Office of Minority Health, DHHS
Rea Panares, M.H.S., Washington Business Group on Health
Carlos Vidal, Ph.D., State University of New York Stonybrook
Malcom Williams, M.P.P., Grantmakers in Health

VIDEO CONFERENCE PARTICIPANTS

Niels Agger-Gupta, Ph.D., California Healthcare Interpreters Association
Sakinah Carter, M.P.H., The California Endowment
Tessie Guillermo, Asian and Pacifica Islander Health Forum
Melba Hinojosa, M.A., RN, MediCal Managed Care, California Department of Health Services
Vivian Huang, California Primary Care Association
Wendy Jameson, M.P.P., M.P.H., California Health Care Safety Net Institute
Beatriz Solis, M.P.H., LA Care Health Plan
Jai Lee Wong, The California Endowment

* observer from sponsoring office

settings, either for themselves or for a child or other family member. All participants had private health insurance, Medicare, Medicaid/MediCal, or Indian Health Service coverage.

In addition, two focus groups were conducted by telephone with African American and Hispanic healthcare providers throughout the United States: one was conducted with nurses, the other with physicians. Participants were asked to provide their opinions and comments on the quality of healthcare services that minority patients receive. They also discussed how their race or ethnicity affected their medical training or professional careers. Providers' perspectives added a rich content for understanding patients' experiences with racism in healthcare, addressing some of the institutional factors that affect quality of care.

An experienced facilitator, who possessed knowledge of cultural and linguistic differences of ethnic minority groups, led each of the nine groups. Facilitators for the consumer groups were matched with regard to race, ethnicity, and primary language. Study staff were present at Washington, DC area and phone-based focus groups.

To supplement qualitative information on the experiences and perceptions of racial and ethnic minority patients, advocates, and their healthcare providers, roundtable discussions were held at two national conferences (the Asian American and Pacific Islander Health Forum [AAPIHF] conference in Alameda, CA and the Indian Health Service [IHS] Research conference in Albuquerque, NM) where racial and ethnic minority health issues were discussed. At both conferences, study staff solicited participants from among conference attendees and invited them to participate in small group discussions (up to 20 people) to discuss participants' perceptions of racial and ethnic healthcare disparities and strategies to eliminate them. At the Indian Health Service Research Conference, a member of the study committee (Dr. Jennie Joe) facilitated a small group discussion that including American Indian tribal leaders, healthcare providers, and IHS staff. At the AAPIHF conference, study staff facilitated three small discussion groups, including representatives of advocacy and community groups, healthcare providers, and others.

B

Literature Review

The study committee conducted an extensive review of literature on racial and ethnic disparities in healthcare (discussed in Chapter 1). In this appendix, summary tables of this literature are presented, along with criteria used in the conduct of this review.

To assess the evidence regarding racial and ethnic differences in health care, the committee conducted literature searches via PUBMED and MEDLINE databases to identify studies examining racial and ethnic differences in medical care for a variety of disease categories and clinical services. Searches were performed using combinations of following keywords:

- Race, racial, ethnicity, ethnic, minority/ies, groups, African American, Black, American Indian, Alaska Native, Native American, Asian, Pacific Islander, Hispanic, Latino.
- Differences, disparities, care.
- Cardiac, coronary, cancer, asthma, HIV, AIDS, pediatric, children, mental health, psychiatric, eye, ophthalmic, glaucoma, emergency, diabetes, renal, gall bladder, ICU, peripheral vascular, transplant, organ, cesarean, prenatal, hip, hypertension, injury, surgery/surgical, knee, pain, procedure, treatment, diagnostic.

This search yielded over 600 citations. To further examine this evidence base and address the study charge that called for an analysis of "the extent of racial and ethnic differences in health care that are not otherwise attributable to known factors such as access to care," only studies that provided some measure of control or adjustment for racial and ethnic differences in insurance status (e.g., ability to pay/insurance coverage or co-morbidities) were included in the literature review. Other "threshold" criteria included:

- Publication in past 10 years (1992-2002; this criterion was established because more recent studies tend to employ more rigorous research methods and present a more accurate assessment of contemporary patterns of variation in care);
- Publication in peer-reviewed journals;
- Elimination of studies focused on racial and ethnic differences in health status (except as it is affected by the quality of health care) and health care access, as well as publications that were editorials, letters, published in a foreign language, were non-empirical, or studies that controlled for race or ethnicity; and
- Inclusion only of studies whose primary purpose was to examine variation in medical care by race and ethnicity, contained original findings, and met generally established principles of scientific research (e.g., studies that stated a clear research question, provided a detailed description of data sources, collection, and analysis methods, included samples large enough to permit statistical analysis, and employed appropriate statistical measures).

In addition, to ensure the comprehensiveness of the review, the committee examined the reference lists of major review papers that summarize this literature (e.g., van Ryn, 2002; Geiger, this volume; Kressin and Petersen, 2001; Bonham, 2001; Sheifer, Escarce, and Schulman, 2000; Mayberry, Mili, and Ofili, 2000; Ford and Cooper, 1995). Articles not originally identified in the initial search were retrieved and analyzed for appropriateness of inclusion in the committee's review. Finally, to ensure that the committee's search was not limited to studies with "positive" findings of racial and ethnic differences in care, searches were conducted for studies that attempted to assess variations in care by patient socioeconomic status and geographic region. These studies were included if the researchers assessed racial or ethnic differences in care while controlling, as noted above, for patient access-related factors.

To assess the quality of this evidence base, the committee ranked studies on several criteria:

- Adequacy of control for insurance status (studies of patients covered under the same health system or insurance plan were considered to be more rigorous than studies that merely assessed the availability of health insurance among the study population);
  - Use of appropriate indicators for patient socioeconomic status (e.g., studies that measured patients' level of income, education, or other indicators of socioeconomic status);
  - Analysis of clinical data, as opposed to administrative claims data (see limitations of administrative claims data noted below);
  - Prospective or retrospective data collection (prospective studies were considered to be more rigorous than retrospective analyses);
  - Appropriate control for patient co-morbid conditions;
  - Appropriate control for racial differences in disease severity or stage of illness at presentation;
  - Assessment of patients' appropriateness for procedures (e.g., studies that provide primary diagnosis and include well-defined measures of disease status, as in studies of cardiovascular care that assess racial differences in care following angiography) or that compare rates of service use relative to standardized, widely-accepted clinical guidelines; and
  - Assessment of racial differences in rates of refusal or patient preferences for non-invasive treatment.

Studies that met the committee's "threshold" criteria are summarized in Table B-1.

As a "second level" analysis of the quality of evidence regarding racial and ethnic disparities in cardiovascular care, the committee identified a subset of studies that permit a more detailed analysis of the relationship between patient race or ethnicity and quality of care, while considering potential confounding variables such as clinical differences in presentation and disease severity. Several criteria were established to identify these studies, using generally accepted criteria of research rigor and quality. To begin, the committee identified only studies using clinical, as opposed to administrative data, for the reasons cited above. Secondly, the committee identified studies that provided appropriate controls for likely confounding variables, and/or employed other rigorous research methods. These criteria included the use of adequate control or adjustment for racial and ethnic differences in insurance status; prospective, rather than retrospective data collection; adjustment for racial and ethnic differences in co-morbid conditions; adjustment for racial and ethnic differences in disease severity; comparison of rates of cardiovascular services relative to measures of appropriateness; and assessment of patient outcomes.

Several caveats should be noted in undertaking this approach. One, studies using clinical data allow researchers to better assess whether disparities in care exist and are significant after potential confounding factors such as clinical variation and the appropriateness of intervention are taken into account, but these studies often are limited to small patient samples in one or only a few clinical settings, therefore sacrificing statistical power and potentially underestimating the role of institutional variables as contributing to healthcare disparities. Second, assessments of racial and ethnic differences in patients' clinical outcomes following intervention must be made with caution. Patients' outcomes following medical intervention reflect a wide range of factors, some of which are unrelated to the intervention itself (e.g., the degree of social support available to patients following treatment) and may vary systematically by race or ethnicity. In addition, a finding of no racial or ethnic differences in patient outcomes (e.g., survival) despite disparate rates of treatment should not be interpreted as demonstrating that disparities in the use of medical intervention are inconsequential. In such instances, researchers should ask whether equivalent rates of intervention might be associated with better patient outcomes among minorities. Finally, this second level of analysis should not be interpreted as suggesting that the larger literature presented above is insufficient to draw conclusions regarding disparities in healthcare. Almost all of the individual studies reviewed earlier possess limitations, but the collective body of this evidence is robust.

Despite these caveats, this second review afforded an opportunity to assess whether racial and ethnic disparities in care remain when racial differences in clinical presentation and other potentially confounding variables are controlled. Studies were considered in this second review only if they met four of six criteria noted above, in addition to the "threshold" criteria that studies employ clinical databases. Thirteen studies were identified through this process (see Table B-2). Of these, only two (Leape et al., 1999; Carlisle et al., 1999) found no evidence of racial and ethnic disparities in care after adjustment for racial and ethnic differences in insurance status, co-morbid factors, disease severity, and other potential confounder as noted above. The remaining studies found racial and ethnic disparities in one or more cardiac procedures, following multivariate analysis. Almost all studies found that adjustment for one or more confounding factors reduced the magnitude of unadjusted racial and ethnic differences in care. Among the five studies that collected data prospectively, however, all found racial and ethnic disparities remained after adjustment for confounding factors.

TABLE B-1 Summary of Selected Literature—Racial and Ethnic
Disparities in Health Care

Analgesia

Source	Procedure/Illness	Sample
Todd, Deaton, D'Adamo, and Goe, 2000	Assessed racial differences in receipt of analgesia among patients seen for extremity fractures in emergency departments.	Retrospective cohort study of 217 patients (127 African American, 90 white) seen in an emergency department in an urban hospital.
Bernabei, Gambassi, Lapane et al., 1998	Assessed adequacy of pain management among elderly and minority cancer patients admitted to nursing homes.	13,625 cancer patients (12,038 white, 1,041 African American, 163 Hispanic, 107 Asian, 276 American Indian) discharged from hospitals to any of 1,492 Medicare-certified/Medicaid-certified nursing homes in five states.

Analyses	Findings	Limitations
Multiple logistic regressions to predict use of analgesia by race, controlling for time since injury, total time in the emergency department, payer status, and need for fracture reduction.	Nearly three-fourths of white patients (74%) received analgesia, compared to 57% of African American patients. The crude risk of receiving no analgesia was 66% higher for black patients than white. After controlling for covariates, whites remained significantly more likely to receive analgesia (risk ratio = 1.7, 95% CI 1.1 to 2.3).	-Moderate sample size. -Racial/ethnic groups other than white and African American not sampled. -One site sampled. -Retrospective study. -Other relevant confounds such as alcohol and drug use not considered. -Few racial/ethnic minority physicians in sample.
Logistic regression to predict unresolved daily pain, adjusting for gender, cognitive status, communication skills, and indicators of disease severity (e.g., explicit terminal prognosis), being bedridden, number of diagnoses, and use of other medications.	More than a quarter of patients in daily pain (26%), as assessed by self-report and independent raters, received no pain medication. After adjustment, African Americans had 63% greater probability of being untreated for pain relative to whites (odds ratio = 1.63, 95% CI 1.18 to 2.26). Older age, low cognitive performance, and increased number of other medications were also associated with failure to receive any analgesic agent.	-Small numbers in racial/ethnic groups. -Retrospective, cross-sectional study. -Data set not specifically focused on pain. -Pain assessed by observational evaluation. -Family members involved in collection of information to varying degrees. -No data regarding analgesic dose or frequency of administration.

TABLE B-1 Continued

Analgesia

Source	Procedure/Illness	Sample
Cleeland, Gronin, Baez et al., 1997	Assessed adequacy of pain management among minority patients receiving care in settings that primarily serve minorities vs. patients who receive care in settings where few minority patients are treated.	281 minority outpatients (106 African American, 94 Hispanic, 16 other minority) with recurrent or metastatic cancer at 9 university cancer centers, 17 community hospitals and practices, and 4 centers that primarily treat minority patients.
Ng, Dimsdale, Rollnik, and Shapiro, 1996	Assessed racial/ethnic differences in physicians prescription of patient-controlled analgesia for post-operative pain.	454 (314 white, 37 Asian, 73 Hispanic, 30 African American) consecutive patients receiving patient-controlled analgesia in post-operative period.

Analyses	Findings	Limitations
Compared treatment of pain among this sample with a larger, primarily white sample from a previous study where participants were treated in settings where fewer than 10% of patients were ethnic minorities. Pain assessed by independent ratings of patients and physicians. Adequacy of analgesia estimated by widely accepted measure of treatment of pain.	Sixty-five percent of patients who reported pain received inadequate pain medication. Patients treated in settings where the patient population was primarily black or Hispanic and those who were treated at university centers were more likely to receive inadequate analgesia (77%) than those who received treatment in settings where patient population was primarily white (52%; $p < 0.003$). In addition, minority patients were more likely to be undermedicated for pain than white patients (65% vs. 50%; $p < 0.001$), and were more likely to have the severity of their pain underestimated by physicians.	-Data regarding race/ethnicity not available for comparison group. -Data collected immediately after data on the non-minority comparison group collected. -No data collected on ability to pay.
Analysis of variance and post-hoc LSD-tests using ethnicity as independent variable. Dependent variables include amount of narcotic prescribed and amount of narcotic self-administered.	No significant differences found in patient rating of pain or amount of analgesia self-administered. Significant differences in the amount of narcotic prescribed among Asians, blacks, Hispanics, and whites ($F = 7.352$; $p < 0.01$). Whites and African Americans were prescribed more narcotic than Hispanics and Asians. After adjustment for age, gender, preoperative use of narcotics, health insurance, and pain site, ethnicity persisted as independent predictor of amount of narcotic prescribed.	-Relatively small numbers of African Americans and Asians. -Sample located at one site. -Retrospective study. -Analyses did not control for patient size or primary language.

TABLE B-1 Continued

Analgesia

Source	Procedure/Illness	Sample
Todd, Lee, and Hoffman, 1994	Assessed racial/ethnic differences in physician's perceptions of pain in patients with isolated extremity trauma.	Prospective study of 207 patients (138 white, 69 Hispanic) admitted to ED at UCLA Medical Center between 1992-1993.
Todd, Samaroo, and Hoffman, 1993	Assessed ethnic differences in receipt of emergency department analgesia for isolated long-bone fractures.	139 patients (108 white, 31 Hispanic) admitted to emergency department at UCLA. Patients with recorded alcohol or drug use excluded.

Analyses	Findings	Limitations
Analysis of Covariance to evaluate influence of confounding variables on the relationship between ethnicity and differences in patient and physician pain assessment. Independent variables included occupational injury, injury location, patient pain assessment, physician sex, injury type, insurance status, and patient ethnicity.	No differences found between non-Hispanic and Hispanic patients in patient pain assessment, physician pain assessment, or disparity between patient and physician pain assessment. Differences remained nonsignificant after controlling for confounds.	-Patients enrolled study primarily in early evening and weekends. -Moderate samples size. -Racial groups other than Hispanic and white not sampled. -Single site sampled.
Logistic regression to evaluate independent influence of race/ethnicity on probability of analgesic administration. Independent variables included race/ethnicity, gender, language, insurance status, occupational injury, fracture reduction, time of presentation, total time in ED, hospital admission.	55% of Hispanic patients and 26% of white patients received no analgesic (crude relative risk = 2.12, 95% CI 1.35 to 3.32, $p = 0.003$). After simultaneously controlling for covariates Hispanic ethnicity was strongest predictor of no analgesia (odds ratio = 7.46, 95% CI 2.22 to 25.04, $p < 0.01$).	-Retrospective study. -No control for covariates such as precise injury, presence of translators. -Single site. -Small sample size. -Small number of Hispanics in sample. -Racial/ethnic groups other than white and Hispanic not sampled.

TABLE B-1 Continued

Asthma

Source	Procedure/Illness	Sample
Krishnan et al., 2001	Race/ethnicity and gender differences in consistency of care with national asthma guidelines within managed care organizations.	5,062 patients (4,328 white, 734 African-American) who participated in the Outcomes Management System Asthma Study between 9/93 and 12/93.
Zoratti, Havstad, Rodriguez et al., 1998	Assessed racial/ethnic differences in treatment for asthma in a managed care setting.	464 African-American and 1,609 white patients treated for asthma in a Southeast Michigan managed care system (27 ambulatory care clinics).

Analyses	Findings	Limitations
Multivariate logistic regression to determine whether race/ethnicity and sex were associated with five indicators of National Asthma Education and Prevention Program (NAEPP) guidelines (medication, self-management education, control of factors related to asthma severity, periodic assessment, and asthma specialist care).	After controlling for age, education, employment, and symptom frequency there were no significant race/ethnicity or sex differences in the use of medication regimen consistent with NAEPP recommendations for patients with moderate or more severe asthma.	-Results may not apply to patients with mild asthma. -Bias in self-report data. -Racial/ethnic groups other than white and African-American not sampled.
Regression analysis to predict use of services, adjusting for age, gender, marital status, and income (as assessed by average income of patients' community of residence).	African-American patients were more likely than whites to access care in emergency rooms ($p < 0.001$), were hospitalized more often ($p = 0.023$), and were less likely to be seen by an asthma specialist ($p = 0.027$), after controlling for income, marital status, gender, and age. Among only low-income patients, African Americans were more likely to be treated in emergency rooms than whites, although no significant differences were found in access to specialty care and hospitalization rates. After adjusting for age, gender, marital status and income, African Americans were more likely to use oral corticosteroids ($p = 0.026$) and were less likely to use inhaled anticholinergic medications ($p = 0.016$).	-Racial/ethnic groups other than African American and white not assessed. -Use of administrative database. -Retrospective cross-sectional study. -Number prescriptions filled used as estimate of actual use. -No adjustment for co-morbidities.

TABLE B-1 Continued

Cancer

Source	Procedure/Illness	Sample
Elston Lafata, Cole Johnson, Ben-Menachem, Morlock et al., 2001	Assessed sociodemographic differences in the receipt of colorectal cancer surveillance care.	251 patients (157 white, 94 minority [largely African American]) treated for colorectal cancer in a managed care organization.
Farley, Hines, Taylor et al., 2001	Racial differences in cervical cancer survival in military health system.	Retrospective examination of 1,553 patient records (65% white, 10% African-American, 8% Filipino, 4% Korean, remaining percentages Japanese, Hawaiian, Indian, Asian, Pacific Islander, unknown, or other) from the Automated Central Tumor Registry for the U.S. Military Health Care System between 1988 and 1999. Patients included were diagnosed with invasive cervical carcinoma.
Merrill, Merrill, and Mayer, 2000	Receipt of surgery or radiation therapy among white and African-American women with cervical cancer.	Data from 8,119 patients (86% white, 14% African-American) with invasive cervical cancer, as obtained from 11 tumor registries in Surveillance, Epidemiology, and End Results (SEER) program.

Analyses	Findings	Limitations
Kaplan-Meier survival analysis to determine cumulative incidence of service receipt; Cox Proportional Hazard models to quantify the effects of baseline clinical and sociodemographic characteristics on risk of service receipt. Analyses adjusted for age, race, gender, site and stage of original disease, type of treatment, comorbidity index, estimated income.	Within 18 months of treatment, over half of the total cohort received a colon examination (55%), nearly three-fourths had received carcinoembryonic antigen (CEA) testing, and nearly six in ten (59%) received metastatic disease testing. Whites were more likely than African Americans, however, to receive CEA testing (RR = 1.47, 95% CI 1.12 to 2.14) and displayed a slight but non-significant trend toward higher rates of colonic examination (RR = 1.43, 95% CI 0.94 to 2.18).	-Racial/ethnic groups other than African American and white not examined. -Retrospective study. -Use of claims data.
Survival analysis performed with Kaplan-Meier survival curves and log rank tests to determine significant differences. Cox proportional hazards regression to assess factors influencing survival. Data regarding age at diagnosis, histology, grade, stage, SES, treatment modality obtained.	No significant difference between the distribution of age, stage, grade or histology between African Americans and whites. No difference between these groups found in type of treatment. Differences in five- and 10-year survival rates were also not statistically significant.	-Small numbers in racial/ethnic minority groups. -Retrospective study. -Administrative data.
Logistic regression to predict receipt of therapy after adjusting for stage and grade of cancer, patient age, nodal status, histology, and presence of multiple cancer primaries.	Overall, 8.03% of whites and 11.64% of blacks did not receive either radiation therapy or surgery. For both blacks and whites, the odds of not receiving treatment increased with older age and distant and unstaged disease (vs. localized disease). Blacks were more likely to be diagnosed unstaged and were less likely to have localized disease; once stage was accounted for, racial differences in treatment status became insignificant. Among those not treated, blacks were more likely to have treatment not recommended than whites (53.68% vs. 40.32 %). Of those cases not	-Racial/ethnic groups other than African American and white not examined. -Administrative data. -Retrospective study. -No controls for hospital characteristics, appropriateness, SES.

TABLE B-1 Continued

Cancer

Source	Procedure/Illness	Sample
Bach, Cramer, Warren, and Begg, 1999	Early stage lung cancer.	10,984 patients (10,124 white, 860 African Americans) age 65 and older with resectable stage I or stage II non-small-cell lung cancer. Patients resided in one of 10 study areas of the Surveillance, Epidemiology, and End Results (SEER) program.
McMahon, Wolfe, Huan et al., 1999	Assessed use of diagnostic and screening procedures among Medicare Part B eligible population.	All Medicare Part B transactions in the state of Michigan from 1986 to 1989 in which procedures were used to diagnose colorectal disease.
Dominitz, Samsa, Landsman, and Provenzale, 1998	Assessed racial/ethnic differences in receipt of treatment and survival among patients with colorectal cancer in Veterans Administration (VA) health system.	3,176 patients (17.9% African American) with a new diagnosis of colorectal cancer.

Analyses	Findings	Limitations
	receiving therapy, few were due to patient refusal (3.76% among whites, 5.88% among blacks).	
Kaplan-Meier method used for constructing survival curves with log-rank statistic used for comparisons. Cox proportional-hazards method used to adjust for confounding variables. Analyses controlled for sex, income, age, stage of disease, type of Medicaid insurance, and comorbidity.	*Rate of surgery:* 64% for black patients vs. 76.7% for white patients ($p < 0.001$). *Five-year survival rate:* 26.4% for black patients vs. 34.1% for white patients ($p < 0.001$). However, there was a nonsignificant difference in survival rates b/w black and white patients who underwent surgery and similar rates for those who did not. This suggests that lower survival rates among black patients is largely explained by the lower rate of surgical treatment.	-Relatively small sample of African Americans. -Racial/ethnic groups other than white and African American not examined. -Retrospective study. -Administrative data.
Series of stepwise logistic regression analyses to predict association between procedure utilization and patient sociodemographic characteristics and residence characteristics.	Assessed contribution of patient age, sex, race, urbanicity of patients' community, per capita income of community, education level of community, and availability of physicians, internists, and gastroenterologists per 100,000 population to prediction of diagnostic procedures. African Americans were more likely than whites to receive barium enema only (odds ratio = 1.38, 95% CI 1.34 to 1.41), were less likely to receive a combination of barium enema and sigmoidoscopy (odds ratio = 0.80, 95% CI 0.78 to 0.83), and were less likely to receive any colonoscopy (odds ratio = 0.83, 95% CI 0.81 to 0.85).	-Racial/ethnic groups other than white and African American not examined. -Administrative data. -Retrospective study.
Logistic regression to predict likelihood of surgical resection, chemotherapy, or radiation therapy, after adjusting for patient demographic characteristics, comorbidities, distant metastases, and tumor location.	No significant racial differences found in rates of receipt of surgical resection (70% among blacks, 73% among whites; odds ratio = 0.92, 95% CI 0.74 to 1.15), chemotherapy (23% for both blacks and whites; odds ratio = 0.99, 95% CI 0.78 to 1.24), or radiation therapy (17% among blacks, 16% among whites; odds ratio = 1.10, 95% CI 0.85 to 1.43). Five-year relative survival rates were similar for black and white patients (42% vs. 39% respectively, $p = 0.16$).	-Racial/ethnic groups other than African American and white not assessed. -Administrative data. -Lack of data on SES.

TABLE B-1 Continued

Cancer

Source	Procedure/Illness	Sample
Howard, Penchansky, and Brown, 1998	Assessed racial/ethnic differences in survival of breast cancer.	246 women (89 African American, 157 white) who sought care for breast cancer in one of three health maintenance organizations (HMOs).
Ball and Elixhauser, 1996	Colorectal cancer.	20,634 discharges b/w 1980 and 1987 from 500 acute care hospitals in the U.S.
Imperato, Nenner, and Will, 1996	Assessed variation by race/ethnicity in rates of radical prostatectomy among male	Pattern analysis of 4,154 Medicare claims for radical prostatectomy to treat pros-

Analyses	Findings	Limitations
Logistic regression to predict stage of disease at time of diagnosis and Cox survival analysis to assess determinants of survival.	No significant racial differences were found in stage of disease, utilization of health services before diagnosis of breast cancer, or receipt of breast examination. African-American patients were more likely to die than whites (30% vs. 18%, $p < 0.04$) and experienced shorter average survival (1.63 years vs. 2.77 years, $p < 0.024$). Two percent of whites and eight percent of African Americans missed two or more appointments following diagnosis; after adjusting for the number of appointments made, African Americans were more likely than whites to miss appointments. Missed appointments and stage of diagnosis were strongly associated with survival, and reduced the impact of race on survival.	-Relatively small sample. -Racial/ethnic groups other than African American and white not examined. -Retrospective review.
Logistic regression to predict diagnostic subgroups, procedure types, in-hospital mortality. Semilogaraithmic ordinary least squares regression for length of stay. *Covariates:* patient demographics, insurance status, clinical factors, and provider characteristics.	Black and white rates of inpatient mortality were equivalent only for the most severely ill. Otherwise, odds of inpatient mortality were 59% to 98% higher for black patients (odds ratio = 1.59 to 1.982, $p < 0.05$ to $p < 0.01$). Procedure type was equivalent only for the sickest patients. Black patients with primary tumor and no evidence of oncologic sequelae were 41% less likely than whites to receive a major colorectal therapeutic procedure (odds ratio = 0.59, $p < 0.001$). When metastasis was recorded black patients with primary tumor were 27% less likely to received a major colorectal therapeutic procedure (odds ratio = 0.726, $p < 0.05$).	-Racial/ethnic groups other than African American and white not examined. -Use of discharge data. -Retrospective study.
Pattern analysis of rates of prostatectomy, relative to incidence of prostate cancer	Rates of radical prostatectomy were lower among African Americans than among whites (b/w ratio ranged from	-Rates for racial/ethnic groups other than white and

TABLE B-1 Continued

Cancer

Source	Procedure/Illness	Sample
	Medicare patients in New York state.	tate cancer between 1991 and 1993.
Harlan, Brawley, Pommerenke et al., 1995	Assessed variations in the use of radical prostatectomy and radiation to treat prostate cancer by geographic area, age, and race/ethnicity.	Data for 67,693 men (9.4% African American) with localized and regional cancer, as obtained from Surveil-lance, Epidemiology, and End Results (SEER) program database between 1984 and 1991.
Optenberg, Thompson, Friedrichs et al., 1995	Assessed long-term survival of black and white prostate cancer patients in Department of Defense (DoD) medical facilities.	1,606 prostate cancer patients (7.5% African American, 92.5% white) who were active duty personnel, dependents, or retirees eligible for care in the military medical system.

Analyses	Findings	Limitations
and Medicare claims for both black and white males.	0.59 in 1991 to 0.86 in 1993; no confidence intervals provided).	African American not examined. -Retrospective study. -Administrative data. -Analyses did not control for income/ SES, comorbidities or other potential confounds.
Chi-square test of association between race and receipt of treatment. Tests for trends calculated using Mantel-Haenszel test.	Black men aged 50 to 69 years were less likely than similarly aged white men to receive prostatectomy. For black and white men aged 70 to 79 years, rates of protatectomy were similar in 1984, but became significantly divergent by 1991, as a larger proportion of white men received the procedure ($p < 0.01$). In 1991, a significantly higher proportion of black men aged 50 to 59 years received radiation. For all age groups in 1991, twice as many blacks as whites (12.5% vs. 6.6%) received no treatment.	-Racial/ethnic groups other than white and African American not examined. -Administrative data. -Retrospective study. -Adjustment not made for comorbidities, SES or other potential confounds.
Multiple life-table regression analysis to determine if stage and grade of cancer, wait time, age or race affect patient survival. Cox proportional hazard function used to compute mortality risk ratios for black and white patients.	Blacks presented at a significantly higher stage of cancer development than whites (26.4% of blacks presenting with distant metastases compared to 12.3% of whites, $p < 0.001$), and demonstrated a greater percentage of recurrence (30.6% vs. 21.4%, $p = 0.02$). There were no significant racial differences in wait time to receive treatment, and no significant differences were found in the type of treatment when stratified by stage of presentation. Overall, stage, grade, and age were found to affect survival, but not race. When analyzed by stage, blacks demonstrated longer survival for distant metastatic disease (mortality risk ratio = 0.644, 95% CI 0.396 to 1.036).	-Racial/ethnic groups other than white and African American not examined. -Administrative data. -Retrospective study.

TABLE B-1 Continued

Cardiovascular Disease

Source	Procedure/Illness	Sample
Petersen et al., 2002	Assessed racial differences in treatment for AMI.	Analysis of 606 black and 4,005 white VA patients with diagnosed AMI discharged from one of 81 VA hospitals.
Bell and Hudson, 2001	Racial and gender differences in emergency room treatment of chest pain.	Analysis of 379 records of patients (229 white, 150 African American) presenting to ER with chest pain during one calendar year at two county hospitals in North Carolina.
Okelo et al., 2001	Rates of recommendation for coronary revascularization when race/ethnicity were unknown by physicians.	Data reviewed for 938 consecutive cardiac catheterizations in 882 patients (26.5% African American, 73.5% white) performed between 1993 and 1995. Cardiologists and cardiothoracic surgeons provided with all clinical and angiographic data without racial identifiers and were asked for revascularization recommendations.

Analyses	Findings	Limitations
Logistic regression to assess use of guideline-based medications, invasive cardiac procedures, and all-cause mortality at 30 days, 1 year, and 3 years.	No differences between African-American and white patients in receipt of beta blockers, but African Amercans were more likely to receive aspirin and were less likely to receive thrombolytic therapy at time of arrival and were less likely to receive bypass surgery, even when only high-risk coronary anatomic subgroups were assessed. No racial differences found in rates of refusal of invasive treatment.	-Racial/ethnic groups other than white and African American not examined. -Retrospective data collection. -Physician, hospital characteristics not assessed.
Logistic regression to assess whether treadmill testing, cardiac catheterization (CC), and echocardiogram (Echo) were recommended or performed. Analysis of covariance to assess wait time to first EKG. Models tested main effects of clinic, gender, race, and insurance, and interactions between gender and race and between insurance and race. Number of cardiovascular related co-morbid conditions also included in models.	*Treadmill:* no significant differences. *CC:* Whites more likely to receive cardiac catheterization (adjusted odds ratio = 2.8317, 95% CI 1.7833 to 4.4963). *Echo:* African Americans more likely to receive Echo (adjusted odds ratio = 0.5927, 95% CI 0.377 to 0.931). *Time to first EKG:* African-American patients waited longer than whites for EKG.	-Racial/ethnic groups other than white and African American not examined. -Relatively small sample. -Retrospective. -Results from diagnostic procedures (e.g., treadmill stress tests) that may have explained variance in CC not available.
Revascularization recommendations compared between African-American and white patients and correlated with clinical data. Logistic regression analyses performed for CABG and PTCA. Independent variables included age, African-American ethnicity, co-morbid disease, LV dysfunction, number of coronary arteries with significant stenosis, and involvement of specific arteries.	After adjustments, African Americans more likely to have a recommendation for PTCA (odds ratio = 1.42, 95% CI 0.96 to 2.11, $p = 0.08$) and less likely to have recommendation for CABG (odds ratio = 0.59, 95% CI 0.37 to 0.94, $p = 0.02$).	-Racial/ethnic groups other than African American and white not examined. -Physician, hospital characteristics not assessed.

TABLE B-1 Continued

Cardiovascular Disease

Source	Procedure/Illness	Sample
Schneider, Leape, Weissman et al., 2001	Assess whether racial differences in cardiac revascularization are due to "overuse" of the procedure in white patients.	Stratified weighted random sample of 3,960 Medicare beneficiaries in 173 hospitals (in five states) who underwent coronary angiography in 1991 and 1992.
Watson, Stein, Dwamera et al., 2001	Influence of race and gender on use of invasive procedures in patients with acute myocardial infarction (AMI).	Prospective study of 838 patients (443 white men, 264 white women, 79 African-American men, 49 African-American women) with AMI seen between January 1994 and April 1995 in five community hospitals in Michigan.
Canto, Allison, Kiefe et al., 2000	Reperfusion therapy for acute myocardial infarction (AMI).	26,575 Medicare patients (25,044 white, 1,531 African American) meeting eligibility criteria for reperfusion therapy.

Analyses	Findings	Limitations
RAND criteria used to determine proportion of coronary artery bypass graft (CABG) and percutaneous transluminal coronary angioplasty (PTCA) procedures that were appropriate, uncertain, or inappropriate. Multivariable logistic regression analysis to assess odds of receiving inappropriate PTCA or inappropriate CABG surgery. Analyses controlled for age, income, clinical characteristics, and state procedure performed.	Rates of inappropriate PTCA ranged from 4% to 24% among study states, and 0% to 14% for CABG surgery. White men had significantly higher adjusted odds than African American men of receiving inappropriate PTCA (odds ratio = 2.42, 95% CI 1.02 to 5.76). No significant differences were found among white women, African-American women, and African-American men. Adjusting for between-hospital effect of race and gender somewhat reduced higher odds of inappropriate PTCA among white men. Inappropriate CABG surgery did not differ by race.	-Retrospective study examining medical record and claims data. -Racial/ethnic groups other than African American not examined.
Multiple logistic regression to identify predictors of cardiac catheterization (CC). Of those undergoing CC, analyses to predict coronary artery bypass grafting (CABG), percutaneous transluminal coronary angioplasty (PTCA), or atherectomy. Analyses adjusted age, hospital of admission, insurance, severity of AMI, and comorbidity. Coronary artery anatomy added as covariate in analyses conducted among patients receiving CC.	Rate of being offered CC (with white men as reference group), was 0.88 (95% CI 0.60 to 1.29, $p = 0.502$) for white women, 0.79 (95% CI 0.41 to 1.5, $p = 0.465$) for black men, and 1.14 (95% CI 0.53 to 2.45, $p = 0.733$) for black women. For those receiving CC, the rate of being offered angioplasty was 1.22 (95% CI 0.75 to 1.98, $p = 0.416$) for white women, 0.61 (95% CI 0.29 to 1.28, $p = 0.192$) for black men, and 0.4 (95% CI 0.14 to 1.13, $p = 0.084$) for black women. The rate of being offered CABG was 0.47 (95% CI 0.24 to 0.89, $p = 0.021$) for white women, 0.36 (95% CI 0.12 to 1.06, $p = 0.065$) for black men, and 0.37 (95% CI 0.11 to 1.28, $p = 0.118$) for black women.	-Racial/ethnic groups other than African American and white not examined. -Small sample of African Americans. -Single geographic location. -No controls for appropriateness or SES.
Bivariate and multivariate analyses of prevalence ratios to predict use of reperfusion therapy by race and gender. Statistical adjustments for age, medical history, clinical	White men were most likely to receive reperfusion therapy (59%), followed by white women (56%), black men (50%), and black women (44%). Prevalence ratios (after statistical adjustment):	-Study excluded patients who were not white or African American. -No controls for socioeconomic status.

TABLE B-1 Continued

Cardiovascular Disease

Source	Procedure/Illness	Sample
Carlisle, Leape, Bickel, Bell et al., 1999	Underuse and overuse of diagnostic testing for coronary artery disease.	356 patients (43% white, 27% African American, 19% Latino, 9% Asian or Pacific Islander) presenting to ER in one of five Los Angeles area hospitals. Patients completed questionnaire asking whether they had received diagnostic testing for coronary artery disease. Patient medical records were also reviewed.
Daumit, Hermann, Coresh, and Powe, 1999	Ethnic differences in use of cardiovascular procedures in patients with end-stage renal disease as they transition to Medicare health insurance.	4,987 patients (3,152 white, 1,835 African American) with end-state renal disease from 303 dialysis facilities between 1986 and 1987. Patients were followed for up to seven years. Data obtained from the Case Mix Severity Study of the US Renal Data System.

Analyses	Findings	Limitations
presentation, and hospital characteristics. Logistic regression to assess whether education, insurance status, gender, age, and race/ethnicity were independent predictors of underuse or overuse.	WW/WM – 1.00 (95% CI 0.98 to 1.03); BW/BM – 1.00 (95% CI 0.89 to 1.13); BW/WM – 0.90 (95% CI 0.82 to 0.98); BM/M – 0.85 (95% CI 0.78 to 0.93). Only level of education was associated with underuse, or inappropriate use of diagnostic testing. Underuse more likely to occur among patients without a college education (odds ratio = 2.2, 95% CI 1.0 to 4.4).	-Retrospective cohort study. -Study limited to patients presenting to ER. -Approximately 50% of potential subjects did not respond or could not be contacted. -Issues of colinearity among education, insurance, and race/ethnicity.
Logistic regression to assess effect of race on receipt of a cardiovascular procedure at baseline. Covariates include age, type insurance at baseline, type of employment, employment status, marital status, region of country, coronary artery disease, history of smoking, cholesterol level, triglyceride level, history diabetes, obesity, cerebrovascular disease, congestive heart failure, history malignant condition, low serum albumin level, and type of dialysis. Logistic regression also used to identify receipt of procedure during follow-up. Cox proportional hazards model used to assess time to receipt of procedure during follow-up for white compared to African American patients.	After adjustment, odds of having a cardiac procedure at baseline were nearly three times greater for white patients than for African-American patients (odds ratio = 2.92, 95% CI 2.04 to 4.18). During follow-up white patients were 1.4 times more likely to have a procedure (adjusted relative risk = 1.41, 95% CI 1.13 to 1.77). In patients with Medicare before end-stage renal disease, the baseline difference in procedure use was eliminated over follow up (odds ratio = 1.05, 95% CI 0.56 to 1.6). Among patients who already had Medicare at baseline, the adjusted odds ratio of procedure use for white compared to African-American patients was 3.0. At follow-up, no difference between ethnic groups seen in procedures after hospitalization for myocardial infarction or coronary disease.	-No controls for hospital characteristics and availability of procedures. -Data obtained from administrative records. -Racial/ethnic groups other than white and African American not included.

TABLE B-1 Continued

Cardiovascular Disease

Source	Procedure/Illness	Sample
Gregory, Rhoads, Wilson et al., 1999	Assess racial differences in rates of cardiac procedures, relative to availability of hospital-based invasive cardiac services.	13,690 New Jersey residents (1,217 African American, 12,473 white) hospitalized with a primary diagnosis of AMI.
Hannan, van Ryn, Burke et al., 1999	Coronary artery bypass graft (CABG) surgery.	1,261 post-angiography patients (680 white non-Hispanic, 314 African American, 267 white Hispanic), stratified by race and gender, who would benefit from CABG in New York state, according to RAND appropriateness and necessity criteria. Patients identified and tracked for three months Data obtained from clinical data, telephone and mail surveys of patients and physicians, and information from NY Cardiac Surgery Reporting System.
Leape, Hilborne, Bell et al., 1999	Assessed use of CABG or PCTA for patients for whom revascularization procedures	631 patients (44% white, 27% African American, 29% Hispanic) at 13 New York City

Analyses	Findings	Limitations
Logistic regression to predict receipt of catheterization and PTCA/CABG, after controlling for patient clinical and demographic factors and availability of cardiac procedures in hospital where patients were first admitted.	For all patients, the likelihood of receiving catherterization within 90 days of AMI was significantly greater among those hospitalized in facilities that provided cardiac services. Blacks were less likely to receive catheterization than whites (b/w odds ratio = 0.74 for those younger than age 65 [95% CI 0.61 to 0.90], 0.68 for those age 65 years and older [95% CI 0.56 to 0.83]) controlling for age, sex, health insurance status (for those younger than age 65), anatomic location of primary infarct, co-morbidities, and the availability of cardiac services. Similarly, blacks were less likely than whites to receive revascularization procedures within 90 days of admission (b/w odds ratio = 0.63 for those younger than age 65 [95% CI 0.52 to 0.76], 0.69 for those age 65 years and older [95% CI 0.54 to 0.86]), controlling for patient demographic and clinical factors and availability of cardiac services.	-Ethnic/racial groups other than African American and white not examined. -Retrospective cohort study. -Use of hospital records. -No controls for SES.
Stepwise logistic regression to predict use of CABG within three months. Statistical adjustments for age, gender, vessels diseased, risk status (low, medium, high), type of insurance, and other clinical characteristics.	African-American and Hispanic patients were significantly less likely to undergo CABG than white non-Hispanics. Odds ratios: white/African-American – 0.64 (95% CI 0.47 to 0.87); white/Hispanic – 0.60 (95% CI 0.43 to 0.84).	-Results may not be representative of NYS (in terms of access by race/ethnicity and gender in the state). -No controls for SES.
Logistic regression to assess	No significant variations found in rates of revascularization among African-American patients, (72%), Hispanic patients (67%) and white patients (75%).	-Moderate sample size.

TABLE B-1 Continued

Cardiovascular Disease

Source	Procedure/Illness	Sample
	were deemed clinically necessary.	hospitals who met RAND criteria for necessary revascularization. Data obtained by hospital record review.
Scirica, Moliterno, Every, Anderson et al., 1999	Racial/ethnic differences in care of patients with unstable angina.	2,948 (77% white, 14% black, 4% Hispanic, 1% Asian, 3% unknown race/ethnicity) consecutive patients with unstable angina admitted to 35 U.S. hospitals in 1996 (GUARANTEE registry). Medical records were reviewed and questionnaire was completed for each patient.
Canto, Herman, Williams, Sanderson et al., 1998	Racial/ethnic differences in presenting characteristics, treatment, and outcomes in patients with myocardial infarction.	275,046 consecutive AMI patients (86% white, 3% Hispanic, 1% Asian and Pacific Islander, < 1% Native American) enrolled in the National Registry of Myocardial Infarction 2 from 1994 to 1996. African-American patients not included in analyses.

Analyses	Findings	Limitations
probability that a patient would receive revascularization as a function of demographic characteristics and type of hospital.	Rates of revascularization were significantly lower, however, among hospitals that did not provide revascularization services (and therefore had to refer patients to other hospitals) than those that did provide revascularization (59% to 76%, difference = 17% [95% CI 8% to 35%]).	-Retrospective study. -Data obtained by record review. -No controls for SES.
Logistic regression to assess independent contribution of demographic, insurance, and clinical factors in distinguishing white from nonwhite patients.	Nonwhites had higher incidence of hypertension and diabetes. Cardiac catheterization was performed less often in nonwhites as compared to whites (36% vs. 53%, $p = 0.001$). In patients meeting criteria for appropriate catheterization (by AHRQ guidelines), fewer nonwhites underwent the procedure (44% vs. 61%, $p = 0.001$) and among these fewer nonwhites had significant coronary stenosis (72% vs. 90%, $p = 0.001$). Angioplasty and CABG received equally often in white and nonwhite patients, among those catheterized who had indications for revascularization.	-Relatively small number of minorities. -Collapse of minorities into one category. -No controls for SES.
Logistic regression to assess factors predicting acute reperfusion strategies, invasive cardiac procedures, and mortality. Variables include demographics, medical history, cardiac risk factors, chest pain, symptom onset to hospital arrival, Killip class, pulse, systolic blood pressure, electrocardiogram, and hospital characteristics.	Hispanics were as likely as whites to receive thrombolytic therapy. Asian and Pacific Islanders were less likely to receive this therapy (odds ratio = 0.84, 95% CI 0.72 to 0.99). Native Americans more likely than whites to receive thrombolytic therapy (odds ratio = 1.18, 95% CI 0.90 to 1.54). All minority groups as likely as whites to receive coronary arteriography. Hispanics were as likely as whites to undergo revascularization procedures, however Asian and Pacific Islanders were less likely to undergo angioplasty (odds ratio = 0.82, 95% CI 0.64 to 1.04) and more likely to have bypass surgery (odds ratio = 1.23, 95% CI 0.96 to 1.57). Native Americans were less likely to undergo both angioplasty	-NRMI-2 not randomized sample of patients. -No available information on SES. -Retrospective study.

TABLE B-1 Continued

Cardiovascular Disease

Source	Procedure/Illness	Sample
Taylor, Canto, Sanderson, Rogers, and Hilbe, 1998	Racial/ethnic differences in management and outcome in patients with Acute Myocardial Infarction (AMI).	Patients from National Registry of Myocardial Infarction 2 (NRMI-2). 275,046 patients included (86% white, 6% black).
Laouri, Kravitz, French et al., 1997	Assessed use of CABG and/or PTCA for patients for whom procedures are deemed clinically necessary following coronary angiography.	671 patients (55% white, 21% Latino, 12% African-American) at six hospitals (four public and two academically affiliated private hospitals) who met explicit clinical criteria for coronary revascularization. Data abstracted from medical records and from patient interviews.
Peterson, Shaw, DeLong et al., 1997	Assessed racial/ethnic differences in use of coronary angioplasty and bypass surgery among patients with	Prospective study of 12,402 white and African-American patients at Duke University Medical Center (10.3% Afri-

Analyses	Findings	Limitations

(odds ratio = 0.72, 95% CI 0.50 to 1.05) and bypass surgery (odds ratio = 0.63, 95% CI 0.38 to 1.04) than whites.

Mortality similar among whites, Hispanics, Asian and Pacific Islanders, and Native Americans.

Logistic regression to assess variables independently predicting utilization of acute reperfusion strategies, invasive cardiac procedures, and mortality. Variables included age, race, sex, payer status, history, chest pain, ST elevation, MI location and type, symptom onset to hospital arrival, Killip class, pulse, systolic BP, contraindications to thrombolysis, census region, and hospital characteristics.

Black patients were less likely to receive intravenous thrombolytic therapy (odds ratio = 0.76, 95% CI 0.71 to 0.80), coronary arteriography (odds ratio = 0.85, 95% CI 0.77 to 0.95), and coronary artery bypass surgery (odds ratio = 0.66, 95% CI 0.58 to 0.75). No significant differences were found in hospital mortality.

-NRMI-2 not randomized sample of patients.
-No available information on SES.
-Retrospective study.

Assessed underuse of coronary revascularization relative to RAND/UCLA criteria for necessity of revascularization procedure. Logistic regression analyses evaluated the effect of gender, ethnicity and type of hospital on CABG or PCTA, or any revascularization, controlling for age, clinical presentation, angiographic findings, and ejection fraction.

African Americans were significantly less likely than whites to undergo necessary CABG (b/w odds ratio = 0.49, 95% CI 0.23 to 0.99), and were less likely to undergo necessary PTCA (odds ratio = 0.20, 95% CI 0.06 to 0.72). Patients at public hospitals were less likely to undergo PTCA than those at private hospitals (odds ratio = 0.10, 95% CI 0.02 to 0.44).

-Moderate sample size.
-Retrospective study.
-No controls for SES, or hospital characteristics.

Logistic regression models to predict the likelihood that a patient would undergo angioplasty or

African Americans were 13% less likely than whites to undergo angioplasty (odds ratio = 0.87, 95% CI 0.73 to 1.03) and 32% less likely to

-Racial/ethnic groups other than white and African

TABLE B-1 Continued

Cardiovascular Disease

Source	Procedure/Illness	Sample
	documented coronary disease. Also assessed whether differences were associated with differences in survival rates.	can American) with documented coronary disease.
Ramsey et al., 1997	Assessed gender and ethnic differences in receipt of percutaneous transluminal coronary angioplasty (PTCA) and aortocoronary bypass surgery (ACBS).	1,228 Mexican-American and white patients hospitalized for myocardial infarction (MI). Data collection part of Corpus Christi Heart Project.
Sedlis, Fisher, Tice et al., 1998	Assessed racial differences in receipt of cardiac procedures in a VA hospital.	1,474 white and 322 African-American patients who had undergone catheterization and were likely candidates for surgery or angioplasty.
Taylor, Meyer, Morse, and Pearson, 1997	Assessed rates of cardiovascular procedures by race in	Abstracted chart reviews from 1,441 patients (1,208 white, 155 African American,

Analyses	Findings	Limitations
bypass surgery. Extension of life associated with bypass surgery calculated by use of proportional-hazards regression model. Risk ratios for black and whites compared after adjusting for base-line prognostic factors. Independent variables included age, sex, severity of disease, other clinical and co-morbid factors, and insurance.	undergo bypass surgery (odds ratio = 0.68, 95% CI 0.56 to 0.82). Racial differences were more marked among patients with severe disease (48% of African Americans with severe coronary disease underwent surgery vs. 65% of whites, $p < 0.001$). Analysis of survival benefit of surgery also revealed racial differences; among patients expected to survive more than one year, 42% of African Americans underwent surgery, compared to 61% of whites ($p < 0.001$). Finally, the adjusted five-year mortality rate among patients revealed that African-American patients were 18% more likely than whites to die (odds ratio = 1.18, 95% CI 1.05 to 1.32).	American not examined. -Single site. -No information about patient preferences. -No controls for SES.
Logistic regression to predict receipt of services, after adjusting for age, sex, previous diagnosis of coronary heart disease, MI, diabetes mellitus, hypertension, occurrence of congestive heart failure during MI, location and type of MI.	Among only patients who had received catheterization to determine extent of disease, Mexican Americans were less likely to receive PTCA, but not ACBS, than whites after adjusting for clinical and demographic characteristics (odds ratio = 0.65, 95% CI 0.43 to 0.99).	-Single geographic location. -No controls for SES, hospital characteristics.
Analyses were generated from surgical referral conference at VA hospital between 1988 and 1996. Racial differences in conference recommendation and patient compliance with recommendations were analyzed using Fisher's exact test.	Therapeutic cardiac procedures (surgery or PTCA) were offered more frequently for white patients (72.9%) than African-American patients (64.3%; odds ratio = 1.497, $p = 0.0022$). This difference could not be explained by simple clinical differences between the two groups. African-American patients, however, were more likely than whites to refuse invasive procedures (odds ratio = 2.026, 95% CI 1.311 to 3.130).	-Racial/ethnic groups other than African American and white not examined. -Single site. -Potential confounds such as SES not assessed.
Logistic regression to assess	No differences found in rates of catheterization procedures between white and "nonwhite" patients during AMI	-Retrospective study. -Potential con-

TABLE B-1 Continued

Cardiovascular Disease

Source	Procedure/Illness	Sample
	military health services system.	78 other) with principle or secondary diagnosis of AMI in 125 military hospitals.
Weitzman, Cooper, Chambless et al., 1997	Assessed rates of performance of cardiac procedures in relation to gender, race, and geographic location.	5,462 patients (815 of these African-American) in four states (North Carolina, Mississippi, Maryland, and Minnesota) hospitalized for myocardial infarction (MI).
Allison, Kiefe, Centor et al., 1996	Assess variations in use of medications among African-American and white Medicare patients hospitalized with Acute Myocardial Infarction (AMI).	Retrospective medical record review of 4,052 patients (3,542 white, 510 African American) hospitalized in all acute care hospitals in Alabama with principle discharge diagnosis of AMI.

Analyses	Findings	Limitations
differences by patient race in rates of catheterization or revascularization procedures, controlling for age, gender, cardiovascular risk factors, and clinical data relevant to admission for AMI.	admission (odds ratio = 0.96, 95% CI 0.69 to 1.34) or between white and black patients (odds ratio = 1.19, 95% CI 0.80 to 1.78). Similarly, no differences were found in rates of revascularization (PTCA or CABG) between white and "nonwhite" patients (odds ratio = 0.90, 95% CI 0.59 to 1.39) or between white and black patients (odds ratio = 1.11, 95% CI 0.65 to 1.89). No differences were found in mortality or rates of readmission within 180 days following initial discharge. However, white patients were significantly more likely than nonwhite patients to be considered for future catheterization (odds ratio = 1.77, 95% CI 1.20 to 2.61).	founds such as SES, disease severity, appropriateness not assessed.
Logistic regression to estimate odds of having diagnostic and therapeutic procedures performed during an MI event by race, gender, and type of hospital.	After controlling for severity of MI and co-morbid conditions, blacks admitted to teaching hospitals were significantly less likely to receive PTCA (b/w odds ratio = 0.4, 95% CI 0.2 to 0.6), CABG (b/w odds ratio = 0.4, 95% CI 0.2 to 0.9) or thrombolytic therapy (b/w odds ratio = 0.5, 95% CI 0.3 to 0.8). Similarly, blacks admitted to non-teaching hospitals were significantly less likely to receive PTCA (b/w odds ratio = 0.5, 95% CI 0.3 to 0.7), CABG (b/w odd ratio = 0.3, 95% CI 0.2 to 0.6) or thrombolytic therapy (b/w odds ratio = 0.5, 95% CI 0.3 to 0.7).	-Racial/ethnic groups other than African American and white not assessed. -Potential confounds such as SES, co-morbidities, appropriateness not assessed.
Logistic regression to assess rate of receipt of thrombolysis, beta-andrenergic blockade and aspirin, controlling for patient age, gender, clinical factors, severity of illness, algorithm-determined candidacy for therapy, and hospital characteristics	After controlling for patient appropriateness for therapy, age, gender, clinical characteristics, and hospital characteristics, white patients were more likely to receive thrombolytics than black patients (odds ratio = 0.51, 95% CI 0.38 to 0.78). No differences were found in receipt of beta-blockers (odds ratio = 1.18, 95% CI 0.91 to 1.53)	-Racial/ethnic groups other than white and African American not examined. -Relatively small sample of African Americans. -Retrospective study. -Data obtained

TABLE B-1 Continued

Cardiovascular Disease

Source	Procedure/Illness	Sample
Herholz et al., 1996	Assessed gender and ethnic differences in receipt of cardiovascular medications on discharge from hospital following myocardial infarction (MI).	Discharge data for 982 patients hospitalized for definite or possible MI; data are from the Corpus Christi Heart Project.
Blustein, Arons, and Shea, 1995	Assessed variations by race, payor, and gender in process of care leading up to revascularization procedures for patients with cardiovascular disease.	5,857 non-Medicare (less than 65 years of age) patients admitted to hospitals in California with a principal diagnosis of acute myocardial infarction (AMI).
Carlisle et al., 1995	Assessed use of coronary artery angiography, bypass graft surgery, and angioplasty among Los Angeles	131,408 patients (89,781 white, 16,509 African American, 19,218 Latino, and 5,900 Asian) discharged from L.A. County

Analyses	Findings	Limitations
(e.g., rural vs. urban, teaching vs. non-teaching).	or aspirin (odds ratio = 1.00, 95% CI 0.81 to 1.24) by patient race.	through record review. -No controls for SES.
Logit regression to predict receipt of medications by gender and ethnicity, after adjusting for age, diagnosis of diabetes mellitus, hypertension, congestive heart failure, serum cholesterol level, and cigarette smoking.	Mexican Americans received fewer medications than whites (odds ratio = 0.62, 95% CI 0.33 to 1.15), even after adjusting for clinical and demographic characteristics. Mexican Americans were less likely to receive almost all major medications, especially antiarrhythmics, anticoagulants, and lipid-lowering therapy.	-Single geographic region. -No controls for SES, hospital characteristics, appropriateness.
Series of chi square and regression analyses to determine likelihood of receipt of services during prehospital, intrahospital (duration of initial hospitalization), interhospital, and posthospital (readmission for revascularization following initial hospitalization) phases. African-American and Hispanic patients grouped together as "minority" due to small numbers.	Authors found differences in likelihood of receipt of procedures during nearly every phase of treatment for different racial and payor groups. Whites, those with private insurance, and those with more severe heart disease were more likely to gain initial admittance to hospitals providing revascularization services. Once hospitalized, whites, males, those with private insurance, and those with more severe disease were more likely to actually receive revascularization. These same patterns were observed among those patients not initially admitted to hospitals offering revascularization but who later received revascularization upon re-admittance or transfer. In logistic regression analyses to assess odds of receiving revascularization during any admission, whites were more likely to receive revascularization (odds ratio = 1.49 [no CI reported]), as were the privately insured.	-Relatively small number of minorities. -Administrative data, lack of clinical detail. -Retrospective study.
Series of logistic regression models to assess relationship between use of invasive procedures and ethnicity, controlling for primary	African Americans were less likely than whites to receive bypass graft (odds ratio = 0.62, 95% CI 0.56 to 0.69) and angioplasty (odds ratio = 0.80, 95% CI 0.72 to 0.88). Latinos	-Retrospective. -Administrative records used. -Proxy used for co-morbidity and income.

TABLE B-1 Continued

Cardiovascular Disease

Source	Procedure/Illness	Sample
	County residents with possible ischemic heart disease.	hospitals following angiography, CABG, or angioplasty. National Hospital Discharge Survey records of 10,348 patients (9,289 white, 159 African American) hospitalized with AMI.
Giles et al., 1995	Assessed race and sex differences in rate of receipt of catheterization, PTCA, or coronary artery bypass surgery (CABS).	
Maynard, Every, Martin, and Weaver, 1995	Implications of less intensive use of revascularization in black patients on long-term survival.	420 black and 10,834 patients hospitalized for acute myocardial infarction in metropolitan Seattle from 1988 to 1994.

Analyses	Findings	Limitations
diagnosis, age, gender, insurance type, income (proxy), co-morbidities, and differences among hospitals in volume of invasive procedures.	were less likely to receive angiography (odds ratio = 0.90, 95% CI 0.85 to 0.95). Asian Americans did not differ from whites in invasive cardiac procedure rates, although all three ethnic groups were less likely to receive procedures than whites when hospital procedure volume was not controlled.	
Logistic regression analysis adjusting for age, type of health insurance, hospital size and type, region, in-hospital mortality, and hospital transfer rates to assess differences in rates of procedures by race. Analyses also performed to match individuals admitted to the same hospital and who did not undergo a procedure. Analyses limited to procedures occurring during initial hospitalization.	Significant differences by race and gender were found after statistical adjustment and patient matching procedure. With white males as the referent, black men were less likely to receive catherterization (odds ratio = 0.67, 95% CI 0.51 to 0.87) or CABS (odds ratio = 0.63, 95% CI 0.44 to 0.90), while black women were less like to receive catheterization (odds ratio = 0.50, 95% CI 0.37 to 0.68), PTCA (odds ratio = 0.42, 95% CI 0.23 to 0.76) or CABS (odds ratio = 0.37, 95% CI 0.22 to 0.62). Among only those patients who underwent catheterization (and therefore had access to a cardiologist), black women were less likely to receive subsequent PTCA or CABS.	-Administrative data. -Retrospective. -No controls for SES. -May only be able to generalize to patients with more severe disease.
Logistic regression to assess racial differences in age-adjusted hospital mortality and use of revascularization. Log rank statistic used to determine differences in survival.	No significant differences found in proportion of black and white patients receiving thrombolytic therapy or cardiac catheterization. After adjusting for use of cardiac catheterization, percent professionals in census block, history of prior coronary surgery, history of angina, use of thrombolytic therapy, sex, and history of congestive heart failure, black patients 40% less likely to undergo revascularization (odds ratio = 0.60, 95% CI 0.45 to 0.81, $p = 0.0008$). After adjustment race was not associated with long-term survival.	-Relatively small sample of African-American patients. -Racial/ethnic groups other than African American and white not assessed. -SES estimated by census blocks.

TABLE B-1 Continued

Analgesia

Source	Procedure/Illness	Sample
Peterson, Wright, Daley, and Thibault, 1994	Racial differences in procedure use and survival following acute myocardial infarction (AMI) within Department of Veterans Affairs.	33,641 (29,119 white, 4,522 African American) male veterans discharged with diagnosis of AMI from January 1988 to December 1990.
Ayanian, Udvarhelyi, Gatsonis et al., 1993	Assessed racial differences in rates of coronary revascularization following angiography and relationship of these differences to hospital characteristics.	27,485 Medicare Part A enrollees (26,389 white, 1,096 African American) who underwent inpatient coronary angiography in 1987.
Whittle, Conigliaro, Good, and Lofgren, 1993	Racial differences in use of cardiovascular procedures in Department of Veterans Affairs.	Retrospective study of 428,300 male veterans (74,570 African American, 353,730 white) discharged from VA hospitals with diagnoses of cardiovascular disease or chest pain between 1987 and 1991.

Analyses	Findings	Limitations
Logistic regression to assess effect of race on use of cardiac catheterization, coronary angioplasty, coronary bypass surgery, and overall coronary revascularization. Likelihood ratios calculated for 30-day, 1-year, and 2-year survival. Analyses adjust for age, cardiac complications, number of secondary diagnoses, previous hospitalization, hospital location, on-site availability of cardiac catheterization and bypass surgery, and year of admission.	After adjustment, as compared to white patient, African Americans 33% less likely to undergo cardiac catheterizations within 90 days of AMI (odds ratio = 0.67, 95% CI 0.62 to 0.72); 54% less likely to undergo coronary bypass surgery within 90 days of AMI (odds ratio = 0.46, 95% CI 0.40 to 0.53), and 42% less likely to undergo angioplasty within 90 days of AMI (odds ratio = 0.58, 95% CI 0.48 to 0.66). The black/white ratio for any cardiac revascularization procedure within 90 days of AMI was 0.46 (95% CI 0.41 to 0.52). African Americans more likely to survive 30 days following AMI compared to whites (adjusted odds ratio = 1.18, 95% CI 1.07 to 1.31). No differences found between races for 1 or 2-year survival rates.	-Racial ethnic groups other than white and African American not included. -Administrative database. -Retrospective study. -No controls for SES.
Logistic regression analyses to predict revascularization, controlling for age, sex, region, Medicaid eligibility, principal diagnosis, secondary diagnoses, and hospital characteristics.	African Americans were less likely than whites to receive a revascularization procedure (w/b adjusted odds ratio = 1.78, 95% CI 1.56 to 2.03). Greater use of revascularization occurred in public, private, teaching, nonteaching, and urban/suburban hospitals, and in hospitals where revascularization procedures were available, as well as in hospitals where such procedures were not available, after controlling for patient demographic and clinical factors. No significant black/white differences in rates of revascularization were found in rural hospitals.	-Racial/ethnic groups other than African American and white not examined. -Relatively small sample of African-American patients. -Administrative data set. -Retrospective study.
Logistic regression to assess association or race with use of procedures controlling for diagnosis, region, age, co-morbidity, marital status, year of diagnosis, whether CABG performed at hospital where diagnosis made.	After adjustment, white patients more likely than African American patients to undergo cardiac catheterization (odds ratio = 1.38, 95% CI 1.34 to 1.42), angioplasty (odds ratio = 1.50, 95% CI 1.38 to 1.64), and CABG (odds ratio = 2.22, 95% CI 2.09 to 2.36).	-Racial/ethnic groups other than African American not examined. -Retrospective study of administrative data set. -No controls for admission practices.

TABLE B-1 Continued

Cardiovascular Disease

Source	Procedure/Illness	Sample

Cerebrovascular Disease

Mitchell, Ballard, Matchar et al., 2000	Assessed rates of tests and treatment for cerebrovascular disease: noninvasive cerebrovascular tests, cerebral angiography, carotid endarterectomy, anticoagulant therapy, and probability of receiving care from a neurologist.	Inpatient hospital records of 17,437 Medicare patients (15,929 white and 1,508 African American) with a principal diagnosis of transient ischemic attack (TIA).
Oddone, Horner, Sloane et al., 1999	Racial differences in use of carotid artery imaging in Veterans Affairs Medical Centers.	803 patients (389 African American, 414 white) hospitalized in one of four VA Medical Centers between April 1991 and January 1995

Analyses	Findings	Limitations
Computed state age- and sex-adjusted rates of CABG for whites and African Americans and evaluated relative to need for care (as indicated by myocardial infarction rate) and supply of physicians (as indicated by the number of thoracic surgeons and cardiologists per 10,000 persons).	Nationally, CABG rate was 27.1 per 10,000 for whites, 7.6 per 10,000 for African Americans. Racial differences were greater in the Southeast, particularly in non-metropolitan areas. Correlation of CABG rates was significantly associated with the density of thoracic surgeons and location in the Southeast for whites, but physician availability and location was not correlated with CAGB rates for African Americans.	-Some veterans in study obtained care outside of VA. -Administrative data set. -Racial/ethnic groups other than white and African American not examined. -Retrospective study. -Limited information on demographic factors.
Logistic regression adjusting for comorbid illness (including hypertension and prior history of stroke), ability to pay (proxy based on dual Medicaid-Medicare eligibility and area of residence), and other clinical and demographic variables.	After adjusting for patient, illness, and provider characteristics, African Americans were 83% as likely as whites to receive noninvasive cerebrovascular testing (95% CI 0.73 to 0.93). Among those receiving noninvasive testing, African Americans were 54% as likely to receive cerebral angiography (95% CI 0.36 to 0.80), and among those receiving angiography, the odds of African Americans receiving carotid endarterectomy was 0.27 (95% CI 0.09 to 0.78). African Americans were 62% as likely to receive anticoagulant therapy, but this difference not statistically significant given small number of African-American subjects. African-American patients were 21% less likely to receive care from a neurologist (95% CI 0.69 to 0.90).	-Racial/ethnic groups other than African American and white not examined. -Retrospective study. -Administrative data.
Logistic regression to determine adjusted odds ratios for receiving any carotid artery imaging. Models adjust for age, comorbidity,	African American patients were less likely to have an imaging study of their carotid arteries (22% vs. 45%, $p = 0.001$). Race remained an independent predictor of imaging after adjusting	-Retrospective study reviewing medical records. -Very small number of African Ameri-

TABLE B-1 Continued

Cerebrovascular Disease

Source	Procedure/Illness	Sample
		with ICD-9 diagnoses of either transient ischemic attack, ischemic stroke, or amaurosis fugax. Record review of clinical data.

Children's Health Care

| Weech-Maldonado et al., 2001 | Parents' ratings and reports of pediatric care under Medicaid Managed Care by race, ethnicity, and primary language. | Reponses for over 9,000 children (842 Hispanic, 1,344 African American, 131 Asian, 330 American Indian, 6,329 white, 111 other) from the National Consumer Assessment of Health Plans Benchmarking Database 1.0 Data from 33 HMOs from Arkansas, Kansas, Minnesota, Oklahoma, Vermont, and Washington state. |

Analyses	Findings	Limitations

linical presentation, antici-pated operative risk, and hospital. | for clinical factors (odds ratio = 1.50, 95% CI 1.06 to 2.13). Whites were significantly more likely to be assessed as appropriate candi-dates for surgery using RAND criteria (18% vs. 4%, p = 0.001) because of higher prevalence of significant ca-rotid artery stenosis. RR of carotid endarterectomy for whites compared to African Americans was 1.34 (95% CI 0.70 to 2.53). | cans received procedure. -Study limited to hospitalized patients. -No controls for SES.

Ordinary least squares regression to assess the effect of race/ethnicity, Hispanic language, and Asian language on ratings and reports of care, control-ling for parent age, gender, education, and child's health status. Care domains examined include doctor/nurse rating, health care rating, health plan rating, timeliness of care, provider communication, staff help-fulness, and plan service. | Compared with whites, Asian/other reported worse care across several domains [getting needed care (β = -8.11, p < 0.05), timeliness of care (β = -18.65, p < 0.001), provider com-munication (β = -17.19, p < 0.001), staff helpfulness (β = -20.10, p < 0.001), plan service (β = -10.95, p < 0.001)]. English-speaking Asian par-ents did not differ significantly from whites on any reports of care. Spanish-speaking Hispanic parents reported more negative care than whites on timeliness of care (β = -9.24, p < 0.01), provider communication (β = -4.37, p < 0.05) staff helpfulness (β = -6.09, p < 0.05), and plan service (β = -6.93, p < 0.001). English-speaking Hispanic parents did not differ from whites on any reports of care. African-American parents scored lower than whites on reports of get-ting needed care (β = -3.52, p < 0.05), timeliness of care (β = -4.53, p < 0.01), and plan service (β = -4.29, p < 0.001). American Indians had worse reports of care than whites for getting needed care (β = -9.12, p < 0.05), timeliness of care (β = -3.52, p < 0.01), provider communication (β = -3.27, p < 0.05), and plan service (β = -4.12, p < 0.01). | -No controls for other SES character-istics such as in-come, occupation -No examination of clinical meaningful-ness of differences in reports and ratings of care. -Mail and tele-phone surveys, data did not iden-tify surveys admin-istered in English vs. Spanish.

TABLE B-1 Continued

Children's Health Care

Source	Procedure/Illness	Sample
Furth et al., 2000	Access to kidney transplant list.	3,284 patients < 20 years of age (1,122 black, 2,162 white) with ESRD who had first dialysis between January 1, 1988, and December 31, 1993.
Hampers et al., 1999	Assess whether language barriers between patients and physicians were associated with differences in diagnostic testing and length of stay.	Prospective investigation of 2,467 patient visits to Emergency Department between September and December 1997 (413 white, 557 African American, 1,284 Hispanic, 124 other, 89 NA). 286 families did not speak English, representing a language barrier for the physician in 209 cases.
Zito, Safer, dosReis, and Riddle, 1998	Psychotropic medication use.	99,217 African-American (60,868) and white (38,349) youths ages five through 14, who were Medicaid recipients in the state of Maryland seen in ambulatory settings.
Hahn, 1995	Use of prescription medications.	Two samples of children: 1) ages one to five ($n = 1,347$), and 2) ages 6 to 17 ($n = 2,155$) who had at least one ambula-

Analyses	Findings	Limitations
Cox proportional hazard analysis to examine independent effect of race on the time from first dialysis for ESRD until first activation on cadaveric transplant waitlist for index transplant controlling for confounding factors (age, gender, cause of ESRD, SES, incident year of ESRD, ESRD network, facility characteristics).	Controlling for confounders, black patients were 12% less likely than white patients to be activated on the kidney transplant wait list (relative hazard = 0.88, 95% CI 0.79 to 0.97). In addition, after controlling for confounders, the relative hazard for black patients in the lowest SES quartile being activated on the wait list was 0.84 (95% CI 0.70 to 1.01) compared to relative hazard of 1.0 (95% CI 0.8 to 1.3) for black patients in the highest SES quartile.	-Racial/ethnic groups other than African American and white not examined. -Administrative data. -Retrospective study. -Potential confounds such as co-morbidities, appropriateness not examined.
Mann-Whitney U tests used to compare total charges among groups. Analysis of covariance used to assess predictors of total charges and length of ED stay. Race/ethnicity, insurance status, provider training, patient care setting, and triage category, patient age, patient vital signs, included in models to isolate effect of language barrier.	The presence of a language barrier accounted for a $38 increase in charges for testing (F = 14.1, $p < 0.001$) and 20 minute longer ED stay (F = 9.1, $p = 0.003$).	-No independent or family verification of language barrier. -No full control for complexity of cases. -No controls for use of professional interpreter or ad hoc interpreter -Single site
Logistic regression to estimate the probability of psychotropic medication use as a function of race and region. The effect of race controlling for region and interaction of race and region were analyzed.	Caucasians were twice as likely to receive psychotropic prescriptions compared with African Americans after adjusting for geographic region (odds ratio = 1.97, 95% CI 1.84 to 2.12). The interaction of race and region was significant (χ^2 = 23.3, df = 7, $p < 0.001$), such that the odds of receiving psychotropic medications differed by geographic region (range 1.23 to 2.60).	-Racial/ethnic groups other than African American and white not examined. -One geographic location. -Administrative data. -Retrospective study. -Potential confounds such as income, service use, and provider specialties not assessed.
Logistic and multiple regression used to assess the probability of receiving a prescription medication and	*For children ages one to five:* 1) Black children (odds ratio = 0.532) were half as likely to receive prescription medication compared with white	-Administrative data.

TABLE B-1 Continued

Children's Health Care

Source	Procedure/Illness	Sample
		tory care visit in 1987. Data were obtained from the Household Component of the National Medical Expenditure Survey (NMES).

Analyses	Findings	Limitations

children (odds ratio = 1.0) ($p < 0.001$). Adding health factors to the model did not change relationships. However, addition number of physician visits reduced differences, such that they were no longer significant. There was no difference in the probability of receiving medication for Hispanic children compared with white children.

2) After controlling for age, maternal education, insurance, poverty status, source of care, geographic location, health status, # bed days, # reduced activity days, and physician visits, black children received the fewest number of medications. The average number of medications for black children was 86.5% compared to that of white children, while Hispanic children averaged 94.1% compared to that of white children.

For children ages six to 17:

1) Black (odds ratio = 0.536) and Hispanic (odds ratio = 0.621) children were less likely to receive any prescription medication compared to white (odds ratio = 1.0) children. The addition of health factors, and number of physician visits did not change these relationships (odds ratio = 0.601, $p < 0.001$, odds ratio = 0.697, $p < 0.01$ respectively).

2) After controlling for age, maternal education, insurance, poverty status, source of care, geographic location, health status, # bed days, # reduced activity days, and physician visits, black children received the fewest number of medications. The average number of medications for black children was 89.7% compared to that of white children, and 92.1% for Hispanic children compared to that of white children.

TABLE B-1 Continued

Diabetes

Source	Procedure/Illness	Sample
Chin, Zhang, and Merrell, 1998	Assessed quality of care and resource utilization among African-American and white patients with diabetes.	1,376 African-American and white Medicare beneficiaries with diabetes (14% African Americans).

Emergency Services

Source	Procedure/Illness	Sample
Lowe et al., 2001	Assessed racial differences in denial of authorization for emergency department (ED) care by managed care gatekeepers.	15,578 African-American and white patients who sought care in an urban hospital emergency department.
Baker, Stevens, and Brook, 1996	Assessed racial differences in emergency department use.	1,049 patients (295 African American, 237 white, 517 Hispanic) registered for non-emergency medical problems in the Harbor-UCLA Medical Center Emergency Department.

Analyses	Findings	Limitations
Linear and logistic regression to assess independent contribution of race to health status, quality of care, and resource utilization, controlling for sex, education, and age. Measures included patient survey, ADA and RAND criteria for quality of care, and Medicare reimbursement.	African-American patients were less likely to have measurement of glycosylated hemoglobin (adjusted odds ratio = 0.65, 95% CI 0.48 to 0.88) lipid testing (odds ratio = 0.66, 95% CI 0.48 to 0.89), ophthalmological visits (odds ratio = 0.72, 95% CI 0.56 to 0.93), and influenza vaccinations (odds ratio = 0.26, 95% CI 0.19 to 0.36). African-American patients were more likely to use the ED (39% vs. 29%, $p < 0.01$) and had fewer physician visits (8.4 vs. 9.7 visits per year, $p < 0.05$). In addition, African-American patients had higher reimbursement for home health services, however, once adjusting for case-mix variables race was not associated.	-Racial/ethnic groups other than African American and white not examined. -Confounds such as hospital characteristics, appropriateness, and comorbidities not examined.
Multiple logistic regression to assess racial differences in authorization for emergency department services.	After adjusting for patients' age, gender, day, and time of ED visit, type of Managed Care Organization (MCO) and triage category, African Americans were more likely to be denied authorization for care (odds ratio = 1.52, 95% CI 1.18 to 1.94). Patients who were covered by a Medicaid MCO (odds ratio = 1.50, 95% CI 1.19 to 1.90) or those covered with MCOs with mixed Medicaid and commercial patient populations (odds ratio = 2.05, 95% CI 1.41 to 2.98) were more likely than those covered by purely commercial MCOs to be denied authorization for care.	-Racial groups other than African American and white not assessed. -Single site.
Logistic regression to assess independent effect of race/ethnicity on ED use.	19% of African Americans, 13.2% of whites and 11.3% of Hispanic patients reported two or more previous ED visits (in preceding three months) ($p = 0.01$ across groups) (unadjusted odds ratio 1.82 for	-Sample obtained at one site, selective enrollment. -Cross-sectional survey.

TABLE B-1 Continued

Emergency Services

Source	Procedure/Illness	Sample

Eye Care

Source	Procedure/Illness	Sample
Devgan, Yu, Kim, and Coleman, 2000	Surgical treatment of glaucoma in African-American Medicare beneficiaries.	Retrospective cohort analysis of 30,495 African-American and 160,792 white patients over 65 years of age undergoing argon laser trabeculoplasty or trabeculectomy surgery between 1991 and 1994.
Wang, Javitt, and Tielsch, 1997	Glaucoma and cataract treatment.	642,048 Medicare beneficiaries (606,069 white, 35,979 black) age 65 and older who used eye care services. Patients with physician-diagnosed glaucoma or cataract who underwent surgical treatment.

Analyses	Findings	Limitations

| | African Americans compared with Hispanics). After adjusting for age, insurance status, regular source of care, and transportation difficulties, ethnicity was not significantly associated with two or more ED visits in the preceding three months (adjusted odds ratio for Hispanics compared with African Americans 1.48, 95% CI 0.95 to 2.3 and adjusted odds ratio for Hispanics compared with whites was 1.22, 95% CI 0.74 to 2.00). | |

| Age and sex adjusted rates of argon laser trabeculo-plasty and trabeculectomy surgery were obtained and compared with surgery rates expected based on disease prevalence. | For each age and age-sex subgroup, the rate of surgical procedures is higher in African Americans compared to whites. The age-sex-adjusted rate ratio was 2.14 (95% CI 2.11 to 2.16). Assuming treatment should be performed in proportion to age-race prevalence, African Americans underwent glaucoma surgery at 47% below expected rate (expected rate: 5.52 procedures per 1,000 person-year of enrollment, adjusted rate: 2.95 procedures per 100 person-year enrollment). | -Administrative data base. -Data does not contain information on beneficiaries who may be enrolled in HMOs or VA hospitals. -Racial/ethnic groups other than African American and white not analyzed. |

| Black-white relative risk of having a physician-diagnosed condition and surgical treatment were compared to the expected value based on population survey data for each specific disease. | Black patients used eye care services at two-thirds the rate of white patients (age gender adjusted RR = 0.67, 95% CI 0.66 to 0.68). Black women were 73% as likely to use services as white women, while black men were 56% as likely to use services. Among users of eye care services, black patients were 2.2 times more likely than whites to be diagnosed with glaucoma, after adjusting for age and gender (RR = 2.17, 95% CI 2.12 to 2.22). In addition, among users of eye care services, blacks had lower than expected rates of treatment for glaucoma (observed RR = 3.2, 95% CI | -Administrative database. -Differential presentation for care based on severity can not be ruled out. -Other clinical confounds may exist. |

TABLE B-1 Continued

Eye Care

Source	Procedure/Illness	Sample

Gallbladder Disease

Source	Procedure/Illness	Sample
Arozullah, Ferreira, Bennett et al., 1999	Racial variation in rate of adoption of laparoscopic cholecystectomy procedure in Department of Veterans Affairs Medical System. Mortality and length of hospital stay also examined.	16,181 patients (14,249 Caucasian and 1,932 African American) diagnosed with gall bladder or biliary disease who underwent either open cholecystectomy or laparoscopic cholecystectomy. Data were collected through: a) record review of claims files, and b) prospectively compiled clinical data from records and interview, for the year before the new procedure was introduced and the first four years of use of the procedure (1991-1995).

Analyses	Findings	Limitations
	3.1 to 3.4 vs. expected RR of 4.3, 95% CI 3.5 to 5.4), but a higher treatment rate for cataract (RR = 1.2, 95% CI 1.2 to 1.3). Among patients with physician diagnosed glaucoma and cataract, black patients were more likely to undergo surgical treatment for these diagnoses than white patients (RR = 1.5 for glaucoma, 95% CI 1.4 to 1.5; RR = 1.2 for cataract, 95% CI 1.2 to 1.3).	
Modified multiple logistic regression model to predict the use of laparoscopic versus open cholecystectomy. Predictors included race, age, marital status, hospital geographic location, co-morbid illnesses, and year of surgery. To examine mortality and length of stay, multiple logistic regression equations used. Predictors included age, gender, marital status, coexisting medical condition, geographic region, year of care, and type of cholecystectomy.	*Claims data* indicate that after controlling for confounding variables, African-American patients who underwent cholecystectomy were 25% less likely as white patients to undergo the laparoscopic procedure (adjusted odds ratio = 0.74, 95% CI 0.66 to 0.83). The shortening of postoperative length of hospital stay (from 9 to < 4.5 days with new procedure) occurred in the first year for white patients and in the fourth year for African-American patients ($p < 0.001$). *Clinical data* indicate that after adjustment, African-American patients were 0.68 times as likely to undergo the laparoscopic procedure (95% CI 0.55 to 0.84).	-Administrative data set. -Racial/ethnic groups other than African American not examined.

TABLE B-1 Continued

HIV/AIDS

Source	Procedure/Illness	Sample
Shapiro, Morton, McCaffrey et al., 1999	Assessed racial/ethnic, gender, and other sociodemographic variations in care (number of care-seeking visits and use of protease inhibitors [PI] or nonnucleoside reverse transcriptase inhibitors [NNRTI]) for persons infected with HIV.	Multistage probability sample of 2,846 individuals, including African-American and Hispanic patients, using data from the HIV Costs and Services Utilization Study.
Bennett, Horner, Weinstein et al., 1995	Assessed quality of care for pneumocyctis carinii pneumonia (PCP) among white, Hispanic and African-American patients with HIV receiving care in either Veterans Administration (VA) hospitals or non-VA systems.	Retrospective chart review of a cohort of 627 VA patients and 1,547 non-VA patients with treated or cytologically confirmed PCP who were hospitalized from 1987 to 1990.
Moore, Stanton, Gopalan, and Chaisson, 1994	Assessed use of anti-retroviral drugs and prophylactic therapy to treat pneumocyctis carinii pneumonia (PCP) in an urban population infected with HIV.	838 African-American, Hispanic, and white patients presenting at an urban HIV clinic from March 1990 through December 1992. Data obtained through interview and record review with six-month follow-up.

Analyses	Findings	Limitations
Logistic regression to predict use of PI and NNRTI, prophylaxis against pneumocyctis carinii pneumonia (PCP), use of antiretroviral medication, hospitalizations, ambulatory visits, and emergency department visits.	Adjusting for insurance status, CD4 cell count, sex, age, method of exposure to HIV, and region of country, African-American and Hispanic patients were 24% less likely than whites to receive PI or NNRTI at initial assessment, although this disparity declined to 8% at the final assessment stage, a difference that remained statistically significant ($p = 0.016$). On average, blacks waited 13.5 months to receive these medications, compared to 10.6 months for whites ($p < 0.001$).	-Potential confounds such as co-morbidities, SES not assessed.
Logistic regression to predict diagnostic procedures (use and timing of bronchoscopy) and use and timing of PCP medications, controlling for insurance status, age, sex, risk group status, severity of PCP illness at admission, use of medications prior to admission, type of hospital, and hospital volume of patients with AIDS.	For all patients, regardless of the type of hospital in which they were treated, use of anti-PCP medications was initiated within two days of admission for 70% to 77% of patients. Approximately 60% of patients underwent a bronchoscopy at some point during hospitalization. Black and Hispanic patients at non-VA hospitals were more likely to die during hospitalization, and were less likely to undergo bronchoscopy in the first two days of admission. No racial differences were found in use of bronchoscopy, receipt of anti-PCP medications within two days of admission, or mortality in VA hospitals.	-Retrospective study. -No controls for SES, co-morbidities.
Logistic regression to predict receipt of antiviral agents or PCP prophylaxis, adjusting for patient income, insurance status, mode of HIV transmission, and place of residence.	No racial differences were found in the stage of HIV disease at the time of presentation. However, 63% of eligible whites, but only 48% of eligible blacks received antiretroviral therapy, and PCP prophylaxis was received by 82% of eligible whites and only 58% of eligible blacks. African-American patients were significantly less likely than whites to receive antiretroviral therapy (odds ratio = 0.59, 95% CI 0.38 to 0.93) or PCP prophylaxis (odds ratio = 0.27, 95% CI 0.13 to 0.56). Whites were more likely to report a usual source of care (59%) than African Americans (34%, $p < 0.001$).	-Single site. -Confounds such as comorbidities not assessed.

TABLE B-1 Continued

Maternal and Infant Health

Source	Procedure/Illness	Sample
Aron, Gordon, DiGiuseppe et al., 2000	Cesarean delivery rates.	25,697 women (19,996 white, 5,701 nonwhite) with no prior history of cesarean delivery admitted to 21 northeast Ohio hospitals from January 1993 through June 1995. Data were obtained from Cleveland Health Quality Choice.
Barfield, Wise, Rust et al., 1996	Civilian vs. military outcomes in prenatal care utilization, birth weight distribution, and fetal and neonatal mortality rates.	2,171,147 births for African-American and white mothers [79,154 in military hospitals (16.2% AA), 2,091,993 in civilian hospitals (9.5% AA)] recorded from 1981 to 1985 in the Maternal and Child Health database compiled by the Community and Organization Research Institute of the University of California – Santa Barbara.

Analyses	Findings	Limitations
Nested (to account for clustering of patients in individual hospitals and provide more robust estimates of variance of group effects) logistic regression used to yield odds ratios for cesarean delivery in non-white patients relative to whites and for patients with government insurance or who were uninsured relative to patients with commercial insurance. Analyses were adjusted for 39 risk factors.	Overall rates of cesarean delivery were similar in white and nonwhite (over 90% African-American) patients. After adjusting for clinical risk factors, non-white women were more likely to deliver via cesarean (odds ratio = 1.34, 95% CI 1.14 to 1.57, $p < 0.001$). Analysis also indicated that insurance status independently influences use of cesarean delivery.	-Results may reflect regional characteristics. -Retrospective study. -No assessment of appropriateness or necessity of cesarean.
Relative risks and Mantel-Haenszel Chi-square analyses for stratified comparisons were calculated.	*Prenatal care utilization:* utilization was lower for black patients than white patients in both military (RR = 0.79, 95% CI 0.75 to 0.82) and civilian (RR = 0.51, 95% CI 0.50 to 0.52) populations. However, the magnitude of the disparity was lower in the military population ($p < 0.001$). *Birth weight:* for military and civilian groups black patients had higher rates of very low birth weight and moderately low birth weight, however, rates were significantly lower in the military group. For example in the very low-birth-weight category, the rate for black births was lower that the rate for black civilian births (RR = 0.68, 95% CI 0.56 to 0.82). For white patients the military rates of very low birth weight (RR = 0.75, 95% CI 0.65 to 0.87) were also significantly lower than their civilian counterparts. *Fetal and neonatal mortality:* For military and civilian groups, mortality was significantly higher for black patients. While fetal mortality rates for white	-Racial/ethnic groups other than African American and white not examined. -Administrative data. -Retrospective study. -Observational study, no control for insurance in civilian group, SES, co-morbidities.

TABLE B-1 Continued

Maternal and Infant Health

Source	Procedure/Illness	Sample
Braveman, Egerter, Edmonston, and Verdon, 1995	Cesarean delivery rates.	217,461 singleton first live births (15,529 African American, 19,142 foreign-born Asian, 62,303 foreign-born Latina, 26,802 U.S.-born Latina, 93,685 white) among women in California in 1991.
Brett, Schoendorf, and Kiely, 1994	Use of prenatal care technologies (ultrasonography, tocolysis, amniocentesis).	Births among non-Hispanic black and non-Hispanic white women in 1990 (3.1 million available for ultrasonography, 3.2 million for tocolysis, 37,000 for amniocentesis). Data were obtained from the National Center for Health Statistics.

Analyses	Findings	Limitations
	patients were similar for military and civilian groups, rates for black military groups were significantly lower than their civilian counterparts (RR = 0.80, 95% CI 0.65 to 0.99).	
Multiple logistic regression to determine adjusted odds ratios of cesarean delivery by race/ethnicity.	After adjusting for covariates (insurance, personal, community, medical, and hospital characteristics), African-American women were 24% more likely to undergo cesarean than whites (adjusted odds ratio = 1.24, 95% CI 1.18 to 1.31). U.S.-born Latinas were also at an elevated risk compared to whites (adjusted odds ratio = 1.07, 95% CI 1.03 to 1.12). Among women residing in 25% or more non-English speaking communities, who delivered high-birth weight babies or who gave birth at for-profit hospitals, cesarean delivery was more likely among nonwhites and was over 40% more likely among black women than white women (odds ratio = 1.51, 95% CI 1.20 to 1.89; odds ratio = 1.42, 95% CI 1.21 to 1.67; odds ratio = 1.42, 95% CI 1.20 to 1.68, respectively).	-Data collected in single region. -Retrospective study.
Logistic regression was used to estimate likelihood of tocolysis and Mantel-Haenszel to estimate use of ultrasonography and amniocentesis. Confounders controlled for include: maternal age, education, marital status, location of residence, birth order, timing of first prenatal care visit, and plural births.	Amniocentesis was used substantially less frequently by black women (adjusted RR = 0.58, 95% CI 0.56 to 0.60). Ultrasonography was received by black women slightly less frequently than white women (adjusted RR = 0.88, 95% CI 0.87 to 0.88). Black women with singleton births were slightly more likely to receive tocolysis than white women (adjusted RR = 1.06, 95% CI 1.04 to 1.09), although the risk of idiopathic pre-term delivery is estimated to be three times higher in black women. Women with plural births received tocolysis two thirds as often as white women (adjusted RR = 0.69, 95% CI 0.62 to 0.75).	-Racial/ethnic groups other than African American and white not examined. -Administrative data. -Retrospective study. -No controls for hospital characteristics, many prenatal care details (e.g., time of procedure), regional differences in practices, appropriateness of procedure.

TABLE B-1 Continued

Maternal and Infant Health

Source	Procedure/Illness	Sample
Kogan, Kotelchuck, Alexander, and Johnson, 1994	Self-reported receipt of prenatal care advice from providers.	8,310 women (6,782 white non-Hispanic and 1,532 black women) who participated in the 1988 National Maternal and Infant Health Survey conducted by the National Center for Health Statistics.

Mental Health

Kales, Blow, Bingham et al., 2000	Impact of race on mental health care utilization among veterans.	Retrospective study of 23,718 patients (859 Hispanic, 3,529 African American, 19,330 white) age 60 and older hospitalized for psychiatric diagnoses treated in Department of Veterans Affairs inpatient facilities in 1994.
Melfi, Groghan, Hanna, and Robinson, 2000	Antidepressant treatment.	13,065 Medicaid patients diagnosed with depression treated between 1989-1994.

Analyses	Findings	Limitations
Logistic regression to assess contribution of race to mothers' report of receipt of advice or instructions during any of their prenatal visits on: breast-feeding, alcohol consumption, tobacco, and use of illegal drugs. Analyses controlled for age, marital status.	After adjustment for covariates, more white women reported receiving advice for alcohol (odds ratio = 1.29, 95% CI 1.10 to 1.51) and smoking cessation (odds ratio = 1.20, 95% CI 1.01 to 1.39). Breast-feeding promotion just missed significance with a trend toward more advice for white women. A significant interaction between race and marital status emerged, such that black single women were 1.4 times more likely than single white women to not receive advice on drug cessation, while there were no racial differences among married women.	-Racial/ethnic groups other than African American and white not examined. -Data self-report.
ANCOVA to test for group differences in inpatient psychiatric variables. Covariates included age, medical co-morbidity, psychiatric co-morbidity, and survival months. Analyses also performed for outpatient variable (outpatient visits).	After adjustment, African-American patients had significantly fewer outpatient psychiatric visits (least-squares means: H = 15.9 visits, AA = 15.3 visits, W = 22.3 visits, W > AA, $p < 0.02$). Similarly, African-American patients with substance abuse disorders had significantly more outpatient psychiatric visits than white patients (least-squares means: H = 19.4 visits, AA = 23.2 visits, and W = 13.2 visits, AA > W, $p < 0.0001$). No significant differences found in inpatient care.	-Administrative database. -Potential confounds such as medication dosing/response, treatment compliance, illness course, personal resources not measured. -Relatively few Hispanics in sample.
Bivariate tests between those who did and did not receive antidepressants and between racial categories. Logistic regressions to examine determinants of receiving antidepressants. Covariates included age, gender, Medicaid eligibility status, year of initial depression, if initial care received	44% of whites and 27.8% blacks received antidepressant treatment within 30 days of 1st indicator of depression ($p < 0.001$). Whites were more likely to receive antidepressants than black patients (odds ratio = 0.495, 95% CI 0.458 to 0.536, $p = 0.0001$) and other/unknown racial category patients (odds ratio = 0.749, 95% CI 0.627 to 0.880, p = 0.0006). Blacks were less likely than whites to	-Racial/ethnic groups other than African Americans and whites not assessed. -Administrative database. -Retrospective study.

TABLE B-1 Continued

Mental Health

Source	Procedure/Illness	Sample
Segal, Bola, and Watson, 1996	Prescription of antipsychotic medications by physicians in psychiatric emergency services.	442 patients (256 white, 107 African American, 47 Hispanic, 10 Asian, 22 "other") seen in psychiatric emergency rooms. Data were obtained through observation of evaluations and record review. Evaluators were primarily psychiatrists (80%) and white (88%).
Chung, Mahler, and Kakuma, 1995	Inpatient psychiatric treatment.	164 adults (76 African American, 88 white) admitted to acute inpatient setting with Axis I diagnosis of major mood or psychotic disorders.

Analyses	Findings	Limitations
from mental health provider, number of comorbid conditions.	receive SSRIs (odds ratio = 0.844, 95% CI 0.743 to 0.959, p = 0.0093) when prior clinical research suggests that blacks are more susceptible than whites to side effects of Tricyclics and therefore should be more likely to receive SSRIs.	-Information not available on severity of depressive disorder.
Analysis of covariance models constructed using least-squares regression or logistic regression to assess the influence of race on five prescription practice indicators. Models controlled for presence of psychotic disorder, severity of disturbance (GAS score), dangerousness, psychiatric history, if physical restraints used, hours spent in the emergency service, clinician's efforts to engage patient in treatment, if optimum time was spent on the evaluation.	More psychiatric medications were prescribed to African Americans than other patients (β = 0.99, p < 0.005). African-American patients received more oral doses (β = 1.21, p = 0.02) and injections (β = 0.54, p = 0.04) of antipsychotic medications. The 24-hour dosage of antipsychotic medication given to African Americans was significantly higher than for other patients (β = 862, p < 0.001). The tendency to overmedicate African-American patients was lower when clinician's efforts to engage the patients in treatment were rated as being higher. Models predicting number of medications, number of oral and injected antipsychotic and 24-hour dosage became non-significant.	-Small number of minorities. -Sites all urban public hospitals in single geographic area. -No controls for SES, hospital characteristics.
ANOVA and Logistic regression to assess effects of race, diagnosis (psychotic vs. nonpsychotic), and socioeconomic status (insurance status) on treatment. Data were obtained through record review.	After controlling for diagnosis and SES, African-American patients had shorter length of stay (F = 9.12, df = 1, 150, p = 0.003). In addition, white patients were 3.8 times more likely than African-American patients to be on one-to-one observational status (95% CI 1.6 to 8.9). Analysis of interactions indicated that among high SES patients, African Americans were 3.5 times more likely to receive urine drug screens, regardless of diagnosis (n = 109, 95% CI 1.2 to 10.1).	-Relatively small sample. -Single site. -Retrospective study. -No assessment of diagnostic validity between the two groups.

TABLE B-1 Continued

Mental Health

Source	Procedure/Illness	Sample
Padgett, Patrick, Burns, and Schlesinger, 1994	Use of inpatient mental health services.	7,768 persons insured by Blue Cross and Blue Shield Association's Federal Employees Plan in 1983, who had at least one inpatient psychiatric day and random sample of 5,000 nonusers of mental health services.

Peripheral Vascular Disease

Guadagnoli, Ayanian, Gibbons et al., 1995	Amputation and leg-sparing surgery for peripheral vascular disease of the lower extremities.	19,236 Medicare patients who underwent amputation or leg-sparing surgery at 3,313 hospitals in the U.S.

Analyses	Findings	Limitations
Logistic regression developed for each ethnic group to predict probability of at least one day of psychiatric hospitalization and number of inpatient days. Predictors included predisposing factors (education, family size, percentage of county black, Hispanic, or white), enabling factors (region of country, salary, high or low option selected for insurance coverage), and need factors (annual medical expenses, family's annual medical expenses, other family member receipt of inpatient psychiatric care.	No significant differences were found among blacks, whites and Hispanics in the probability of a psychiatric hospitalization or in number of inpatient psychiatric days.	-Administrative data. -Retrospective study. -No assessment of diagnostic validity.
Logistic regression to assess odds of amputation and surgery for black relative to white patients, controlling for case-mix, region, and hospital characteristics.	Black patients were more likely to undergo all forms of amputation than were white patients (unadjusted odds ratio = 1.47 to 2.24). White patients were twice (unadjusted odds ratio = 0.51) as likely to undergo lower-extremity arterial revascularization and almost three times (unadjusted odds ratio = 0.35) more likely to undergo angioplasty than black patients. Among patients with diabetes, black patients were 58% more likely than white patients to undergo above the knee amputation (adjusted odds ratio = 1.58, 95% CI 1.32 to 1.90). Black patients who did not have diabetes were twice as likely to undergo the procedure (adjusted odds ratio = 2.13, 95% CI 1.87 to 2.41).	-Racial/ethnic groups other than African American and white not examined. -Administrative data. -Retrospective study. -No controls for potential confounds such as SES, disease severity, appropriateness.

TABLE B-1 Continued

Peripheral Vascular Disease

Source	Procedure/Illness	Sample

Pharmacy

Source	Procedure/Illness	Sample
Morrison, Wallenstein, Natale et al., 2000	Differences in white and nonwhite neighborhoods in pharmacy stocking of opioid analgesics.	Random sample of 30% (347) of New York City pharmacies. Pharmacists surveyed via telephone.

Physician Perceptions

Source	Procedure/Illness	Sample
Thamer, Hwang, Fink et al., 2001	Racial and gender differences in nephrologists recommendations for renal transplantation using hypothetical patient scenarios.	271 nephrologists (72% white, 14% Asian, 5% African American) surveyed as part of the Choices for Health Outcomes in Caring for ESRD (CHOICE) Study. Survey administered between

Analyses	Findings	Limitations
	Among patients with diabetes, blacks were 48% and 32% less likely to undergo percutaneous transluminal angioplasty (adjusted odds ratio = 0.52, 95% CI 0.40-0.67) and lower-extremity bypass surgery (adjusted odds ratio = 0.68, 95% CI 0.59 to 0.79), respectively. Among those who did not have diabetes, black patients were 71% less likely to undergo angioplasty (adjusted odds ratio = 0.29, 95% CI 0.23 to 0.37) and 44% less likely to undergo lower-extremity bypass surgery (adjusted odds ratio = 0.56, 95% CI 0.50 to 0.63).	
Generalized linear model to assess relationship between racial/ethnic composition of neighborhoods and opioid supplies of pharmacies. Analyses controlled for proportion of elderly persons at census-block level and crime rates at the precinct level.	Overall, two-thirds of pharmacies that did not carry any opioids were in predominantly nonwhite neighborhoods. After adjustment pharmacies in predominantly nonwhite neighborhoods (< 40% of residents white) were significantly less likely to have adequate opioid supplies than were pharmacies in predominantly white neighborhoods (at least 80% residents white) (odds ratio = 0.15, 95% CI 0.07 to 0.31). Among 176 pharmacies with inadequate stock, reasons were as follows: 54%—little demand for medications, 44%—concern about disposal, 20%—fear of fraud and illicit drug use, 19% —fear of robbery, 7%—other (e.g., problems with reimbursement).	-No controls for differences in pharmacy supplies across neighborhoods. -Sample from one site. -Possible reporting errors by pharmacists. -Pharmacists only questioned about opioids recommended as appropriate first-line medications.
Scenarios presented patient's age, race (white, African American, Asian), gender, living situation, treatment compliance, diabetic status, residual renal function status, HIV	Asian males less likely than white males to be recommended for transplantation (odds ratio = 0.46, (95% CI 0.24 to 0.91). Females were less likely than males to be recommended (adjusted odds ratio = 0.41, 95% CI 0.21 to 0.79). No differences between African-American and white patients were found.	-Survey data in lieu of treatment data. -Potential bias in response rate. -No controls for patient SES.

TABLE B-1 Continued

Physician Perceptions

Source	Procedure/Illness	Sample
		June 1997 to June 1998. Response rate 53%.
Weisse, Sorum, Sanders, and Syat, 2001	Racial and gender differences in pain management.	111 surveyed primary care physicians from Northeast regions of U.S. who were presented vignettes depicting patients with medical complaints, two painful (kidney stone, back pain) and one control (sinusitis). Race and gender of fictitious patients varied. Questions following vignettes assessed physicians' aggressiveness in treating symptoms.

Effect of race and SES on

Analyses	Findings	Limitations

status, weight, and cardiac ejection fraction. Responding physicians asked if they would recommend transplantation given presence of certain criteria. Multiple logistic regression to assess independent effect of nephrologist and patient factors on decision to recommend transplantation. Analyses adjust for patient and neurologist demographics, clinical characteristics, nephrologist training, and organizational affiliations.

Analysis of variance to assess impact of patient gender and race on treatment decision (hydrocodone dosage). Physician age and years in practice included as covariates.

Kidney stone pain: Decision to treat with hydrocodone did not vary by race. Among physicians who opted to treat with medication, dose of hydrocodone selected did not differ by patient race (white = 308 mg, African American = 271 mg), patient gender, or physician gender. Interaction between physician gender and patient race was found (F $_{1,85}$ = 9.65, p = 0.003). Male physicians prescribed higher doses to white patients than to African Americans, while female physicians prescribed higher doses to African-American patients.

Back pain: Decision to treat with hydrocodone did not vary by race. Similarly, dose selected did not differ by patient race (white 188 = mg, African American = 233 mg), patient gender, or physician gender. No interactions were observed.

Sinus Infection: Decision to treat with antibiotic did not differ by patient race or gender. White patients were prescribed a longer course of antibiotics (X = 13.7 vs. 9.2 days, $F_{1,87}$ = 4.90,

-Small sample size.
-Convenience sample.
-Physicians in Northeast, limiting generalizability.
-Approximately 50% of solicited physicians participated.
-No controls for physician prescribing habits.
-Racial/ethnic groups other than white and African American not investigated.
-Few racial/ethnic minority physicians in sample.

TABLE B-1 Continued

Physician Perceptions

Source	Procedure/Illness	Sample
van Ryn and Burke, 2000	physician perceptions of patients.	618 patient encounters at eight New York state hospitals.
	Assessed physicians' recommendations for managing chest pain, using vignettes of "patients" that varied only in gender and ethnicity.	

Patients Perceptions

Doescher et al., 2000	Racial and ethnic differences in patients' perceptions of their physicians (trust and satisfaction).	32,929 patients surveyed through the Community Tracking Survey, a nationally representative sample surveyed 1996-1997.

Analyses	Findings	Limitations
	$p = 0.03$) and were prescribed refills more often ($X_1^2 = 107$ vs. 4.05, $p = 0.04$).	
Logistic regression used to regress physician percep-tion variables on patient race and SES, controlling for each other and patient age, sex, sickness, depression, mastery, social assertive-ness, as well as physician age, sex, race, and specialty.	Black patients rated less positively than white patients on several dimen-sions including physicians' assess-ment of patient intelligence (odds ratio = 0.51, p 0.01), feelings of affiliation toward the patient (odds ratio = 0.68, p 0.05) and beliefs about patient's likelihood of risk behavior (odds ratio = 0.58, p 0.02) and adherence with medical advice (odds ratio = 0.62, p 0.01).	-Potential for social desirability in responses. -Finding limited to one state and nar-row sample of patients. -Use of single-item measures. -Differences in care not measured.
Logistic regression analysis to assess the effects of "patient" race and gender, while controlling for physi-cians' assessment of the probability of coronary	Physicians were less likely to recom-mend cardiac catheterization for women than men (odds ratio = 0.60, 95% CI 0.4 to 0.9) and African Ameri-cans than whites (odds ratio = 0.60, 95% CI 0.4 to 0.9). Analysis of race-sex interaction revealed that African-American women were significantly less likely to be referred for catheter-ization than white men (odds ratio = 0.4, 95% CI 0.2 to 0.7).	-Representativeness of sample: partici-pants recruited at national meeting. -Hospital character-istics where physician's prac-ticed unknown. -Underemphasis of subgroup analysis.
Analyses adjusted for socio-economic factors.	After adjustment, patients from mi-nority groups reported less positive perceptions of physicians than white patients on both scales.	-Racial/ethnic subgroups not assessed. -Physician race/ ethnicity or other characteristics not assessed. -Potential for re-sponse bias.

TABLE B-1 Continued

Radiographs

Source	Procedure/Illness	Sample
Selim, Gincke, Ren, Deyo et al., 2001	Racial and ethnic differences in use of lumbar spine radiographs.	401 patients (315 white, 22 African American, 4 nonwhite Hispanic, 1 "other") with low back pain (LBP) receiving ambulatory care services in VA clinics in Boston area. Patients completed Medical Outcome Study Short Form Health Survey (SF-36), LBP questionnaire, comorbidity index, and straight leg raising (SLR) test.

Rehabilitative Services

Harada, Chun, Chui, and Pakalniskis, 2000	Assessed sociodemographic and clinical characteristics associated with use of physical therapy (PT) in acute hospitals, skilled nursing facilities, or both.	Records of 187,900 hip fracture patients (94% white, 4% African American, 3% "other") derived from Medicare administrative databases.
Horner, Hoenig, Sloane et al., 1997	Assessed racial differences in utilization of inpatient rehabilitative services among elderly stroke patients.	2,497 African-American and white Medicare patients hospitalized following stroke at any of 297 acute-care hospitals in five states.

Analyses	Findings	Limitations
Logistic regression to assess race, age, education, income, comorbidities, pain intensity, radiating leg pain, SLR, 2 summary scores from the SF-36 (physical component summary, mental component summary) as predictors of obtaining lumbar spine radiographs during 12 months of follow-up.	At higher levels of back pain, nonwhite patients received more spine films than did white patients (74% vs. 50%, $p < 0.01$). Among patients with positive straight leg raising test, nonwhite patients had more spine films than white patients (23% vs. 11%, $p < 0.01$). After controlling for clinical characteristics, race was no longer an independent predictor of lumbar spine radiograph use.	-Relatively small sample. -Small number of African-American and Hispanic participants. -Potential bias in self-report data. -Nonwhite patients combined in analyses. -Generalizability of population— elderly male veterans in Boston area.
Logistic regression to predict PT by pattern of use. Independent variables included age, gender, comorbidity index, surgery type, fracture type, urinary incontinence, and hospital characteristics.	African-American patients were less likely than whites to receive acute physical therapy only (b/w odds ratio = 0.81, 95% CI 0.73 to 0.89), were less likely to receive therapy in both acute care and skilled nursing facilities (b/w odds ratio = 0.70, 95% CI 0.65 to 0.76), and were more likely to receive no physical therapy at all (b/w odds ratio = 1.30, 95% CI 1.18 to 1.43).	-Relatively few minority patients. -Administrative data. -Retrospective study. -Analysis limited to acute hospitalization.
Logistic regression to predict utilization of physical and occupational therapy by race.	After adjusting for clinical and socioeconomic factors associated with use of physical and occupational therapy, no racial differences were found in the likelihood of use of therapy (RR = 1.06, 95% CI 0.89 to 1.27) or time to initiate therapy (African Americans = 6.6 days, whites = 7.4, $p = 0.42$). Similarly, no racial differences were found in length of physical or occupational therapy in days or as a proportion of hospital stay.	-Administrative data. -Retrospective study.

TABLE B-1 Continued

Rehabilitative Services

Source	Procedure/Illness	Sample
Hoenig, Rubenstein, and Kahn, 1996	Racial and other sociodemographic and geographic differences in use of physical and occupational therapy in elderly Medicare patients with acute hip fracture.	2,762 African-American and white Medicare patients (9% African American) treated in 297 randomly-selected hospitals from five states.

Renal Care and Transplantation

Ayanian, Cleary, Weissman, and Epstein, 1999	Effect of patient preferences on access to renal transplantation.	1,392 patients (384 African-American women, 354 white women, 337 African-American men, 317 white men) with end-stage renal disease who had recently begun to receive maintenance treatment with dialysis in Southern California, Alabama, Michigan, and the mid-Atlantic region of the U.S.

Analyses	Findings	Limitations
Multivariate logistic regression to predict utilization of physical or occupational therapy by race, socio-demographic variables, severity of hip fracture, geographic region, and other factors. Data obtained through record review.	After controlling for clinical factors, African-American patients (odds ratio = 1.56, 95% CI 1.04 to 2.34) and dual eligible Medicare/Medicaid patients (odds ratio = 1.36, 95% CI 1.05 to 1.76) were less likely to receive high-intensity physical or occupational therapy. No racial differences were found in time to initiation of therapy.	-Small number African Americans. -Retrospective study.
Measures included interviews and data from the renal networks and the United Network for Organ Sharing. Logistic regression to estimate: 1) the adjusted relative odds of referral for evaluation at a transplant center; and 2) placement on a waiting list for a transplant or receipt of transplant within 18 months after start of dialysis, for African-American and white men and women. Analyses control for patient preference and expectations, perceptions of care, region, age, education, income, insurance, employment, marital status, car ownership, type facility, cause of renal failure, health status, and co-morbidities.	African-American patients were slightly less likely than white patients to report wanting a kidney transplant (76.3% African-American women vs. 79% of white women, $p = 0.13$; 80.7% African-American men vs. 85.5% white men, $p = 0.04$). However, compared to preferences, African-American patients were much less likely than white patients to have been referred to a transplant center for evaluation (50.5% of African-American women vs. 70.7% of white women; and 53.9% for African-American men vs. 76.2% for white men; $p < 0.001$ for each comparison), and to have been placed on a waiting list or to have received a transplant within 18 months after initiating dialysis (31.9% African-American women vs. 56.5% for white women, and 35.3% for African-American men vs. 60.6% for white men, $p < 0.001$ for each comparison).	-Racial/ethnic groups other than African American and white not examined. -Potential bias in patient recall.

TABLE B-1 Continued

Renal Care and Transplantation

Source	Procedure/Illness	Sample
Kasiske, London, and Ellison, 1998	Racial/ethnic differences in early placement on kidney transplantation waiting list.	41,596 patients registered with 238 UNOS centers on the national OPTN kidney and kidney-pancreas waiting list between April 1, 1994, and June 30, 1996.
Barker-Cummings, McClellan, Soucie, and Krisher, 1995	Use of peritoneal dialysis as initial treatment for end-stage renal disease (ESRD).	10,726 patents who began treatment for end-stage renal disease at dialysis centers in North Carolina, South Carolina, and Georgia and who reported to ESRD Network between January 1, 1989, and December 31, 1991.

Use of services and procedures—General

Jha, Shlipak, Hosmer et al., 2001	Hospital mortality.	39,190 male patients (28,934 white and 7,575 black) admitted to 147 VA hospitals nation-wide for one of six diagnoses (pneumonia, angina, congestive heart failure, chronic obstructive pulmonary disease, diabetes, chronic renal failure).

Analyses	Findings	Limitations
Logistic regression to assess patient and center characteristics on listing before dialysis or registration after being placed on maintenance dialysis.	White patients more likely to be placed on waiting list before vs. after initiating maintenance dialysis than non-white patients. Independent predictors of listing before dialysis included being African American (odds ratio = 0.465, $p < 0.001$, reference: white), Hispanic (odds ratio = 0.588, $p < 0.001$, reference: white) and Asian/other (odds ratio = 0.548, $p < 0.001$, reference: white), in addition to factors including age, prior transplant, level of education, employment status, insurance status, receiving insulin, listed for kidney-pancreas vs. kidney only, and listed in a center with high volume.	-Retrospective study utilizing administrative data. -Analyses did not include measures for hospital characteristics of appropriateness.
Logistic regression (backward stepwise procedure) to assess relationship between ethnicity and initial dialysis modality, controlling for patient characteristics.	African Americans were 57% less likely than whites to be initially treated with peritoneal dialysis (odds ratio = 0.43, 95% CI 0.39 to 0.47). After controlling for confounding characteristics (age, education, social support, home ownership, functional status, albumin level, hypertension, history of MI, peripheral neuropathy, and comorbid diabetes) the odds ratio of initial treatment for African Americans compared with whites was 0.45 (95% CI 0.38 to 0.52).	-Racial/ethnic groups other than African American and white not assessed. -Potential confounds such as hospital characteristics, appropriateness not examined.
Principle outcome was mortality at 30 days. Secondary outcomes were in-hospital and 60-day mortality. Analysis included logistic regression for inpatient mortality and Cox Proportional hazard models for 30-day and 6-month mortality to estimate the	Mortality at 30 days was 4.5% in black patients and 5.8% in white patients (RR = 0.77, 95% CI 0.69 to 0.87, $p = 0.001$). Mortality for black patients was lower for each of the six diagnoses. Adjustments for patient and hospital characteristics had a small effect (RR = 0.75, 95% CI 0.66 to 0.85, $p < 0.001$). Black patients also had lower in-hospital and 6-month mortality.	-Racial/ethnic groups other than African American and white not examined. -Administrative data. -Retrospective study. -Confounders such as illness severity,

TABLE B-1 Continued

Use of services and procedures—General

Source	Procedure/Illness	Sample
Tai-Seale, Freund, and LoSasso, 2001	Effect of mandatory enrollment in managed care (MC) on service use among African American compared to white Medicaid beneficiaries.	Data from Medicaid eligibility, claims, and MC encounter data from two counties in one state where one county implemented "freedom-of-choice" waiver enrolling its Medicaid beneficiaries in MC, and one county not involved in the waiver. In the waiver county, 3,490 adults and 3,414 children from pre-period (12 months prior to enrollment); 4,082 adults and 3,834 children in post-period. In non-waiver county, 2,087 adults and 2,093 children in pre-period and 1,200 adults and 1,200 children in post-period. Approximately half sample in each group was African American.
Andrews and Elixhauser, 2000	Ethnic differences in receipt of major therapeutic procedures during hospitalization.	Data from 1.7 million (88% white, 12% Hispanic) hospital discharges. Data from 1993 discharge abstracts from Healthcare Cost and Utilization Project State Inpatient Database for California, Florida, and New York.
Weinick, Zuvekas, and Cohn, 2000	Racial and ethnic magnitude of disparities in use of health care services from 1977 to 1996.	Data from three national databases (1977 National Medical Care Expenditure Survey, 1987 National Medical Expenditure Survey, 1996 Medical Expenditure Panel Survey).

Analyses	Findings	Limitations

independent association of race with mortality.

Count data models adjusted for nonrandom selection within difference-in difference (DD) econometric approaches. Services assessed include physician visits, emergency department visits, and inpatient admissions. Difference-in difference method used to identify the program effect of mandatory enrollment in managed care on use of services.

African-American beneficiaries had fewer visits to physicians than white beneficiaries after mandatory enrollment. This held for both adults (DD = -1.937, p < 0.01) and children (DD = -0.813, p < 0.01). No differences found for inpatient admissions. African-American children had a significant increase in use of emergency rooms (DD = 0.116, p < 0.01).

In analyses controlling for racial differences in trends of service use that were unrelated to managed care, but may have biased difference-in-difference estimates, results indicate that African-American adults (DD = -2.463, p < 0.01) and children (DD = -1.098, p < 0.01) had lower levels of relative service use. Increases in emergency department visits for African-American children not evident. Decrease inpatient service use found for African-American adults (DD = -0.039, p < 0.05).

admissions practices not assessed.

-Racial/ethnic groups other than African American and white not assessed.
-Use of administrative data.
-Using different samples in pre- and post-waiver periods.
-Data from two counties in one state.
-Disproportional enrollment of African Americans in HMOs.

Logistic regression to assess effect of ethnicity on likelihood of receiving therapeutic procedure for 63 conditions. Analyses controlled for age, gender, disease severity, health insurance, income of patient's community, and hospital characteristics.

Hispanics less likely than non-Hispanics to receive major procedures for 38% of 63 conditions and more likely to receive procedures for 6.3% of conditions.

-Administrative database.
-Data could not examine differences between Hispanic subgroups.

Outcomes analyzed included usual source of care, probability of having at least one ambulatory care (AC) visit, and average number of visits for those indicating AC services. Other variables

In 1996, blacks were 2.1 percentage points more likely than whites to lack a usual source of care (p < 0.10) and Hispanics were 9.9 percentage points more likely than whites to lack a usual source of care (p < 0.001). Disparities increased from 1977 to 1996,

-Administrative data bases.
-Retrospective study.
-Need and appropriateness of services not examined.

TABLE B-1 Continued

Use of services and procedures—General

Source	Procedure/Illness	Sample
White-Means, 2000	Use of services (paid care-giver, therapist, mental health, dentist, foot doctor, optometrist, chiropractor, ER visit, doctor visits, prescription medications) by disabled elderly.	Data are from the National Long Term Care Survey. 527 black and 4,007 white disabled elderly Medicare recipients.
Khandker and Simoni-Wastila, 1998	Prescription drug utilization.	487,922 black and 341,274 white Georgia Medicaid enrollees in 1992. 76% of black and 84% of white enrollees received prescriptions through Medicaid on an outpatient basis.
Harris, Andrews, and Elixhauser, 1997	Influence of race (African American and white) and gender on likelihood of hav-	Discharge abstract data on 1,727,086 discharges (87.9% white, 12.1% African American, 63.6% female, 36.4%

Analyses	Findings	Limitations

examined included insurance coverage, family income, age, sex, marital status, education, health status, region of country, and residence in or outside of metropolitan area. Used regression-based difference-indifference approach to examine change in disparities over time, controlling for variables listed above.

particularly among Hispanics. Adjusted analyses indicate that the disparity for Hispanics increased by 6.5 percentage points ($p < 0.01$). The disparity for blacks decreased 3.2 percentage points ($p < 0.05$) during this time period.

50-75% of disparities would remain if disparities in income and insurance coverage were eliminated.

Regression analysis to estimate relative influence of health conditions and financial resources on racial patterns of community long-term care services. Models include measures of medical conditions and disabilities, income, insurance status, regional and rural residence, whether unpaid caregivers provide in-home services, and sociodemographic characteristics (gender, education).

Given similar medical conditions, black patients are less likely to use services, particularly prescription medications and physician services. Black patients who live in rural areas, small cities, and western states or who have more joint and breathing problems are more likely to use services. Differences in personal attributes (i.e., income, health) do not fully explain racial differences in use of prescriptions and physician services.

-Racial/ethnic groups other than African American and white not examined.
-Administrative data.
-Retrospective study.

Model estimating black-white differences in use and level of use of prescription drugs controlling for age, sex, and Medicaid eligibility characteristics.

Black children used 2.7 fewer prescriptions compared to white children. Black adults used 4.9 fewer prescriptions, and black elders used 6.3 fewer prescriptions than white elders (all significant at the 99% level). White Medicaid enrollees had higher use and spending than black enrollees across most high-volume therapeutic drug categories.

-Racial/ethnic groups other than African American and white not examined.
-Administrative data.
-Retrospective study.
-SES and clinical factors not examined as potential confounds.

Logistic regression to assess independent effect of race and gender on likelihood of having a major procedure

African Americans were less likely than whites to receive major therapeutic procedures in 37 of 77 (48.1%) conditions. They were more likely

-Racial/ethnic groups other than white and African

TABLE B-1 Continued

Use of services and procedures—General

Source	Procedure/Illness	Sample
	ing a major therapeutic or diagnostic procedure.	male) from the Hospital Cost and Utilization Project (HCUP-2) for 1986. Hospitals include national sample of 469 facilities.
Giacomini, 1996	Gender and ethnic differences in hospital-based procedure utilization.	Retrospective analysis of data on 7,249 hospital discharges in California between 1989 and 1990.

Analyses	Findings	Limitations
(identified using ICD-9-CM codes). Analyses controlled for influence of personal (age, expected pay source, indicators of clinical condition) and hospital-level characteristics (e.g., bed size, public ownership, teaching hospital, urban location).	than whites to receive a major therapeutic procedure in 9.1% of conditions. There was no significant difference in 42.8% of disease categories (alpha = 0.05). Similarly, African Americans were less likely to receive a major diagnostic, without therapeutic, procedure in 20.8% of conditions, more likely to receive diagnostic procedure in 13% of disease categories. There were no significant differences between races in 66.2% of categories.

Females were less likely than males to receive major therapeutic procedures for 32 of 62 (52%) conditions. Females were less likely to receive a major diagnostic, without therapeutic, procedure in 26% of conditions.

Patterns emerged with respect to conditions for which there were race and gender differences. For example, African Americans had lower rates than whites and women had lower rates than men for many trauma categories. | American not examined. -Retrospective study. -Administrative data. |
| Logistic regression to estimate likelihood of obtaining procedure as function of ethnicity and gender. Analyses controlled for insurance status, age, principal diagnosis, and number of co-morbidities. Odds ratios calculated for following procedures: heart transplant, kidney transplant, extracorporeal shockwave lithotripsy, hip replacement, carotid endarterectomy, CABG, PTCA, pace- | White patients were more likely than African Americans to receive kidney transplantation (odds ratio = 3.05, 95% CI 2.27 to 4.17), defibrillator implant (odds ratio = 2.86, 95% CI 1.28 to 6.25), CABG (odds ratio = 2.44, 95% CI 2.08 to 2.78), endarterectomy (odds ratio = 2.27, 95% CI 1.41 to 3.70), and angioplasty (odds ratio = 2.00, 95% CI 1.79 to 2.22).

Whites were more likely than Latino patients to receive angioplasty (odds ratio = 1.72, 95% CI 1.56 to 2.22), kidney transplantation (odds ratio = 1.58, 95% CI 1.20 to 2.08), and CABG | -Administrative data. -Retrospective study. -Potential confounds including measures of SES, appropriateness of services, hospital characteristics not assessed. |

TABLE B-1 Continued

Use of services and procedures—General

Source	Procedure/Illness	Sample
Gornick, Eggers, Reilly et al., 1996	Assessed racial differences in mortality and use of services among a Medicare population.	26.3 million Medicare beneficiaries (24.2 million whites, 2.1 million African Americans) aged 65 years or older.
Phillips, Hamel, Teno et al., 1996	Assessed racial differences in use of: operation, dialysis, pulmonary artery catheterization, endoscopy, bronchoscopy, and hospital charges.	9,105 hospitalized adults (79% white, 16% African American, 3% Hispanic, 1% Asian) in five geographically diverse teaching hospitals, with one of nine illnesses associated with average 6-month mortality of 50%. Data collected through chart review and interviews with patients and physicians.

Analyses	Findings	Limitations

maker implant, and automatic cardioverter-defibrillator implant.

(odds ratio = 1.49, 95% CI 1.35 to 1.67).

Whites were more likely than Asian patients to receive endarterectomy (odds ratio = 2.08, 95% CI 1.18 to 3.85) and angioplasty (odds ratio = 1.30, 95% CI 1.15 to 1.47).

Asians were more likely than whites to receive hip replacement (odds ratio = 0.47, 95% CI 0.29 to 0.77).

Males' odds of receiving most procedures exceeded those of females.

Analyses: Multiple regression to predict utilization rates by race-specific median income, age, gender, and interaction of race and income.

Findings: B/w differences found in:
mortality: 1.19 men ($p < 0.001$), 1.16 women ($p < 0.001$)
hospital discharges: 1.14, $p < 0.001$
ambulatory care visits: 0.89, $p < 0.001$
bilateral orchiectomy: 2.45, $p < 0.001$
amputations of lower limbs: 3.64, $p < 0.001$
Adjusting for differences in income reduced differences, but not significantly.

Limitations:
-Racial/ethnic groups other than African American and white not examined.
-Administrative data.
-Retrospective study.
-Factors such as clinical, hospital characteristics not assessed as potential confounds.

Analyses: Logistic regression to assess independent effect of race on procedure use, controlling for age, gender, education, income, type insurance, severity of illness, functional status, study site, and other confounding variables

Findings: Black patients utilized significantly fewer resources than patients of other races (odds ratio = 0.70, 95% CI 0.6 to 0.81). The median adjusted difference in hospital cost was $2,805 lower for black patients (95% CI $1,672 to $3,883 less). Results remained significant after adjusting for physician's perceptions of patients' prognosis.

Limitations:
-Highly selective sample.
-Data on SES variables not available for all subjects.

TABLE B-1 Continued

Use of services and procedures—General

Source	Procedure/Illness	Sample
Wilson, May, and Kelly, 1994	Assessed racial differences in receipt of total knee arthro-plasty among older adults with osteoarthritis.	Records of nearly 300,000 Medicare recipients who underwent total knee arthro-plasty between 1980 and 1988.
Escarce, Epstein, Colby, and Schwartz et al., 1993	Racial differences in use of medical procedures among Medicare enrollees.	1986 physician claims data for 1,204,022 Medicare enrollees (1,109,954 whites and 94,068 African Americans). Indi-viduals enrolled in HMOs excluded.

Vaccination

Schneider et al., 2001	Magnitude of racial differ-ences in influenza vaccination in managed care vs. fee-for-service insurance.	Data from 1996 Medicare Current Beneficiary Survey. 13,674 Medicare beneficiaries (12,414 white, 1,260 African American).

Analyses	Findings	Limitations
Natural logarithm transformation method to estimate confidence intervals for white-to-black ratios of rates of total knee replacement.	The prevalence of symptomatic osteoarthritis of the knee was lower among whites than blacks, although this difference was non-significant. African Americans, however, were less likely than whites to receive total knee arthroplasty (odds ratios ranged from 1.5 to 2.0 for women, 3.0 to 5.1 for men). This disparity persisted at each of five levels of income strata.	-Racial/ethnic groups other than African American and white not examined. -Administrative data. -Retrospective study. -Clinical, SES, hospital factors, appropriateness not explored as confounds.
Mantel-Haenszel method to calculate white-black relative risks, adjusting for age and sex.	Whites more likely than African Americans to receive 23 of 32 services (white-black RR > 1.0, $p < 0.05$). For example, whites were 1.5 to 2.0 times as likely to receive eight of the study services, 2.0 to 3.0 times as likely to receive three of the services, and more than 3.0 times as likely to receive coronary bypass, coronary angioplasty, and carotid endarterectomy. African Americans were more likely than whites to receive seven services (white-black RR < 1.0, $p < 0.05$). For example, African Americans more than 1.5 times as likely to receive laser trabeculoplasty, glaucoma surgery, and retinal photocoagulation.	-Racial/ethnic groups other than African American and white not assessed. -Administrative data. -Retrospective study. -Potential confounds such as SES and clinical and hospital characteristics not assessed.
Percentage of respondents (adjusting for SES, clinical comorbidities, and care-seeking attitudes) who received vaccination and magnitude of racial disparity in vaccination was calculated, comparing patients with managed care.	Both whites and African Americans had higher rates of vaccination under managed care, however racial disparity was not reduced under managed care. After adjustment, the racial disparity in fee for service was 24.9% (95% CI 19.6% to 30.1%). The disparity in managed care was 18.6% (95% CI 9.8% to 27.4%). Both disparities were statistically significant, however the	-Racial/ethnic groups other than African American and white not examined. -Potential bias in self-report data.

TABLE B-1 Continued

.Use of services and procedures—General

Source	Procedure/Illness	Sample

Women's Health

Source	Procedure/Illness	Sample
Brown, Perez-Stable, Whitaker, Posner et al., 1999	Hormone Replacement Therapy (HRT).	8,986 women (50% white, 20.2% Asian, 14.7% African American, 8.6% Latina, 6.3% Soviet immigrant) seen in the general internal medicine, family medicine, and gynecology practices at UCSF between January 1, 1992, and November 30, 1995.
Marsh, Brett, and Miller, 1999	Hormone replacement therapy (HRT).	25,203 sampled visits made by women (age 45-64, 16.4% by black and 83.6% by white women). Data were obtained from the National Health Care survey.

Analyses	Findings	Limitations
and those with fee-for-service insurance.	absolute percentage point difference in racial disparity between the managed care and fee-for-service groups (6.3%, 95% CI -4.6% to 17.2%) was not.	

Analyses	Findings	Limitations
Logistic regression was used to calculate odds of prescribing HRT for each ethnic group using whites as the reference group. Predictor variables were age, income, and clinical diagnosis.	Compared to white women, all other groups were less likely to be prescribed HRT after adjusting for age, income, diabetes, hypertension, CHD, and osteoporosis. Asians (odds ratio = 0.56, 95% CI 0.49 to 0.64), African Americans (odds ratio = 0.70, 95% CI 0.60 to 0.81)), Latinas (odds ratio = 0.70, 95% CI 0.58 to 0.84), and Soviet immigrants (odds ratio = 0.14, 95% CI 0.10 to 0.20) were each less likely to receive a prescription for HRT than were white women. Women with osteoporosis were also more likely to receive HRT.	-Single site. -Retrospective review. -Data not available on variables such as education, menopausal symptoms, hysterectomy status, etc. -Physician recommendations or patient characteristics not assessed.
Logistic regression used to examine whether any previously identified racial differences in HRT could be attributed to known confounders (age, source of payment for visit, drugs other than HRT, whether physician had previously seen patient, physician or clinic specialty type, site of care, region of practice, obesity, duration of visit, physician sex).	While physician visit rates were equal for black and white women, the rate of visits per year in which HRT was prescribed to white women (odds ratio = 0.38, 95% CI 0.32 to 0.45) was more than twice the rate for black women (odds ratio = 0.17, 95% CI 0.12 to 0.23) in this age group.	-Racial/ethnic groups other than African American and white not examined. -Retrospective study. -Limited information on patient characteristics.

TABLE B-1 Continued

Women's Health

Source	Procedure/Illness	Sample
Burns, McCarthy, Freund, Marwill et al., 1996	Mammography.	3,187,116 women (7% black, 93% white) ages 65 and older receiving Medicare who resided in one of the following states, Alabama, Arizona, Connecticut, Georgia, Kansas, New Jersey, Oklahoma, Pennsylvania, Oregon, or Washington. Women had received bilateral mammography. Data were obtained from HCFA database for 1990.

Analyses	Findings	Limitations
Logistic regression to predict mammography use according to age, number of primary care visits, income, state of residence for black and white women in each state.	In every state, at each primary care visit level (one, two, or three or more visits) black women had mammography less often than white women (even across income levels). Age, income, and state adjusted logistic models reveal that among white women, primary care use has a significant effect on use of mammography: *for one visit* odds ratio = 2.73, 95% CI 2.70 to 2.77, *for two visits* odds ratio = 3.98, 95% CI 3.93 to 4.03, *for three or more visits* odds ratio = 4.62, CI 4.58 to 4.67. Results for black women reveal an analogous, but weaker effect: *for one visit* odds ratio = 1.77, CI 1.67 to 1.87, *for two visits* odds ratio = 2.49, CI 2.36 to 2.63, *for three or more visits* odds ratio = 3.15, CI 3.04 to 3.25.	-Racial/ethnic groups other than African American and white not examined. -Administrative data. -Retrospective study.

TABLE B-2 Selected Studies Exerting Control Over Key Clinical
Characteristics

Author	Year	Type of Data	Insurance	Prospective/ Retrospective	Adjust for: Comorbidities?
Petersen et al.	2002	Clinical	VA healthcare system	Retrospective	Yes
Conigliaro et al.	2000	Clinical	VA healthcare system	Retrospective	Yes
Carlisle et al.	1999	Clinical records and ED logs	Statistical adjustment for type of insurance	Retrospective	No
Daumit et al.	1999	Clinical	ESRD Medicare	Prospective	Yes
Hannan et al.	1999	Clinical	Statistical adjustment for type of insurance	Prospective	Yes
Leape et al.	1999	Clinical and laboratory data from medical records	Statistical adjustment for type of insurance	Retrospective	No
Scirica et al.	1999	Clinical	Statistical adjustment for type of insurance	Prospective	Yes
Canto et al.	1998	Clinical	Statistical adjustment for payor status	Retrospective	Yes

Disease Severity	Approriateness	Assessed Outcomes?	Find Disparities?
Yes	Yes	Yes – no overall differences in mortality found.	Yes, black patients with AMI were equally likely as whites to receive beta-blockers, more likely than whites to receive aspirin, but were less likely to receive thrombolytic therapy at time of arrival and were less likely to receive bypass surgery, even when only high-risk coronary anatomic subgroups were assessed. No racial differences in refusal rates for invasive treatment.
Yes	Yes	No	Yes, especially when CABG was deemed "necessary."
No	Yes	No	No, only lack of post-high school education was significant predictor of underuse.
Yes	Yes	Yes	Yes, but diminished with insurance eligibility.
Yes	Yes	No	Yes, African-American patients less like to undergo CABG than whites, considering RAND criteria.
Yes	Yes	No	No significant racial or ethnic differences after accounting for hospital type and necessity of revascularization.
No	Yes	No	Yes, among patients meeting criteria for appropriate catheterization, fewer nonwhites received catheterization.
Yes	No	Yes	Non-African-American minorities less likely to receive beta-blocker TX at discharge, but as likely to receive intravenous thrombolytic therapy (except Asian/Pacific Islanders) and undergo coronary arteriography and revascularization procedures as whites. No differences in hospital mortality.

TABLE B-2 Continued

Author	Year	Type of Data	Insurance	Prospective/ Retrospective	Adjust for: Comorbidities?
Taylor et al.	1998	Clinical	Statistical adjustment for payor status	Retrospective	Yes
Laouri et al.	1997	Clinical and laboratory data from medical records	Not assessed, but patients sampled from both public (where patients are likely insured) and private hospitals (patients likely uninsured).	Retrospective with patient follow-up	Yes
Maynard et al.	1997	Clinical	Statistical adjustment for payment by Medicaid	Prospective	Yes
Peterson et al.	1997	Clinical data	Statistical adjustment for type of insurance	Prospective	Yes
Taylor et al.	1997	Clinical data	Statistical adjustment for payment type of insurance	Prospective	Yes

Disease Severity	Approriateness	Assessed Outcomes?	Find Disparities?
Yes	No	Yes	Yes, African Americans less likely to receive intravenous thrombolytic therapy, coronary arteriography, and CABG than whites. No differences in hospital mortality.
Yes	Yes	No	Yes, significant underuse of revascularization procedures among African Americans and patients at public hospitals.
Yes	No	Yes	Despite less intensive use of revascularization procedures in African Americans, long-term survival after AMI was similar to whites.
Yes	Yes	Yes	African Americans less likely than whites to receive bypass surgery, but no differences found in angioplasty. Differences in treatment most pronounced among patients with severe disease. Differences in treatment associated with lower survival among African Americans.
Yes	Yes	Yes	African Americans less likely than whites to receive bypass surgery, but no differences found in angioplasaty. Differences in treatment most pronounced among patients with severe disease. Differences in treatment associated with lower survival among African Americans.

C

Federal-Level and Other Initiatives to Address Racial and Ethnic Disparities in Healthcare

The following list represents a sample of Federal and non-Federal programs, initiatives, and collaborations related to racial/ethnic disparities in healthcare. This list is not intended to represent a comprehensive inventory of Federal programming; rather, it presents some examples of efforts intended to reduce and/or eliminate disparities.

EXECUTIVE OFFICE OF THE PRESIDENT

Office of Management and Budget

Guidance on Aggregation and Allocation of Data on Race for Use in Civil Rights Monitoring and Enforcement. Purpose of these guidelines is to: a) establish guidance for agencies that collect or use aggregate data on race, and b) establish guidance for the allocation of multiple race responses for use in civil rights monitoring and enforcement. The guidelines do not mandate the collection of race data, but standardize its collection if agencies choose to gather it.

DEPARTMENT OF HEALTH AND HUMAN SERVICES

HHS-Wide Initiatives

Minority HIV/AIDS Initiative. This initiative, in collaboration with the Congressional Black Caucus, seeks to improve the nation's effectiveness in preventing and treating HIV/AIDS in African American, Hispanic, and other minority communities. This initiative began in 1999 with $156 million and was increased to $251 million in 2000. The funds are distributed in the following areas: 1) providing technical assistance and infrastructure support, 2) increasing access to prevention and care, and 3) building stronger linkages to address the needs of specific populations. Grants are provided to community-based organizations, research institutions, minority-serving colleges and universities, healthcare organizations, and state and local health departments. Agencies involved include Centers for Disease Control and Prevention, Health Resources and Services Administration, Indian Health Services, National Institutes of Health, Office of Minority Health, Office of Minority Health-Resource Center, Office on Women's Health, and the Substance Abuse and Mental Health Services Administration.

HHS and the American Public Health Association announced in 2000 a partnership to eliminate racial and ethnic health disparities. The partnership includes a three-phase plan to develop guidelines for collaboration to develop a detailed, comprehensive national plan, and to implement the plan by 2002.

Office of the Secretary

Office of Minority Health

Healthy People 2010. A set of health objectives for the nation to achieve over the next decade. The first goal of Healthy People 2010 is to help individuals of all ages increase life expectancy and improve their quality of life. The second goal of Healthy People 2010 is to eliminate health disparities among different segments of the population. Products of the initiative include, for example, the publication *A Community Planning Guide Using Healthy People 2010*, a guide for building community coalitions, creating a vision, measuring results, and creating partnerships dedicated to improving the health of a community.

The Cross Cultural Health Care Program (CCHCP) was created in 1992 to serve as a bridge between communities and healthcare institutions to ensure access to healthcare that is culturally and linguistically appropriate. This program facilitates cultural competency training for providers and medical staff, interpreter training for community interpreters and bilingual healthcare workers, outreach to underrepresented communities, community-based research, interpreter services, translation services, and publications and videos relating to cross-cultural healthcare.

Office for Civil Rights

The Office has engaged in a number of efforts related to disparities in care. It has addressed redlining issues (limiting or eliminating services in specific geographic areas), conducted compliance review of home health-care agencies nationwide to ascertain compliance with civil rights statutes, and investigated how managed care plans establish their service area and how they target their marketing activities. For example, Region II (New York) has developed a self-assessment tool for providers to assist them in ensuring that their facility is able to meet the challenge of servicing a diverse population. The New York Regional Office is also investigating allegations of racial disparities in the provision of healthcare services by some healthcare providers in two counties in New York (e.g., poor quality of care for minorities, lack of access to more prominent medical facilities, language barriers to healthcare), and is collecting and analyzing data pertaining to specific healthcare facilities in an effort to gain a better understanding of the root causes of disparities. In addition, Region V (Chicago) has conducted investigations focused on disparities in kidney transplant programs.

Agency for Healthcare Research and Quality

Measures of Quality of Care for Vulnerable Populations. This initiative will develop and test new quality measures for use in the purchase or improvement of healthcare services for priority populations. For example, one such project will develop a quality of care measure for hypertension in a population of Hmong refugees and pilot test the instrument.

Assessment of Quality Improvement Strategies in Health Care. A recently funded study will create a partnership of six health providers to evaluate the effectiveness of nurse management compared to usual care for congestive heart failure patients in Harlem.

Translating Research into Practice (TRIP). Initiated in 1999, this funding is aimed at generating knowledge about approaches that effectively promote the use of empirically derived evidence in clinical settings that will lead to improved healthcare practice and sustained practitioner behavior change. A priority for the FY2000 TRIP initiative is to determine to what extent general strategies need to be modified to improve quality of care for minority populations.

Understanding and Eliminating Minority Health Disparities Initiative will support the development of Centers of Excellence that will conduct research to provide information on factors that influence quality, outcomes, costs, and access to healthcare for minority populations.

Centers for Disease Control and Prevention

Racial and Ethnic Approaches to Community Health (REACH 2010). This five-year demonstration project seeks to eliminate disparities in health in the following priority areas: infant mortality, cervical cancer, cardiovascular disease, diabetes, HIV/AIDS, and immunizations. The two-phase project will support community coalitions in the design, implementation, and evaluation of community-driven strategies to eliminate health disparities. Phase I is a 12-month planning period during which needs assessments and action plans are developed. Phase II is a four-year period during which action plans will be carried out. An evaluation logic model will be used to guide the collection of data.

National Program of Cancer Registries. This program provides funding to states/territories to enhance existing registries and create new registries. FY2001 funding will focus on training and technical assistance to improve collecting race and ethnicity data and evaluating the completeness and accuracy of data for racial and ethnic minority populations.

Alaska Native Colorectal Cancer Education Project is being developed and will involve screening tests and the provision of specific language to Alaska Natives for use with healthcare providers when discussing colorectal cancer.

Hispanic Colorectal Cancer Outreach and Education Project is a partnership with the National Alliance for Hispanic Health to increase awareness and screening for colorectal cancer. The CDC is also investigating psychosocial and cultural influences that impact prevention attitudes, behaviors, and adherence to screening guidelines among Puerto Ricans and Dominicans.

National Comprehensive Cancer Control (CCC) Program seeks to develop coordinated efforts with health agencies to increase the number and quality of cancer programs and to reduce the burden of cancer in minority populations.

National Breast and Cervical Cancer Early Detection Program (NBCCEDP) is a 10-year-old program that funds all 50 state health agencies, DC, 12 tribal organizations, and 6 territories to conduct breast and cervical cancer early detection programs. The program works to ensure that women receive screening services, needed follow-up, and assurance that tests are preformed in accordance with current guidelines.

National Training Center initiative trains providers serving American-Indian women to enhance cultural sensitivity and client-provider interactions. The CDC is also developing a CD-ROM to educate Ohio providers about various cultural perspectives on breast care and interpersonal communication with patients.

Research on *prostate cancer screening behaviors* among African-American men, in collaboration with Loma Linda University, will examine the relationship between what primary care providers report telling their patients about prostate cancer and how the men perceive the messages.

The CDC has proposed the addition of questions on "reactions to race" to the 2002 *Behavior Risk Factor Surveillance System*. As questions regarding the effects of racism on disparities in health status are raised, the CDC has proposed the addition of race questions to the survey in order to begin to measure racism and its impact on health.

Centers for Medicare and Medicaid Services

Reducing Health Care Disparities National Project. This project focuses on working at the state level to reduce disparities. Its objectives are to improve health status and outcomes in racial/ethnic populations and reduce disparity between healthcare received by beneficiaries who are members of a targeted racial and ethnic group and all other beneficiaries living in each state.

Excellence Centers to Eliminate Ethnic/Racial Disparities (EXCEED) initiative involves the awarding of grants that will help understand and address factors that contribute to ethnic and racial inequities in healthcare. For example, projects involve topics such as racial and ethnic variations in medical interactions, improving the delivery of effective care to minorities, and understanding and reducing native elder health disparities.

Health Resources and Services Administration

Measuring Cultural Competence in Health Care Delivery Settings. This Project in coordination with the Lewin Group seeks to develop a measurement model of cultural competence for healthcare delivery settings. The objectives are to advance the conceptualization of measurement of cultural competence in healthcare settings, identify specific indicators and measures that can be used to assess cultural competence in healthcare, and assess the feasibility and practical application of these measures. Products of the project will include: a framework for measuring cultural competence in healthcare settings; a synthesis and assessment of existing measures; and a report recommending domains, indicators, measures, measurement uses, and data sources regarding competence measurement.

Community Access Program (CAP). The CAP helps healthcare providers develop integrated, community-wide systems that serve the uninsured and underinsured. CAP grants are designed to increase access to healthcare by eliminating fragmented service delivery, improving efficiencies among safety net providers, and by encouraging greater private sector involvement. Currently, CAP grants support 76 communities in urban and rural areas and on tribal lands. A new application competition in the fall of 2001 will support 40 more communities. Partners in the CAP coalitions include local health departments, public hospitals, community health centers, universities and state governments. The partners use CAP funds to create and expand collaboration in three main areas—coordinated intake and enrollment systems, integrated management information systems, and referral networks and coordination of services. The agency also will use FY 2001 funds to provide training and technical assistance to all CAP grantees and to support a national evaluation of the program.

The *Provider's Guide to Quality and Culture* serves as a source for health professionals seeking resources on cultural issues within the context of quality of care. The Guide emerged out of the Quality Center of the Bureau of Primary Health Care and was developed by Management Sciences for Health, a nonprofit organization focused on the improvement of global health. The Guide responds to four of the six national aims articulated by the National Institute of Medicine's (IOM) *Crossing the Quality Chasm* report (safety, effectiveness, patient-centeredness, and equity).

The *Oral Health Initiative*, an initiative of HRSA and HCFA, seeks to eliminate disparities in access to oral healthcare and improvement of oral health. The goals of the initiative are to: a) integrate dental health activities within the two agencies; b) partner with public agencies and private dental professional educational and advocacy organizations; and c) promote the application of dental science and technology to reduce disparities.

Indian Health Service

The Indian Health Service has a number of programs in place to improve healthcare access and quality, as well as increase community awareness of disease prevention and treatment. For example, the *Southwest Native American Cardiology Program* was developed in 1993. This program was developed to provide direct cardiovascular care to Native Americans at reservation clinics within the Navajo, Phoenix, and Tucson Areas as well as provide tertiary care for complex cardiovascular disease in Tucson. The *National Diabetes Program* was initiated to develop, document, and sustain a public health effort to prevent and control diabetes in American Indian and Alaska Native communities. Other programs, such as the *Elder Care Initiative*, serve to promote the development of high-quality care for American Indian and Alaska Native elders. The activities of the initiative are focused on information and referral, technical assistance and education, and advocacy. This is accomplished in partnership with a variety of tribal, state, federal, and academic programs.

National Institutes of Health

A trans-NIH working group, consisting of each NIH institute and center director, was initiated in 1999 to develop a *strategic research agenda on health disparities.* The objectives of the working group are to: develop a five-year Strategic Research Agenda; recruit and train minority investigators to advance community outreach activities; form new and enhance current partnerships with minority and other organizations that have similar goals to close health gaps; define, code, track, analyze, and evaluate progress more uniformly across the agency; and enhance public awareness.

The *National Center on Minority Health and Health Disparities (NCMHD)* at the National Institutes of Health was established in 2000. The new Center will conduct and support research, training, dissemination of information, and other programs about minority health conditions and about populations with health disparities. The goals of the Center are to assist in the development of an integrated cross-discipline national health research agenda; to promote and facilitate the creation of a robust minority health research environment; and to promote, assist, and support research capacity building activities in the minority and medically underserved communities.

Substance Abuse and Mental Health Services Administration

Community Action Grant Program—Hispanic priority. Awards are made to Hispanic community-based organizations to support the development and implementation of substance abuse prevention, addictions treatment, and mental health services for Hispanic adults and adolescents. For example, among the new grants is a program that is working toward a specialized dual-diagnosis model for Hispanic/Latino clients with co-occurring mental and addictive disorders.

Specialized HIV/AIDS outreach and substance abuse treatment, a grant program to support community-based substance abuse treatment programs targeted to minority populations at risk for HIV/AIDS.

SAMHSA developed a *pocket guide and desk reference* for clinicians, which has been translated into Spanish, to help providers assess and treat substance abuse conditions. Physicians and nurses serving these communities are being trained at regional meetings, an effort coordinated by the Interamerican College of Physician Surgeons.

SAMHSA established a multi-disciplinary panel to develop *standards of mental healthcare for Latinos.* The panel developed a report that includes Standards from the Consumer Perspective, Clinical Guidelines for Providers, and Provider and System Competencies for Training. The standards are being piloted to develop performance indicators and best practices.

SAMHSA has made available new funds to help improve access, addictions treatment, and mental health services in racial/ethnic minority communities in order to reduce disparities in services.

American Indian and Alaskan Native Planning Grants provide funds to communities to support the development of local substance abuse treatment system plans to deliver integrated substance abuse, mental health services, primary care, and other public health services.

Activities of *The Special Programs Development Branch* have included: the collection of data on access to and quality of mental health services within ethnic and minority communities; working with representatives of consumer, advocacy, professional, and provider organizations serving minority communities to improve mental health treatment; developing guidelines and measures to assist state and local governments in making services and systems of care responsive to diverse cultural needs; and examining the impact of managed care on access, quality, and cost of mental health services for ethnic and minority populations.

DEPARTMENT OF VETERANS AFFAIRS

The Department has instituted several *Centers for Excellence* in healthcare that focus on healthcare issues unique and prevalent in the minority community. For example, the Centers for Excellence in Hepatitis C, Treatment and Prevention have been established in California and Florida. The Center has developed culturally sensitive literature on hepatitis C for distribution in minority communities and has been translated into Spanish, Cherokee, and Navajo.

The Department has initiated several investigations to examine disparities in care in areas including prostate cancer, cardiac procedures, osteoarthritis care, and delivery of care to American Indians and Hispanic Americans.

OTHER PROGRAMS/INITIATIVES TO
ADDRESS HEALTHCARE DISPARITIES

The *Cambridge Health Alliance* is a network of three hospitals, the Cambridge Public Health Department, community based programs, physician practices, neighborhood health centers, and a managed Medicaid health plan. The communities serviced by the Alliance have large and diverse minority populations, with 26% of residents living below 200% of the federal poverty line. Among the many intergrated services included are multilingual interpreter services, public health, and preventive services.

D

Racial Disparities in Healthcare: Highlights from Focus Group Findings

Meredith Grady
Tim Edgar

Westat
1650 Research Boulevard
Rockville, Maryland
June 2001

STORIES OF RACIAL DISCRIMINATION IN HEALTHCARE PRACTICE

Racial discrimination occurs on many levels, in a variety of contexts, intertwined with income, education level, and other sociodemographic factors. It can be subtle or disturbingly overt. During the eight focus groups, participants were asked to talk about their own personal experiences with racism in healthcare. When asked whether discrimination exists in receiving quality healthcare, one African-American participant summed up the collective response in this way: "The medical world just reflects the real world." Throughout the following section, participants' stories and opinions are presented in their own words, providing evidence of healthcare inequity that participants attributed directly or indirectly to racial or ethnic discrimination, their lack of English-language proficiency, or both.

Effect of Stereotyping

Participants often felt that the quality of health care services they received stemmed from misperceptions and stereotypes, not the reality of who they are. They said they often feel that health care providers treat them differently and assume they are less educated, poor, or deserving of less respect because of their race or culture. A Hispanic physician, speaking of the perceptions of his colleagues, corroborated participants' opinions that health care providers make assumptions about their patients based on race or ethnicity. "As soon as they look at the patient and see he's African American or Latino, they assume automatically that he doesn't have insurance at all."

The following quotes provide examples of encounters that participants had with healthcare providers who made stereotypical assumptions about their education or culture.

My name is . . . [a common Hispanic surname] and when they see that name, I think there is . . . some kind of a prejudice of the name. . . . We're talking about on the phone, there's a lack of respect. There's a lack of acknowledging the person and making one feel welcome. All of the courtesies that go with the profession that they are paid to do are kind of put aside. They think they can get away with a lot because "Here's another dumb Mexican." (Hispanic participant)

I've had both positive and negative experiences. I know the negative one was based on race. It was [with] a previous primary care physician when I discovered I had diabetes. He said, "I need to write this prescription for these pills, but you'll never take them and you'll come back and tell me you're still eating pig's feet and everything. . . . Then why do I still need to write this prescription." And I'm like, "I don't eat pig's feet." (African-American participant)

My son broke my glasses so I needed to go get a prescription so I could go buy a pair of glasses. I get there and the optometrist was talking to me as if I was like 10 years old. As we were talking, they were saying, "What do you do," and as soon as they found out what I did [professionally], the whole attitude of this person changed towards me. I don't know if they come in there thinking, "Oh this poor Indian does not have a clue." I definitely felt like I was being treated differently. (Native-American participant)

One participant spoke about a relative who did not want to take her husband's name after marriage for fear of being negatively stereotyped.

My granddaughter, she's a doctor herself. She graduated in Mexico and then she came here. She [studied here] so she could become a doctor here. She married a Mexican guy named [a common Hispanic surname]. You know what she did? She took off [a common Hispanic surname] and kept [another surname], her father's name. (Hispanic participant)

Language Barriers

Many participants in the Chinese- and Spanish-speaking focus groups voiced concern about being treated unfairly because of their lack of English-language proficiency. As a result, they perceived that healthcare providers treat them differently and were concerned that they receive lower quality care.

If you speak English well, then an American doctor, they will treat you better. If you speak Chinese and your English is not that good, they would also kind of look down on you. They would [be] kind of prejudiced. (Chinese participant)

When they see he can't explain himself, they look at him as if [they are] belittling him. They treat him with a lot of inferiority... the doctor, nurses, receptionists. You can tell when the person is not liked by the doctors or the staff. I have seen a lot of discrimination in that manner. (Hispanic participant)

I have a desire to improve my English so I can go to an American doctor and get better treatment. (Chinese participant)

Healthcare providers were also concerned about not being able to communicate adequately with their patients because of a language barrier. One African-American nurse spoke of "seeing the fear in their eyes" and knowing how upset and frustrated patients were in trying to communicate what was wrong with them. A Hispanic nurse acknowledged the language problem, stating that for "new immigrants that do not speak the language properly . . . it is the biggest obstacle they encounter."

Non-English-speaking participants, especially those in the Hispanic group, recounted many examples of personal situations in hospitals and other settings where they were forced to deal with serious health conditions without the benefit of interpreters or patient healthcare staff willing to assist them. They said they encountered healthcare staff who ignored them and avoided trying to help them. Others pointed out instances where they or their family members have received poor quality healthcare services and have been treated disrespectfully because they speak little or no English.

A long time ago my husband was in pain. I had to call an ambulance and they took him to the hospital. We waited three hours. I would ask the nurse to please treat him because he could not stand the pain. She would say, "We're going to call him, we're going to call him." I saw black people being called in, but they never called him back. I asked for some medication in the meantime. They never came out with the medicine. . . . Well, we left. [My husband] told me it must have been because we are Hispanic and don't speak English. They would call and call in black people. . . . I think if we would've been black or American we would have been treated faster. (Hispanic participant)

[My wife] was treated badly. They wouldn't take care of her. They were changing her IV and the nurse was very rough in the way she would take the needle out and put it back in. I felt bad. I had to go and tell them with the little English I speak what was happening. So, they changed the nurse. That's the way it is. All the situations we are experiencing are because we can't communicate in English. (Hispanic participant)

My son was in a bed and another boy was with his mother. Of course, they didn't speak English. The lady didn't know . . . she wanted to know where they were taking the boy. She asked for the girl who was interpreting for her. One of the nurses said, "I don't know why they send these people here without anybody to interpret for them. We'll come back later," and they left . . . but they didn't do anything about finding out where the interpreter was. (Hispanic participant)

I had eye surgery two or three years ago. The specialist was black. There were Hispanics out front. I told them I had an appointment with the doctor. They asked me if I spoke English . . . one said to the other in Spanish, "Go inside with her." "No, you go." I asked them who was going to go with me because the doctor was waiting for me. Once we were inside, he would speak [only to the interpreter] directly. I felt rejected. (Hispanic participant)

Five years ago my son got double pneumonia. The doctors wanted to operate [on] him. . . . They called my husband and he said he had to talk with the specialist who was treating my son to see what he had to say about the surgery. We called . . . and the specialist said my son would not be able to resist that type of surgery. My husband called the hospital and told me not to sign any papers. I didn't speak English. I didn't know anything. They put the paper in front of me to sign. They insisted I sign the paper. My husband told me not to sign anything and [that] he was on his way [to pick us up]. In the end my son didn't have the surgery and he didn't die like they said he would. Three days after they said he needed the surgery he got better. The surgery was not necessary. (Hispanic participant)

I called a pharmacy to see if my daughter's medicine was ready and they put me on hold. They put the phone down and said, "She's a Spanish speaker," and they put me on hold. She left me waiting a long time until I hung up. (Hispanic participant)

The Role of Economics

Oftentimes, participants noted, a person's perceived or actual socioeconomic status can be an obstacle to obtaining quality healthcare services. Participants were concerned that they may receive a lower standard of care because healthcare providers make assumptions about the type of treatment or medication that they can afford because they are racial or ethnic minorities.

I know there have been a couple of times the doctor wanted to prescribe a certain medication but because of how much it was, he prescribed something else. Not what was best, but what I could afford. (African-American participant)

Often times, the system gets the concept of black people off the 6 o'clock news, and they treat us all the same way. Here's a guy coming in here with no insurance. He's low breed. (African-American participant)

A lot of black people don't have money so I guess you would say that it's hard [to get quality healthcare.] A lot of black people don't have any insurance. (African-American participant)

Lack of Respect

Many participants unequivocally believed that the lack of respect healthcare providers have for them leads to lower quality healthcare services than persons of other ethnicities, especially whites, receive. They spoke of instances where the office staff would not "look them in the eye" when they spoke to them or greeted other patients with a more pleasant attitude. Others felt a lack of respect when they were rushed during appointments and sensed that providers or their staff did not want to take the time to help them, answer their questions, or explain medical procedures to them.

They wouldn't accept the appointment over the phone; they just put me on hold. I went in there and she looked at me and I told her I'd been calling trying to make an appointment. She said, "Well, you see this stack of paper, you think you're the only one?" She either thought I was Mexican or she recognized I was Indian, but she would not make that appointment. She just got smart with me and all. I told my husband about it. He's big and white. She got to him just like that. No problem. She got the appointment and got him through. She wouldn't do it for me. (Native-American participant)

I felt that because of my race that I wasn't serviced as well as a Caucasian person was. The attitude that you would get. Information wasn't given to me as it would have [been given to] a Caucasian. The attitude made me feel like I was less important. I could come to the desk and they would be real nonchalant and someone of Caucasian color would come behind me and they'd be like, "Hi, how was your day?" (African-American participant)

I don't have a problem with taking more time to be able to understand each other, but they get really annoyed when you don't understand them. Basically, they get really annoyed if you talk too much because they know they don't understand your language. When I go to the doctor I ask a lot of questions, so they can get really aggravated with me. I don't know if they would do the same thing to a white person. (African-American participant)

Others felt they must wait for long periods of time before receiving medications and other medical assistance, while whites are cared for first.

I would call [for the nurse] when I was feeling pretty bad. They wouldn't come until I finally had to yell, "Help me, I'm in pain! I need something to calm the pain!" They had to call someone and she gave it to me. There were American [patients] there. They would even close the curtains for them. (Hispanic participant)

If your bell was on and the Caucasian lady, she doesn't even have to have her bell on. She was being attended to because they knew they better . . . do a certain quality [of service]. Whereas the same quality should have been given to the black people, but their bell would be on and they still would have to wait. (African-American participant)

Improper Diagnosis or Treatment

More troubling are instances that participants mentioned where the quality of medical treatment was compromised by discriminatory attitudes or practices that participants believed led to either misdiagnosis or improper treatment.

When I was growing up, my parents didn't have health insurance. We would go to the Indian Health Service. You'd go there to the clinic and I think sometimes you wonder about the quality of the medical personnel that was examining you. My younger sister had appendicitis. It burst, and they told her she had a stomach flu. I don't know how they were hiring the medical personnel at that time. It's changed now, but back then I don't think we had some of the best medical officers or nurses. (Native-American participant)

Being in a group practice seeing predominantly African-American patients, I have patients who have seen mainly white physicians in the past. When they come in to visit with us and speak with us, something as simple as [asking them to] sit up on a table and they got a question. "What are you going to do?" "I'm going to examine you." "Oh, my other doctor never did that." (African-American physician)

Of course, in psychiatry we see this [discrimination]. One area we see is in terms of diagnosis. Patients are inappropriately diagnosed and medications prescribed for the patients. We see errors in that. Minority patients will often be diagnosed inappropriately as being schizophrenic. (African-American physician)

When I ask [my Hispanic patients] if the other doctor ever examines you, they say, "No, they give me a prescription." It's amazing. A lot of times these patients have these problems that are missed by the other doctors. (Hispanic physician)

In some instances, participants noted, racial and ethnic minority patients have difficulties gaining access to the specialists they need. One physician noted that specialists mistreat racial and ethnic minority patients to avoid having to provide treatment for them.

I'm in private practice and we refer a lot. We kind of know what specialists to avoid because we hear the patients coming back and telling about what type of treatment they're getting from these specialists. A lot of the specialists in these institutions act like they don't want to see the minority patient at all. When the minority patient ends up there maybe because they're on [a particular] plan... they are mistreated. (African-American physician)

In contrast to situations described by participants in which healthcare providers sought to limit their access to healthcare services, two female participants described being pressured to have surgical procedures that, in retrospect, were deemed unnecessary by other doctors.

> The first thing they wanted to do was a hysterectomy. I was 36 years old and they never really examined me. I was just telling them the symptoms and it scared me and I left. . . . I guess they were trying to stop the population birth, whatever, because [the hospital] back then was for people who didn't have insurance. (African-American participant)

> My Ob-Gyn is Caucasian. I have fibroid tumors and the doctor I've been going to, he's been my Ob-Gyn for 14 years and for the last 2 years he told me I have to have this hysterectomy. I had a girlfriend at the office recommend me to a female African-American physician. . . . A week later she called me at home and said to me, "There's nothing wrong with you. The fibroid is there but if it's not bothering you, if it's not broke, don't fix it. You don't need to have a hysterectomy." (African-American participant)

To overcome discriminatory attitudes from healthcare providers, one participant suggested that it is necessary for minorities to be "strong" and not "humble in your voice and tone" to have a better chance at getting the care they wanted.

> I believe that African Americans do get a lower quality of care. I think if you're educated, if somebody's not treating you right then you kind of push past some of the stuff, but for somebody that doesn't have a good feeling about themselves, whether it's because of race or literacy, that makes it very hard for them to get the care that they need. (African-American nurse)

CHALLENGE OF IDENTIFYING RACIAL AND ETHNIC DISCRIMINATION

Some participants found it difficult to identify obvious examples of discrimination they encountered in their healthcare experiences, although they were certain that discrimination exists in healthcare settings. As one African American participant aptly described, "It's hard to identify discrimination because they don't show it. They'll be sweet and smooth, all the way through it." Participants mentioned experiencing discrimination in many situations, but because of the subtleties often inherent in discrimination, it was challenging to identify overt examples. They often said, "You just know," or "You can feel it" when describing incidences of discrimination.

Overall, participants felt that racial discrimination could not easily be separated from other forms of discrimination. The quotes that appear in the following section illustrate participants' concerns about not receiving appropriate healthcare services, but they also show that the link between one's race or ethnicity and poor treatment can be very complex. While the underlying issues (e.g., economics, improper diagnosis) mentioned here parallel those discussed in an earlier section, the claims made in the following quotes only *suggest* that a lower quality of healthcare stems from racial or ethnic discrimination. The evidence for this causal relationship tends to be circumstantial.

Patients' Appearance

Some participants hinted that attention to appearance, (e.g., being well-dressed) might counteract discriminatory tendencies. One Hispanic participant said he felt it was important to "be presentable," otherwise the healthcare staff would likely make him wait for hours before helping him. Another said:

> *I've noticed that, outward appearance has a lot to do with the rapport that you have with your provider. They talk to you a little different, they treat you a bit differently. You can walk in, you're all battered and crummy looking, and their whole personality changes. You walk in looking half-way decent, and they're very pleasant, and they react and act completely different.* (African-American participant)

Patients' Economic/Insurance Status

Some participants provided examples of how they or their family members received poor healthcare services because of their lack of insurance or perceived inability to pay for these services. They believed that they were being treated differently by the healthcare system, although they did not make a direct link to race or ethnicity.

> *I went back [to IHS] after I found out everything that needed to be done. I went back to the clinic and chewed out the doctor. Then she said, "Wait a minute. Wait a minute. Do you realize how much it's going to cost you? It's like buying a new car." I said "I don't care at this point. It's my life. I don't care how much money I have to pay out of my pocket." Then she says, "Wait a minute. Let's send you to a specialist." I said, "Why didn't you tell me this to begin with? Now that I'm making my move, now you're telling me, OK, now you can do this and that for me?" I said, "No thank you. This is it." (Native-American participant)*

> *My niece went to this hospital and they wouldn't wait on her because she didn't have insurance. They told her she would have to go to the county hospital. So I had to take her to the county hospital. She was bleeding all the way. It was just terrible, because she didn't have insurance.* (African-American participant)

It's almost like "Oh well, this person doesn't have insurance. Let's just give them the IHS treatment." (Native-American participant)

I have a son and he's considered disabled. He had MediCal before. I got it before I got insurance through my job, and I had to wait 100 days before I got the insurance through my job. So I noticed there's a longer waiting period... other people are coming in after me and have later appointments, but they have private insurance, so they're seen before me and my son. And it wasn't just the waiting period; the treatment was different. Now that I have private insurance, as soon as I get there, [they see me]. (Hispanic participant)

An Ob/Gyn who had a large Medicaid population, not just black and Hispanic, but a large Medicaid population . . . they told the doctor they wanted him to have more deliveries at other hospitals. [He refused.] The hospital then, at that point, decided they would stop taking all Medicaid period because this doctor would not leave. For an entire year this hospital wouldn't pay Medicaid just so this doctor wouldn't deliver there anymore. (African-American physician)

Healthcare Setting

Native Americans, because of their unique access to healthcare through the Indian Health Service (IHS), spoke often about the poor quality of care at the IHS clinics. More than participants in the other groups, they defined their ability to get quality healthcare services by the setting in which they received care and not by their race. They did not blame poor healthcare on individual providers as much as they did on the IHS system.

If you go into IHS for a problem, they don't investigate your problem to the extent that a private place does. [Private offices] go through everything like an ultrasound, blood work, the whole nine yards, and they pinpoint the problem. IHS, they give you a temporary solution or shot and it comes back up a month later. (Native-American participant)

I think the way that race plays into it is because we all go to the Indian Health Service because we're Indian. That's where we start out with our healthcare. (Native-American participant)

I've had experiences where I had no choice but to go to the Indian Health Service. You go in there, they rush through you. They misdiagnosed several things with me, and you're just rushed through. I've dealt with accidents, and to get your accidents paid for and stuff, IHS takes forever to get those reports through. It took like 2 years, and that's a very long time. I don't know where they get that, but I don't think that's right. (Native-American participant)

Attitude of Healthcare Providers

Some participants were surprised and disappointed by the uncaring attitude exhibited by some of their healthcare providers or administrative staff. In some cases, they felt staff were unwilling to help them, and information about their health was delayed or not provided to them. In other situations, doctors seemed more interested in insurance payment issues and less concerned with providing appropriate care for their patients.

The doctor comes in and says, "Why is he on oxygen?" I was recovering from surgery. He's looking at the chart and he says, "The insurance doesn't cover it. Take it off." Just like that. I'm right there, and I'm thinking "Wow, that's pretty harsh if it comes from a doctor." That was unfair I thought. (Hispanic participant)

First of all, they didn't send me back the results for 5-6 months. I can't get an answer on the phone when I call. I have to call like 10 times and they put me on hold and say they'll transfer me. They never transfer me. They hang up on me. (Hispanic participant)

A few participants did not think their physicians took the time necessary to listen to them or examine them properly. They felt that their overall health needs were being ignored.

[The doctor] just walks in and has other patients to see, [she asks] "What's wrong with you now?" and that's it. Sometimes I will go into other things that I have felt and it's like, "Oh, just take vitamins." What if there's something else wrong? They're not trying to find out what's wrong. Maybe I have cancer or something. (Hispanic participant)

They just come in, look at the chart, say, "OK, are you taking your medications? See you in 3 months." . . . if they find the chart. Sometimes they can't even find mine. (Hispanic participant)

Other Stories About Misdiagnosis or Improper Treatment

Some participants spoke of going to the hospital or doctor and receiving misinformation or improper service from healthcare providers. In some cases, participants said their healthcare providers misdiagnosed their condition or were too passive in their treatment approach. A few participants questioned whether some providers they went to were qualified to make an accurate diagnosis of their health problem. Again, the concerns expressed in these specific instances were linked to race and ethnicity by implication only.

At the hospital, they sent me over to a doctor, who was not an [eye] specialist. He diagnosed me with cataracts and said I needed surgery the next day. Thanks to a miracle from God, I did not end up blind. [Afterwards] eight days went by that I was blind in that eye. . . . Jose took me to another doctor. The [second] doctor told us I needed surgery the next day. It's a miracle from God that I can see. The other doctor left me with silicone. They put the entire amount that comes in the packet when they should have only put half. Why did the man who wasn't an eye specialist tell me I had cataracts, when what I had was a detached retina? (Hispanic participant)

My daughter was young and I took her to the hospital. She had stomach pains... I went to this private doctor and hospital and they sent us home with some medicines. . . . The next day I sent her to school. The school called me up and said, "You [have] got to come pick up this child because she can't even walk." So I said, "OK, I'm going to County General because they will make sure this child's taken care of." I'm not going back playing with these people [at the private office]. I took her to County General. They had her in there for 5 hours checking everything. I found out that she had walking pneumonia. (African-American participant)

In my country, if they find you have a fibroma they remove it. They don't wait for it to grow. Maybe if they had taken them out this wouldn't have happened to me. (Hispanic participant)

INSTITUTIONAL DISCRIMINATION IN HEALTHCARE

In discussions with African-American and Hispanic physicians and nurses, they spoke not only about the discrimination their patients experience at the provider-patient level, but also cited examples of how healthcare institutions perpetuate discrimination in their policies and methods of practice. Providers felt institutions mandate policies that have a significant negative impact on the provision or access to services for racial and ethnic minority patients.

It's very difficult to recruit Hispanics [for clinical trials] who cannot understand the consent form. I felt there was some resistance [to spending extra time counseling Spanish-speakers]. [I was told] it was just not really necessary, that I can just give them a synopsis of what is in that consent form. I said, "Wait a minute. This is a very important piece of paper. Why should it be different? You don't give a synopsis to English-speakers." So you can see sometimes the double standard there. (Hispanic nurse)

They would not take certain doctors from certain ZIP codes, but we found out what was going on and that subsequently has changed a few years ago. Because they didn't want [minority] patients, they just excluded people from certain ZIP codes, from certain sections of the city. (African-American physician)

Providers also cited examples of discrimination that they have had to contend with personally during their medical training or professional career.

There are those that don't get promoted because of their race or whatever. The reason [may be because] they're not well liked by administration or it may be just that they don't want that person in that setting because of their race—that is out there. Racism is alive and well, and those of us who think that it's not are living in some kind of dream world. (African-American nurse)

The local medical society . . . it's got the good old boy attitude. It's the same old doctors that have been running it, and they're still running it. The new guys kind of have trouble getting in. (Hispanic physician)

I heard an Anglo doctor complaining that his daughter is having trouble getting into medical school. Then another doctor jumps in, another Anglo, "Oh, don't worry about it. I know the admissions coordinator. . . I'll get her in. I'll give him a call and she'll be in." When does a Hispanic or black student have those advantages, the connections? I certainly didn't have any connections, and I still don't have any connections. I couldn't get my son into medical school if I tried. (Hispanic physician)

INCLUSION OF AND RESPECT FOR CULTURE IN HEALTHCARE EXPERIENCES

While some participants did not feel it was essential that providers and patients be of the same race or ethnic background, many participants felt that a cultural match between healthcare providers and patients is helpful in communicating more easily. One African-American physician summed up responses saying, "Basically, you're comfortable with what you're familiar with. That's the bottom line." Participants felt that it is easier to develop a rapport or discuss treatment options with healthcare providers of their own race who already understand their language and cultural idiosyncrasies.

I don't think necessarily you have to be an African American to provide good care to African Americans, but if you're not you really need to be aware of the culture and some of the issues in that culture, and really look at how you feel about dealing with people from that culture. (African-American nurse)

For me, my doctor is a thin doctor, but she knows that I like Mexican food so she knows it's hard for me to lose weight. She understands the way my parents brought me up, the culture, the background, so she knows. In other words, we understand each other because we're both Hispanic. (Hispanic participant)

If someone, the doctor for example, is of the same ethnicity, Hispanic, he understands the idiosyncrasies more. For example, for women, in our country there are certain taboos. It is more difficult to talk about private things. So, a doctor of our same race will understand those things more. (Hispanic participant)

I feel I could relate better to the African American [doctor]. He knows black folks better. If you're talking about high blood pressure, diabetes, sometimes these are things that traditionally do not happen to white folks. To the extent with the ills that we suffer, I believe he would be better suited for me. (African-American participant)

I think there are just certain aspects of the culture that one may know a little bit more about by just being part of the culture. For example, with Hispanic patients, it's more of a touchy feely—especially my relationship with older women. There's always a lot of hugging or kissing, whereas with the men—none of that— there's only hand shaking. When it comes to my African-American women, there is some touchy feely stuff, but, again, there is more distance. I think just being aware of the cultural attitudes makes it slightly different. (Hispanic physician)

In instances where healthcare providers or administrative staff are of a different race or ethnicity than the patients they are treating, participants expressed a desire for more patience and respect from their providers. They felt that doctors and nurses who are treating a high proportion of patients from a particular racial or ethnic group should be familiar with relevant customs that may impact patients' healthcare decisions.

One thing—the elders—they're stubborn. You got to have a lot of patience with them because they think they're all right and they don't want to go to a doctor. It takes a lot just to get them to go. Have patience and be courteous towards them and respect them. (Native-American participant)

A lot of Native Americans are shy. I think that would be good for a doctor to make sure the patient understands the treatment they're going to provide or the cause of their illness and make sure they understand what's going on. (Native-American participant)

Our culture is very different. The Americans have a different way of treating people. We are more affectionate, sweet. We have a lot of time to give, they are very quick. (Hispanic participant)

I think if [doctors] have a basic knowledge of the culture and are sensitive of that, culture is just the traditional part of healing. There was one doctor at IHS. My brother injured his leg, went in, had an x-ray. . . . I remember at the end of the visit, and this was the only time I heard one of the doctors there say, "If you want to go visit your medicine man, feel free to do that." (Native-American participant)

Yeah, I had to have surgery and also my mom. In both cases this is the same doctor, a specialist, and when he explained about my mom, for example, he even took me in the room. He showed her and me, he even on a piece of paper showed how the liver and all this, what they had to do and this and that, and explained in language that we understood and took the time. It took him maybe a little more than 20 minutes, and that counts for something in my book you know. (Hispanic participant)

If they're going to practice in a Native-American setting, they should understand how traditional medicine can lead to healing the patient. (Native-American participant)

Understand what the past healthcare history has been to Native Americans. Maybe just having an understanding of how Native-American healthcare has been across the U.S., not just here in the Southwest, but everywhere. I think that would make [healthcare providers] effective because then they would know what's happened in the past and not repeat the same mistakes. (Native-American participant)

CONCLUSION

The stories and recollections of participants across the eight focus groups provide supporting evidence for the concern that racial and ethnic minorities are less likely to receive appropriate medical services, and that they experience a lower quality of healthcare than do nonminorities. While racial and ethnic discrimination is not always easy to recognize or recall, participants offered many concrete examples of discriminatory situations they encountered. This research adds to the growing body of literature examining racial and ethnic disparities in healthcare and provides evidence of both interpersonal and institutional discrimination. Perhaps, through continued research and awareness, healthcare delivery will become more respectful and culturally appropriate for racial and ethnic minority patients in the future.

E

Committee and Staff Biographies

Alan Nelson, M.D., *Chair,* is an internist-endocrinologist who was in private practice in Salt Lake City, Utah until becoming chief executive officer of the American Society of Internal Medicine (ASIM) in 1992. Following the merger of ASIM with the American College of Physicians (ACP) in 1998, Dr. Nelson headed the Washington Office of ACP-ASIM until his semi-retirement in January 2000, and currently serves as Special Advisor to the EVP/CEO of the College. Dr. Nelson was appointed to the Medicare Payment Advisory Commission (MedPAC) in May 2000. He was president of the American Medical Association in 1989-90 and was president of the World Medical Association from 1991-1992. Dr. Nelson received his M.D. degree from Northwestern University. He is a Master of the American College of Physicians and a member of the Institute of Medicine.

Risa Lavizzo-Mourey, M.D., M.B.A., *Co-Vice Chair,* is the Senior Vice President at the Robert Wood Johnson Foundation. Prior to joining the foundation, she was the Director of the Institute on Aging, Chief of the Division of Geriatric Medicine, and the Sylvan Eisman Professor of Medicine and Health Care Systems at the University of Pennsylvania as well as the Associate Chief of Staff for Geriatrics and extended care for the Philadelphia Veterans Administration Medical Center. Dr. Lavizzo-Mourey's research is at the interface of geriatric medicine and health policy, focusing specifically on disease and disability prevention as well as health care issues among persons of color. She earned her medical degree at Harvard Medical School followed by a Masters in Business

Administration at the University of Pennsylvania's Wharton School. Dr. Lavizzo-Mourey was formerly the Deputy Administrator of the Agency for Health Care Policy and Research, now known as the Agency for Heath Care Research and Quality within the U.S. Department of Health and Human Services. She was also a member of the White House Health Care Policy team. Dr. Lavizzo-Mourey is a Master of the American College of Physicians-American Society of Internal Medicine and a member of the Institute of Medicine.

Martha N. Hill, Ph.D., *Co-Vice Chair,* is Interim Dean, Professor, and Director, Center for Nursing Research, at The Johns Hopkins University School of Nursing. Her research has focused on hypertension care and control in urban African American Communities. Dr. Hill has also worked in the area of diabetes control in African Americans, patient and provider compliance with recommendations, strategies for patient education and behavior change, and health promotion and disease prevention. Her most recent work includes research on barriers to hypertension care and control, and dispelling myths about urban Black men with hypertension. Dr. Hill received her master's degree from the University of Pennsylvania and her doctorate degree in behavioral sciences from the Johns Hopkins School of Hygiene and Public Health. She is a fellow of the American Academy of Nursing, the Society of Geriatric Cardiology, the Society for Behavioral Medicine, and was the 1997-1998 president of the American Heart Association. Dr. Hill is a member of the Institute of Medicine.

Joseph R. Betancourt, M.D., M.P.H., is Senior Scientist, Institute for Health Policy and Director for Multicultural Education, Multicultural Affairs Office at Massachusetts General Hospital-Harvard Medical School. Dr. Betancourt's primary interests include cross-cultural medicine, minority recruitment into the health professions, and minority health/health policy research. His research has focused on developing a framework for cultural competence as a health policy initiative and quality measure (funded by the Commonwealth Fund), and exploring root causes for racial/ethnic disparities in heath (funded by HCFA and the NIH). Dr. Betancourt is a graduate of the New Jersey Medical School, Cornell Medical Center, and the Harvard School of Public Health. He serves on the New York Academy of Medicine's Racial/Ethnic Disparities Working Group and the Greater New York Hospital Association's Steering Committee on Racial/Ethnic Disparities.

M. Gregg Bloche, M.D., J.D., is Professor of Law and Co-Director of the Georgetown-Johns Hopkins Joint Program in Law and Public Health. Dr. Bloche writes and lectures on the law, policy, and ethics of health care provision. His recent and current scholarship addresses efficiency and fairness issues, the interplay between medical markets and the law, patients' rights, and socio-economic and racial disparities in medical care. Professor Bloche received a 1997-2000 Robert Wood Johnson Foundation Investigator Award in Health Policy Research to support his work on the legal and regulatory governance of managed care organizations. He received his J.D. from Yale Law School and his M.D. from Yale University School of Medicine. Dr. Bloche has been a consultant to the Institute of Medicine, South Africa's Truth and Reconciliation Commission (on human rights in the health sector), the Federal Judicial Center, the American Association for the Advancement of Science, the World Health Organization, and other private and public bodies. He serves on the boards of Physicians for Human Rights, Mental Disability Rights International, the *International Journal of Law and Psychiatry*, and other non-profit groups. In addition to his academic publications, he has contributed commentaries and op-eds. to nationally broadcast programs.

W. Michael Byrd, M.D., M.P.H., is Senior Research Scientist and Instructor in the Division of Public Health Practice at the Harvard School of Public Health, and Instructor and Staff Physician at Beth Israel Deaconess Hospital. His work focuses on health policies that impact African-American populations and other disadvantaged minorities. He also has expertise in the medical and public health history of African Americans. Dr. Byrd obtained his M.D. degree from Meharry Medical College and M.P.H. from the Harvard School of Public Health. Before entering academic medicine approximately 15 years ago, Dr. Byrd spent a decade in practice as an OB/GYN in Fort Worth, Texas. Dr. Byrd's previous academic appointments include assistant professorships at Meharry Medical College and SUNY Downstate Medical School, and service as senior attending physician at the teaching hospitals of both medical centers.

John F. Dovidio, M.A., Ph.D., is Charles A. Dana Professor, Department of Psychology and Interim Provost and Dean of the Faculty at Colgate University. Dr. Dovidio's research interests are in stereotyping, prejudice, and discrimination; social power and nonverbal communication; and altruism and helping. He received his M.A. and Ph.D. in social psychology from the University of Delaware. Dr. Dovidio shared the 1985 and 1998 Gordon Allport Intergroup Relations Prize with Samuel L. Gaertner for their work on aversive racism and ways to reduce bias. Dr. Dovidio has been Editor of *Personality and Social Psychology Bulletin,* and he is currently Associate Editor of *Group Processes and Intergroup Relations.* He is a Fellow of the American Psychological Association and of the American Psychological Society, has been President of the Society for the Psychological Study of Social Issues (SPSSI), Division 9 of APA, and is currently Secretary-Treasurer of the Society for Experimental Social Psychology.

José J. Escarce, M.D., Ph.D., is a Senior Natural Scientist at RAND, where he is co-director of the Center for Research on Health Care Organization, Economics and Finance. His research interests and expertise include health economics, managed care, physician behavior, access to medical care, and technological change in medicine. Dr. Escarce has studied racial differences in the utilization of surgical procedures and diagnostic tests by elderly Medicare beneficiaries, and was lead investigator of a study of racial differences in medical care utilization among older persons that was based on the 1987 NMES. He was co-investigator of a study that used interactive videodisc technology to assess the impact of patient race and gender on physician decision making for patients with chest pain. Dr. Escarce is currently working on several projects that address sociodemographic barriers to access in managed care. Dr. Escarce earned a Master's degree in physics from Harvard University, obtained his medical degree and doctorate in health economics from the University of Pennsylvania, and completed his residency at Stanford University.

Sandra Adamson Fryhofer, M.D., M.A.C.P., is a general internist engaged in private practice in Atlanta, Georgia, and the 2000-2001 president of the American College of Physicians-American Society of Internal Medicine. She is also a Clinical Associate Professor of Medicine at Emory University School of Medicine. Dr. Fryhofer has spent much of her career as an advocate for general internal medicine with a special interest in women's health. She can be found throughout the country presenting lectures and serving on panels to offer her expertise on subjects such as menopause, hormone replacement therapy, oral contraceptives, lipid disorders, and treatment of depression in the primary care settings. Dr. Fryhofer received her medical degree and internal medicine training from Emory University School of Medicine, where she is a member of Alpha Omega Alpha honor society. Dr. Fryhofer has been an active member of ACP-ASIM's Educational Policy Committee, diplomat of the American Board of Internal Medicine and active member of the Subcommittee on Clinical Competence in Women's Health.

Thomas Inui, Sc.M., M.D., is Senior Scholar at the Fetzer Institute. Dr. Inui's special emphases in teaching and research have included physician/patient communication, health promotion and disease prevention, the social context of medicine, and medical humanities. He completed his M.D. and Masters of Science in Public Health degrees at The Johns Hopkins University. Previously, he has served as Paul C. Cabot Professor of

Ambulatory Care and Prevention, Director of the Primary Care Division, and Faculty Dean at Harvard Medical School; Professor of Health and Social Behavior at the Harvard School of Public Health; Medical Director for Research and Education at Harvard Pilgrim Health Care; Division Head for General Internal Medicine, Department of Medicine, University of Washington; and Chief of Medicine at the U.S. Public Health Service Indian Hospital in Albuquerque, New Mexico. Dr. Inui is a member of the Institute of Medicine.

Jennie Joe, Ph.D., M.P.H., is Professor of Family and Community Medicine and Director of the Native American Research and Training Center at the University of Arizona. An anthropologist, her research has focused on the availability and use of services in Indian health clinics, provision of health care for the American Indian disabled, and treatment and prevention of diabetes among American Indian youth. Dr. Joe's most recent work includes cross-cultural perspectives in preventing and controlling cancer, recommendations for health care providers working with native families, and the emergence of a Type II diabetes epidemic in youth. Dr. Joe received her M.P.H. and Ph.D. degrees from the University of California, Berkeley.

Thomas McGuire, Ph.D., is Professor of Health Economics at Harvard Medical School. His work has focused on financing and cost effectiveness of behavioral health care and the industrial organization of health care. His most recent research includes an analysis of physician behavior in managed care environments, the use of risk-adjusted premiums to affect incentives to managed care plans to supply the appropriate quality of care, and the economics of health care disparities. Dr. McGuire received his Ph.D. in economics from Yale University. He was the recipient of the Kenneth J. Arrow Award for Best Paper in Health Economics in 1997, and received a Robert Wood Johnson Foundation Investigator Award in Health Policy in 1994. Dr. McGuire is a member of the Institute of Medicine.

Carolina Reyes, M.D., is Vice President of Planning and Evaluation at The California Endowment. Her research has focused on evaluating the effectiveness of programs in health care settings and describing clinical patterns associated with Intimate Partner Violence as well as assessing the quality of maternal health care services. Dr. Reyes is currently a Senior Scholar with the Agency for Healthcare Research and Quality. She received her Medical Degree from Harvard Medical School. Dr. Reyes completed her residency in Obstetrics and Gynecology and her fellowship in Maternal-Fetal Medicine at the Los Angeles County-USC Women's and Children's Hospital. She is an appointed member of the U.S. Secretary of Health and Human Services' Advisory Committee on Infant Mortality. She also serves as Senior Medical Advisor for the National Alliance of Hispanic Health.

Donald Steinwachs, Ph.D., is Chair and Professor of the Department of Health Policy and Management in The Johns Hopkins School of Hygiene and Public health. He is also Director of The Johns Hopkins University Health Services Research and Development Center. His research includes studies of medical effectiveness and patient outcomes for individuals with medical, surgical, and psychiatric disorders; the impact of managed care on access, quality, utilization, and cost; and developing methods to measure the effectiveness of systems of care. Dr. Steinwachs has particular interest in the role of routine management information systems as a source of data for evaluating the effectiveness and cost of health care. He received his M.S. in systems engineering from the University of Arizona and his Ph.D. in Operations Research from The Johns Hopkins University. Dr. Steinwachs is past President of the Association for Health Services Research and is the Director of the Johns Hopkins and University of Maryland Center for Research on Services for Severe Mental Illness (SMI). He also serves as a consultant to federal agencies and private foundations, and serves on the board of directors of Mathematica Policy Research. Dr. Steinwachs is a member of the Institute of Medicine.

David R. Williams, Ph.D., M.P.H., is Professor of Sociology and Senior Research Scientist at the Institute for Social Research at the University of Michigan. His prior academic appointment was at Yale University. Dr. Williams is interested in social and psychological factors that affect health, and especially in the trends and the determinants of socioeconomic and racial differences in mental and physical health. He received an MPH from Loma Linda University and a Ph.D. in sociology from the University of Michigan. Currently, he is on the editorial board of five scientific journals. He has served on two committees of the National Research Council and as a member of the Department of Health and Human Services National Committee on Vital and Health Statistics (and chair of its subcommittee on Minority and Other Special Populations). He has also held elected positions in professional organizations, such as the Secretary-Treasurer of the Medical Sociology Section of the American Sociological Association. Dr. Williams is a member of the Institute of Medicine.

Health Sciences Policy Board Liaison

Gloria E. Sarto, M.D., is Professor and past Chair of the Department of Obstetrics and Gynecology (OB/GYN) at the University of New Mexico

School of Medicine in Albuquerque, New Mexico. Her research interests include studies of genetic disorders and reproductive dysfunction. Dr. Sarto is President of the Society for the Advancement of Women's Health Research and is on the Professional Advisory Board of the Epilepsy Foundation of America. She is a member of the Board of Governors and Board of Directors of the National Center for Genome Resources and chairs the Advisory Council for OB/GYN of the American College of Surgeons. She co-chaired the Panel on Young Adulthood to Perimenopausal Years for the Office of Research on Women's Health Conference, *Opportunities for Research on Women's Health* in 1991, and has participated as a Task Force member in the NIH/ORWH series of workshops, *Beyond Hunt Valley,* 1996-97. Dr. Sarto was a member of the National Advisory Council on Child Health and Human Development, NIH; the Clinical Research Panel of the National Task Force on the NIH Strategic Plan; and the Committee on Research Capabilities of Academic Departments of Obstetrics and Gynecology, Institute of Medicine of the National Academy of Sciences. Additionally, she has been Vice President of the American Board of Obstetrics and Gynecology and Director of its Division of Maternal-Fetal Medicine. Dr. Sarto has published extensively on a wide array of women's health topics, including reproductive medicine and sexually transmitted diseases. She currently is on the editorial boards of *Perinatal Press, Journal of Reproductive Medicine,* and *Women's Health Letter.*

IOM Staff Biographies

Andrew Pope, Ph.D., is director of the Board on Health Sciences Policy at the Institute of Medicine. With expertise in physiology and biochemistry, his primary interests focus on environmental and occupational influences on human health. Dr. Pope's previous research activities focused on the neuroendocrine and reproductive effects of various environmental substances on food-producing animals. During his tenure at the National Academy of Sciences and since 1989 at the Institute of Medicine, Dr. Pope has directed numerous reports; topics include injury control, disability prevention, biologic markers, neurotoxicology, indoor allergens, and the enhancement of environmental and occupational health content in medical and nursing school curricula. Most recently, Dr. Pope directed studies on NIH priority-setting processes, fluid resuscitation practices in combat casualties, and organ procurement and transplantation.

Brian D. Smedley, Ph.D., is a Senior Program Officer in the Division of Health Sciences Policy of the Institute of Medicine. Previously, Dr. Smedley served as Study Director for the IOM reports, *Promoting Health:*

Intervention Strategies from Social and Behavioral Research, and *The Unequal Burden of Cancer: An Assessment of NIH Research and Programs for Ethnic Minorities and the Medically Underserved*. Dr. Smedley came to the IOM from the American Psychological Association, where he worked on a wide range of social, health, and education policy topics in his capacity as Director for Public Interest Policy. Prior to working at the APA, he served as a Congressional Science Fellow in the office of Rep. Robert C. Scott (D-VA), sponsored by the American Association for the Advancement of Science, and as a postdoctoral research fellow in the Education Policy Division of the Educational Testing Service in Princeton, New Jersey. Dr. Smedley received a Ph.D. degree in clinical psychology from the University of California, Los Angeles, where he was a Ford Foundation predoctoral and dissertation fellow.

On a personal note, Dr. Smedley would like to acknowledge his godfather, Dr. Charles H. Wright of Detroit, Michigan. Dr. Wright was an obstetrician whose tireless efforts to increase awareness of the rich history of African peoples and their descendents in America and throughout the world resulted in the creation of the Charles H. Wright Museum of African-American History in Detroit, among many other such institutions. Dr. Wright died on March 7, 2002, shortly before this report was released.

Adrienne Y. Stith, Ph.D., is a Program Officer in the Division of Health Sciences Policy of the Institute of Medicine. Prior to working at the Institute of Medicine, she served as the James Marshall Public Policy Scholar, a fellowship sponsored by the Society for the Psychological Study of Social Issues and the American Psychological Association. She worked in the areas of ethnic health disparities, mental health services for children in schools, and racial profiling. Dr. Stith is also a licensed clinical psychologist, receiving her doctorate in 1997 from the University of Vermont. She completed a postdoctoral fellowship in Adolescent Medicine and Pediatric Psychology at the University of Rochester Medical Center, in Rochester, New York. She provided services to children and adolescents in community mental health centers, schools, primary care settings, teen clinics, and foster care, and worked with pregnant teens as well as children with chronic illness. While at the University of Rochester, her research examined stress and social support in children residing in foster care.

Daniel J. Wooten, M.D., is Professor of Surgery/Anesthesia, James H. Quillen College of Medicine at East Tennessee State University and Scholar-in-Residence at the Institute of Medicine. Dr. Wooten was Executive Associate Dean for Academic and Faculty Affairs at the Quillen College of Medicine for approximately five years before he accepted the appointment at the National Academy of Sciences. From 1974 to 1995 Dr.

Wooten was Chairman, Department of Anesthesiology at the Charles R. Drew University of Medicine and Science, Vice Chair of the Department of Anesthesiology at UCLA and chief-of-service Department of Anesthesiology at King/Drew Medical Center in Los Angeles, CA. He has extensive experience in inner-city health care delivery systems and the institutional infrastructures necessary to support them. Rural medicine, community health and rural primary care health education have been his most recent challenges in northeast Tennessee at the James H. Quillen College of Medicine. Dr. Wooten completed his doctor of medicine degree at Meharry Medical College. He served his internship in internal medicine at George W. Hubbard Hospital in Nashville, completed his residency training in anesthesiology and a fellowship in critical care medicine at the University of Pittsburgh Health Science Center.

Thelma L. Cox is Senior Project Assistant in the Division of Health Sciences Policy. During her eleven years at the Institute of Medicine, she has also provided assistance to the Division of Health Care Services and the Division of Biobehavioral Sciences and Mental Disorders. Ms. Cox has worked on numerous IOM projects, including: Designing A Strategy for Quality Review and Assurance in Medicare; Evaluating the Artificial Heart Program of the National Heart, Lung, and Blood Institute; Study of FDA Advisory Committees, Federal Regulation of Methadone Treatment; Legal and Ethical Issues Relating to the Inclusion of Women in Clinical Studies; Social and Behavioral Science Base for HIV/AIDS Prevention and Intervention; The Unequal Burden of Cancer: An Assessment of NIH Research and Programs for Ethnic Minorities and the Medically Underserved; and, Exploring the Biological Contributions to Human Health: Does Sex Matter? Ms. Cox has received the National Research Council Recognition Award and has been the recipient of two IOM Staff Achievement Awards.

Paper Contributions

Pages 417-738 are not printed in this book
but are on the CD-ROM attached to the inside back cover.

Index